SAUNDERS

# MATH SKILLS *for*
## Health Professionals

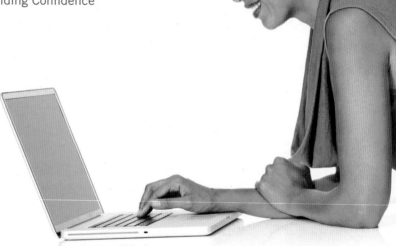

SAUNDERS

# MATH SKILLS *for*
# Health Professionals

SECOND EDITION

## *Rebecca Wallace Hickey, RN, MEd, AHI*

Secondary Health Tech Instructor
Butler Technology and Career Development Schools
Hamilton, Ohio
Adjunct Professor, Allied Health
University of Cincinnati–Blue Ash Campus
Cincinnati, Ohio

ELSEVIER

# ELSEVIER

3251 Riverport Lane
St. Louis, Missouri 63043

Previous edition copyrighted 2010

**International Standard Book Number:** 978-0-323-32248-5

Executive Content Strategist: Kellie White
Content Development Manager: Billie Sharp
Content Development Specialist: Elizabeth McCormac
Publishing Services Manager: Julie Eddy
Project Manager: Jan Waters
Design Direction: Renee Duenow

Printed in India.

Last digit is the print number:   9   8   7   6   5

Working together
to grow libraries in
developing countries

www.elsevier.com • www.bookaid.org

*"Families are the compass that guides us.*
*They are the inspiration to reach great heights,*
*and our comfort when we occasionally falter."*

—Brad Henry

To the men in my life: Gerry, Ryan, Shawn, Kevin and Ben
Thank you for your constant love, support, and humor throughout this process.

*"Creativity is especially expressed in the ability to make connections,*
*to make associations, to turn things around and express them in a new way."*

—Tim Hansen

To my parents, Fred and Barbara:
Thank you for all your encouragement,
especially when I didn't want to be a square peg forced to fit into a round hole.

# Contributors and Reviewers

## CONTRIBUTORS

**BENJAMIN CORY BEAMAN, BS**
Science Instructor
Butlertech Career Development Schools
Hamilton, Ohio

**NICOLE R. CASSIDY, BS, MSED**
Instructor, Mathematics
D. Russel Lee-Butler Technology and Career
    Development Schools
Hamilton, Ohio

## REVIEWERS

**KATHY BURLINGAME, MSN, CRN**
Instructor
Galen College of Nursing
Louisville, Kentucky

**ASHLEY PITLYK, PhD**
Lead Scientist
Booz Allen Hamilton
St. Louis, Missouri

**DEBORAH RAVESTEIN, BS**
ABLE Instructor, Medical Math Instructor,
    Developmental Education Instructor
Miami Valley Career Technology Center
Dayton, Ohio

# Preface for Students

We use math every day. Most people do not realize how often math concepts creep into our daily lives. As this textbook was being developed, I strived to take the math concepts we use every day and illustrate that these are the same concepts that are used in health care math. In addition, I tried to provide a broad scope to include a variety of problems that people in *all* health careers will encounter.

For those of you who do not like math, reflect on what it is about math that you do not like. What are your strengths? What are your weaknesses? Many students say that they do not like math because they do not feel confident in their knowledge level or because they never succeeded at math in the past. "Practice the Skill" exercises are provided for you to assess your level of knowledge. Once you recognize your strengths and weaknesses, you will be able to focus on those areas.

After you have completed each chapter in this text, ask yourself the following questions to help measure your success: Which exercise was your strongest skill and why? Which exercise was your weakest skill and why? If you feel you need additional practice, here are a few suggestions:

- Talk to your instructor regarding which concepts are the hardest.
- Form a study group.
- Create your own practice problems and have someone check them for you.
- Contact your school counselor or advisor to arrange tutoring services.

Remember, new math strategies are being developed on a regular basis. For example, students have taught me mnemonics to remember conversions and a different way to set up and work proportion problems. Confidence in your abilities will increase your accuracy with mathematical computations. I hope that you find this text challenging and it provides you with approaches for applying your knowledge in the health career of your choice.

Please note that the examples and practice problems in this book are meant to teach specific concepts and they may not necessarily reflect actual medical or insurance fees or wages.

# Preface for Instructors

*Saunders Math Skills for Health Professionals* began with my idea of creating a textbook that could be used in all health career disciplines as a stand-alone text or review manual for students who are weak in math. Math—just the word brings groans and negative feedback from many students, as well as a few health care instructors. During the development of this book, I included strategies that I use in the classroom to present the material in a positive, realistic manner, with a splash of humor. I want students to see that math can be fun!

Each chapter includes the following helpful features:

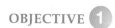

- Chapter Outline: Brief outline that helps to highlight the key topics in the chapter.
- Learning Objectives: Measurable objectives that emphasize the expected learning outcomes. Throughout the text, an Objective icon is placed next to sections that discuss the objective indicated by the number next to the icon.
- Key Terms: Key terms are listed at the beginning of the chapter. Definitions can be found throughout the chapter and in the glossary.
- Chapter Overview: Introduction to the chapter content and why it is important to understand the material.
- Practice the Skill: Exercises for students to assess their knowledge about the topic at hand. (Answers to the odd-numbered questions can be found at the end of the book. In addition, all answers are provided on the Evolve website that accompanies the textbook.)
- Building Confidence with the Skill: Exercises that appear after several topics have been discussed in the chapter and include all topics discussed so far in the chapter. (Answers to the odd-numbered questions can be found at the end of the book. In addition, all answers are provided on the Evolve website that accompanies the textbook.)
- Master the Skill: Exercises that are found at the end of each chapter, designed to test the student's knowledge of the information presented throughout the chapter. (Answers are provided on the Evolve website that accompanies the textbook.)

In addition, special boxes appear throughout the text that include the following:

- Strategy: Provide a systematic process for solving the featured math concept.
- Math Trivia: Include useful and fun tips on when and how math is applied.
- Math Quick Tips: Remind students of math rules.
- Human Error: Remind students to check their work and ask themselves such questions as, "What are the common errors? Did I perform the proper computation? Did I write down the problem correctly?"
- Math in the Real World: Take information that the students use in their everyday lives and demonstrate how the same concept can be applied in health care.

"Example" problems are included throughout each chapter to help illustrate the topic at hand. Because there is more than one way to solve a math problem, I tried to focus not on the result but on the process of finding the result. Many examples will have more than one explanation of how to solve the problem. In my mind, either way is correct as long as the students can explain how they obtained the answer and used proper mathematical concepts.

Like students, many instructors either enjoy math or become frustrated with it. Instructors who teach in health care programs frequently say, "I know how to work the problem; I just don't know how to explain it." I have tried to make the instructor's resources that accompany this text user-friendly to allow the instructor to be successful in delivering the material and the student to be successful in learning it. For an instructor, nothing is more frustrating than appearing to be unprepared for class. I hope these resources help instructors to feel confident in their math abilities and prepared when students challenge their methodology for solving a problem.

Instructor's resources available on the Evolve website that accompanies this book include the following:

- Lesson plans
- PowerPoint presentations
- Test bank
- Complete set of answers to "Practice the Skill" boxes, "Building Confidence with the Skill" boxes, and "Master the Skill" boxes

# Acknowledgments

Behind every author stands a great support system—the unsung heroes. I would like to take this opportunity to thank my unsung heroes:

My students, who over the years have supplied me with different strategies for teaching medical math. Even though they may not all enjoy math, they have learned how to appreciate it.

Ben Beaman and Nicole Cassidy, for their contributions to this textbook. I have greatly enjoyed the different activities we have developed together. Thank you for working with me on this endeavor.

The wonderful staff at Elsevier—Billie Sharp, Betsy McCormac, Kellie White, and all the behind-the-scenes staff. This has been a journey of peaks and valleys. Thank you for your knowledge, support, and reality checks.

My coworkers and the many reviewers who helped me take this book from a dream to reality.

—Rebecca Wallace Hickey, RN, MEd, AHI

*"Education is not an affair of 'telling' and being told, but an active and constructive process."*

—John Dewey

# Contents

## CHAPTER OUTLINE

## LEARNING OBJECTIVES

*Upon completion of this chapter, the learner will be able to:*

1. Define the key terms that relate to basic mathematical computations.

2. Perform calculations using basic addition, subtraction, multiplication, and division.

3. Perform calculations with both positive and negative integers.

4. Demonstrate when exponents can be used.

5. Perform calculations involving parenthesis, and multiplication/division with exponents.

6. Solve mathematical computations using the "order of operation" theory.

7. Identify greatest common factors, least common multiple, and prime numbers.

## KEY TERMS

OBJECTIVE  1

Addend
Addition
Arithmetic
Associative Property of Addition
Associative Property of Multiplication
Base of an Exponent
Borrow
Carry
Common Multiple
Commutative Property of Addition
Commutative Property of Multiplication
Computation
Compute
Difference
Digit

Directed Number
Distributive Property
Divide
Dividend
Divisible
Division
Divisor
Equation
Evaluate
Exponent
Factor
Greatest Common Factor (GCF)
Identity Property of Addition
Identity Property of Multiplication
Least Common Multiple (LCM)

| | |
|---|---|
| Mental Math | Power of 10 |
| Minuend | Prime Number |
| Multiple | Product |
| Multiplicand | Quotient |
| Multiplication | Reciprocal |
| Multiplier | Remainder |
| Negative Numbers | Subtraction |
| Number Sentence | Subtrahend |
| Operations | Sum |
| Order of Operations | Symbol |
| Place Value | Whole Number |
| Positive Numbers | Zero Pair |
| Power | Zero Property |

**OBJECTIVE 1**

Math, just the term, initates one of two responses: "I love math" or "I never was very good at math." Why do people avoid using math? The answer depends on the person's level of confidence in recognizing mathematical computations and how to solve the equation. Most people perform some type of mathematical computation every day. Examples include:

- Leaving a tip
- Balancing a checkbook
- Figuring out discounts
- Adding up the total cost of a purchase
- Figuring out how much it will cost to fill up the gas tank

Yet, when I point this out during class, a student usually responds, "Yeah, but that's not medical math." True, but the principles and formulas are the same. What is medical math? When is math used in health care? Here are a few examples:

- Figuring out medication dosages
- Measuring intake and output
- Measuring laboratory values
- Collecting deductibles or copayments at the time of service
- Performing an inventory of office equipment
- Ordering nonreusable equipment
- Preparing the office staff payroll
- Billing an insurance company for payment of services rendered
- Creating a budget for a company or for personal use

This chapter is a review intended for students to renew their mathematical knowledge and build confidence in their abilities. Maybe you have been out of the educational arena for a while, or possibly math was never your strongest subject in school or you have forgotten some basic mathematical rules. This chapter will help you strengthen your math skills. Some of your classmates may use **mental math** to solve some problems, but pencil and paper will be needed to figure out many problems. In this age of technology, you may be tempted to use a computer. However, even with calculators, the user must be able to properly input the calculations into the device. Avoid the temptation. Refresh your knowledge of mathematical rules and **order of operations**, and then use the calculator to check your answers in this section. A machine is only as accurate as the person programming the information.

# REVIEW OF BASIC MATHEMATICAL OPERATIONS

In this section we will be using **whole numbers** and the different **operations** in which we manipulate them. As a reminder, the order of the numbers represents the different place values of each **digit** (Figure 1-1). Many students prefer to rewrite math problems in a vertical format so that the number **place values** match up.

| 9 | 8 | 7 | 6 | 5 | 4 | 3 | 2 | 1 | 0 |
|---|---|---|---|---|---|---|---|---|---|
|   |   |   |   |   |   |   |   |   | Ones |
|   |   |   |   |   |   |   |   | Tens |   |
|   |   |   |   |   |   |   | Hundreds |   |   |
|   |   |   |   |   |   | Thousands |   |   |   |
|   |   |   |   |   | Ten thousands |   |   |   |   |
|   |   |   |   | Hundred thousands |   |   |   |   |   |
|   |   |   | Millions |   |   |   |   |   |   |
|   |   | Ten millions |   |   |   |   |   |   |   |
|   | Hundred millions |   |   |   |   |   |   |   |   |
| Billions |   |   |   |   |   |   |   |   |   |

**Figure 1-1**   Review the place value using the following number: 9,876,543,210.

## MATH QUICK TIPS 1-1

The answer to an addition problem is the **sum.**

The answer to a subtraction problem is the **difference.**

The answer to a **multiplication** problem is the **product.**

The answer to a division problem is the **quotient.**

## Addition

## MATH TRIVIA 1-1

Do you remember **addition** terminology?

| 75 | > | **Addend** |
|---|---|---|
| + | > | **Symbol** (in this case addition) |
| 25 | > | Addend |
| 100 | > | Sum |

Have you ever added a column of numbers by regrouping in ascending order? Or have you changed the problem by adding some of the smaller numbers together to form a larger number (so that you had fewer numbers to add together)? Did you come out with the correct answer? The answer is yes because of the following mathematical properties:

**Associative Property of Addition**: The sum stays the same when the *grouping* of addends is changed.

*Example:*

$(8 + 2) + 4 = 10 + 4 = 14$

$8 + (2 + 4) = 8 + 6 = 14$

**Commutative Property of Addition**: The sum stays the same when the *order* of the addends is changed.

*Example:*

$8 + 2 + 4 = 14$

$2 + 4 + 8 = 14$

$4 + 8 + 2 = 14$

Remember, there can be more than one way to solve a math problem. The goal is to come up with the same solution.

## PRACTICE THE SKILL 1-1

Compute the following addition problems without the use of a calculator.

1.
```
   9,187
+    425
```

2.
```
  69,215
+    560
```

3.
```
  73,566
+  4,439
```

4.
```
     342
+  9,745
```

5.
```
  90,457
+ 32,665
```

6.
```
     164
     390
+  1,456
```

7.
```
   6,000
     430
+    759
```

8.
```
     749
     896
+    613
```

9.
```
   1,156
     243
+    784
```

10.
```
   7,894
     191
+    654
```

11.
```
     457
      35
+    786
```

12.
```
   5,792
     336
      45
+      6
```

13.
```
     972
  32,468
     891
       6
+     45
```

*(Continued)*

## PRACTICE THE SKILL 1-1
*Continued from p. 4*

Identify the proper place value for the bolded, red number in each problem.

**14.** 7,896,013 _____

**15.** 892,456,032 _____

**16.** 8,945 _____

**17.** 5,437,890,002 _____

**18.** 765,420,301 _____

**19.** 45,678 _____

**20.** 356,781,010 _____

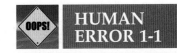

### HUMAN ERROR 1-1

*When adding, did you remember to **carry** your extra digit over one place value?*

## Subtraction and Borrowing

What is the opposite operation of addition? **Subtraction!** Subtraction is used when you want to separate quantities. As with addition, it may be easier to compute the answer if the subtraction problems are rewritten in a vertical fashion. One step of subtraction commonly forgotten is borrowing. If you have a number that cannot be subtracted without resulting in a negative number, you will need to **borrow**.

## STRATEGY 1-1

**1.** We cannot subtract 9 from 8 as a positive number.

**2.** We must borrow 10 from the tens column.

**3.** This changes the 8 to 18 and the 7 to 6.

**4.** Now we can perform the subtraction problem.

*Example:*
$$
\begin{array}{r}
78 \\
-\ 69 \\
\hline
\end{array}
$$

### HUMAN ERROR 1-2

*When setting up your problem, make sure you have lined your numbers up according to their place value. You should start solving your problem by subtracting from the one's column and working to the left.*

**Incorrect Example:**
$$
\begin{array}{r}
2{,}435 \\
-820 \\
\hline
\end{array}
$$

**Correct Example:**
$$
\begin{array}{r}
2{,}435 \\
-\ \ 820 \\
\hline
\end{array}
$$

Let's try a few practice problems *without* the use of a calculator.

1.  $\begin{array}{r} 567 \\ -\ 472 \\ \hline \end{array}$ 

3.  $\begin{array}{r} 45 \\ -\ 28 \\ \hline \end{array}$ 

5.  $\begin{array}{r} 17{,}899 \\ -\ 15{,}922 \\ \hline \end{array}$

2.  $\begin{array}{r} 12{,}457 \\ -\ \ \ 869 \\ \hline \end{array}$ 

4.  $\begin{array}{r} 897 \\ -\ 339 \\ \hline \end{array}$ 

6.  $\begin{array}{r} 23{,}457 \\ -\ \ 7{,}540 \\ \hline \end{array}$

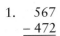 Excellent! Did you remember to borrow? Now let's move on to a series of numbers.

It is easy to add a series of numbers together. When you're faced with a series of numbers you need to subtract, however, it is easier to subtract in groups of two unless you are using a calculator.

*Example:*

$453 - 221 - 47 - 2 =$

First, let's subtract:   $453 - 221 = 232$
Next:                    $232 - 47 = 185$
Next:                    $185 - 2 = 183$
Your final difference is 183.

---

## ? MATH TRIVIA 1-2

Do you remember subtraction terminology?

| | | |
|---|---|---|
| 75 | > | **Minuend** |
| – | > | Symbol (in this case subtraction) |
| <u>25</u> | > | **Subtrahend** |
| 50 | > | Difference |

---

## PRACTICE THE SKILL 1-2

**Compute the following subtraction problems without the use of a calculator.**

1. $\begin{array}{r} 78,507 \\ -\ \ 6,442 \\ \hline \end{array}$

2. $\begin{array}{r} 13,660 \\ -\ \ 2,589 \\ \hline \end{array}$

3. $\begin{array}{r} 789,196 \\ -147,809 \\ \hline \end{array}$

4. $\begin{array}{r} 67,889 \\ -32,455 \\ \hline \end{array}$

5. $\begin{array}{r} 8,920,491 \\ -5,208,383 \\ \hline \end{array}$

6. $\begin{array}{r} 472 \\ 274 \\ -\ \ 47 \\ \hline \end{array}$

7. $\begin{array}{r} 765 \\ 122 \\ -\ \ 14 \\ \hline \end{array}$

8. $\begin{array}{r} 972 \\ 852 \\ -\ \ 21 \\ \hline \end{array}$

9. $\begin{array}{r} 7,894 \\ 654 \\ -\ \ 191 \\ \hline \end{array}$

10. $\begin{array}{r} 567 \\ 457 \\ -\ \ 22 \\ \hline \end{array}$

## Multiplication

If you had the choice, when working with a series of the same number, would you rather add or multiply to obtain your answer? Look at the following example. Which method do you think is easier?

*Example:*

$4 + 4 + 4 + 4 + 4 = 20$

| | | |
|---|---|---|
| 4 | > | The digit |
| <u>× 5</u> | > | The number of times we are adding 4 |
| 20 | > | The answer |

As with addition, there are mathematical properties that allow us to manipulate the factors within the computation and still arrive at the same answer.

**Commutative Property of Multiplication:** The product stays the same when the *order* of the factors is changed.

*Example:*

$10 \times 3 = 3 \times 10$

$25 \times 3 = 3 \times 25$

**Distributive Property:** When one of the factors of a product is written as a sum, multiplying each addend before adding does not change the product.

*Example:*

$3 \times (6 + 14) = (3 \times 6) + (3 \times 14)$

$3 \times 20 \quad = 18 + 42$

$60 \quad\quad = 60$

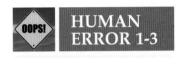

## HUMAN ERROR 1-3

*Remember when multiplying two or more digits, it is helpful to add a 0 to hold the place value.*

Hint: *Add a 0 to hold the place value.*

# MATH TRIVIA 1-3

Do you remember multiplication terminology?

|  |  |  |
|---|---|---|
| 75 | > | **Multiplicand** |
| × | > | Symbol (in this case multiplication) |
| 25 | > | **Multiplier** |
| 1,875 | > | Product |

# PRACTICE THE SKILL 1-3

Compute the following multiplication problems without the use of a calculator.

1.　14
　 × 7

2.　24
　 × 6

3.　12
　×15

4.　44
　×18

5.　576
　 × 6

6.　789
　 × 9

7.　225
　 × 40

8.　15
　× 35

9.　81
　× 98

10.　457
　×221

11.　328
　×122

12.　865
　×437

## Division

As subtraction is the opposite of addition, **division** is the opposite of multiplication. With division, the goal is to **divide** the information into smaller portions. If a number does not divide evenly, what is left is called a **remainder**.

**MATH TRIVIA 1-4**

Do you remember the terminology for division?

| | | |
|---|---|---|
| 75 | > | **Dividend** |
| ÷ | > | Symbol (in this case division) |
| <u>25</u> | > | **Divisor** |
| 3 | > | Quotient |

*Example:*

$$\frac{125}{5}$$

12 divided by 5 is 2 with a remainder of 2 (12 − 10 = 2).
Bring down your 5 to make a new number of 25.
25 divided by 5 is 5.
Answer is 25.

 **HUMAN ERROR 1-4**

*Remember when dividing, that if the divisor cannot be divided into the dividend, then a zero should be placed in the answer and moved to the next place value.*

*Example:*

$$\frac{27}{2}$$

2 divided by 2 = 1
Bring down the 7.
7 divided by 2 = 3 with a remainder of 1.
Answer is 13 with remainder of 1.

Can you check the answer? Yes, by doing a reverse operation. To check division problems, multiply your quotient by the **divisor** and add the remainder. The resulting product should be equal to the dividend.

 **HUMAN ERROR 1-5**

*Most incorrect answers come from inaccurately performing addition, subtraction, multiplication, and division, not because the person did not know what he or she was doing. Take your time—the key to math is accuracy.*

 **PRACTICE THE SKILL 1-4**

**Compute the following division problems without the use of a calculator.**

1. 125 ÷ 15 = _____

2. 72 ÷ 9 = _____

3. 450 ÷ 9 = _____

4. 574 ÷ 22 = _____

5. 124 ÷ 12 = _____

6. 500 ÷ 75 = _____

7. 43,791 ÷ 8 = _____

8. 565 ÷ 5 = _____

9. 34,791 ÷ 44 = _____

10. 8,762 ÷ 445 = _____

11. 81 ÷ 9 = _____

12. 6,432 ÷ 8 = _____

# POSITIVE AND NEGATIVE NUMBERS

OBJECTIVE **3**

One common use of **negative numbers** (Figure 1-2) in everyday life is to describe temperature during the winter months. In many of the northern states, for example, it is not uncommon for the temperature to range from 10 degrees above zero to −20 degrees below zero on the Fahrenheit scale in January and February. When it gets down to −10° F, life can be miserable.

What do negative numbers have to do with medical math? Negative numbers are used to determine:

• Temperature
• Weight loss
• Body fat
• Cell count
• Cash flow
• Profit or loss margins

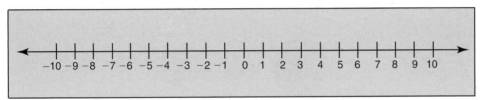

**Figure 1-2**  Negative and positive numbers on the same number line.

As a reminder, **positive numbers** are greater than 0 and are usually symbolized with a plus (+) sign when used in a **number sentence** that has negative numbers. If all **integers** are positive, the + sign is not used, and it is assumed that all numbers are positive. Negative numbers are less than 0 and are preceded by a minus (−) symbol.

You can remember this by always placing the positive numbers first.

*Example:*
Add 14 and −8.
Because 14 is the larger number, the **equation** becomes: $14 + (−8) = 14 − 8 = 6$.

*Example:*
Add −20 and −8.

Because both integers are negative, we should add the two numbers together and assign the negative sign.

*Example:*
What is the difference of −6 and 4 degrees?
We can determine the answer by adding $6 + 4 = 10$.
This could also be accomplished with mental math: −6 is 6 degrees below 0; add that to the 4 degrees above 0 and the difference is 10 degrees $(6 + 4)$. The difference would be $4 − (−6)$, which would be the same as $4 + 6$.

When trying to compute a list of positive and negative numbers, place the positive numbers first followed by the negative numbers. The order of the numbers within the two groups does not matter. Next, add all the positive numbers together and determine a sum. Then determine the sum of the negative numbers. Last, take the two sums and perform the required operation.

*Example:*

$25 + (-13) = 25 - 13 = 12$

*Example:*

Add the following numbers: 12, 10, 5, –12, –5, 15

| List the positive numbers first and find the sum: | $12 + 10 + 5 + 15 = 42$ |
| List the negative numbers and find the sum: | $(-12) - 5 = -17$ |
| Perform the proper computation. | $42 - 17 = 25$ |

**Figure 1-3**   Symbols play a major role in addition of positive and negative numbers.

Remember, as with the temperature, the larger the negative number, the farther away from 0 the number is.

When you are multiplying or dividing, if the numbers in the computation are both positive or both negative, the answer will be a positive number. If the numbers in the computation are a combination of positive and negative, the answer will be a negative number (Figure 1-3).

## MATH QUICK TIPS 1-2

Like symbols = POSITIVE answer
+ multiplied by + = Positive
– multiplied by – = Positive
Unlike symbols = NEGATIVE answer
+ multiplied by – = Negative
– multiplied by + = Negative

*Example:*
+ times + = Positive
– times – = Positive
+ times – = Negative

These are important rules to remember as we discuss order of operations later in this chapter.

## PRACTICE THE SKILL 1-5

Compute the following problems without the use of a calculator.

**1.** $(-6) + 14 =$ _____

**2.** $(-81) + (-8) =$ _____

**3.** $(-456) + 67 =$ _____

**4.** $(-435) + 76 =$ _____

**5.** $457,621 + (-334,211) =$ _____

**6.** $(-3) + (-34) =$ _____

**7.** $(-557) + (-892) =$ _____

**8.** $80 + (-36) =$ _____

**9.** $(-45) + 65 =$ _____

**10.** $334 + (-433) =$ _____

**11.** $(-6) - 2 =$ _____

**12.** $(-14) - (-4) =$ _____

**13.** $(-81) - 57 =$ _____

**14.** $21 - 3 + (-7) =$ _____

**15.** $(-54) + (-22) - 6 =$ _____

**16.** $(-6) \times (-56) =$ _____

**17.** $345 \times (-22) =$ _____

**18.** $(-67) \times 3 =$ _____

**19.** $897 \times (-2) =$ _____

**20.** $5,423 \times (-43) =$ _____

**21.** $56 \div (-9) =$ _____

**22.** $459 \div (-3) =$ _____

**23.** $5,674 \div (-22) =$ _____

**24.** $(-4577) \div 7 =$ _____

**25.** $89,243 \div (-3) =$ _____

## MATH TRIVIA 1-5

Zero Pair occurs when a positive and negative number are either added or subtracted, result in a zero as the answer.

*Example:*
$-1 + 1 = 0$ or $1 - 1 = 0$

## BUILDING CONFIDENCE WITH THE SKILL 1-1

Complete the following math computations without the use of a calculator.

**1.**  $\begin{array}{r} 120 \\ \div\ 15 \end{array}$

**2.**  $\begin{array}{r} 45 \\ \div\ 5 \end{array}$

**3.**  $\begin{array}{r} 4352 \\ \div\ 15 \end{array}$

**4.**  $\begin{array}{r} 540 \\ \div\ 15 \end{array}$

**5.**  $\begin{array}{r} 2695 \\ \div\ 3 \end{array}$

**6.**  $\begin{array}{r} 47 \\ \times\ 4 \end{array}$

*(Continued)*

# BUILDING CONFIDENCE WITH THE SKILL 1-1
*Continued from p. 11*

*Continued from p. 11*

| 7. | 56 × 8 |
|---|---|

8.  921 × 12

9.  782 × 15

10.  421 × 56

11.  237
    431
    + 782

12.  577
    899
    + 78

13.  887
    453
    + 231

14.  421
    1987
    520
    1989
    925
    1964
    113
    + 1965

15.  310
    1991
    702
    1993
    517
    + 1995

16. $(-24) + 43 =$ _____

17. $(-21) + 5 =$ _____

18. $(-53) - (-35) =$ _____

19. $(-112) - 21 =$ _____

20. $547 - (-443) =$ _____

Identify the digit that corresponds with the place value: 8,721,045,683

21. Hundred _____

22. Hundred thousand _____

23. Million _____

24. Ten _____

25. Thousand _____

OBJECTIVE 4

# EXPONENTS

Many of us had to memorize multiplication tables in grade school. We were drilled on multiplication tables—remember 50 problems in 2 minutes? Building on that concept, if you think about it, **exponents** are simplified multiplication problems. Determine how many times the same **base** number appears in the problem. Write the base number, and the exponent becomes the number of times it is repeated in the problem.

Many of us remember exponents with terms like *base*, **power**, *squared*, and *cubed*. The base is the number that will be multiplied to itself, and the exponent is the number of times by which it is to be multiplied. The square root of a number is a number when multiplied by itself, gives you the original number.

*Example 1:*

$4 \times 4 \times 4 = 4^3$

$5 \times 5 \times 5 \times 5 \times 5 \times 5 = 5^6$ or 5 to the 6th power

*Example 2:*

$4 \times 4 \times 4 \times 3 \times 3 = 4^3 \times 3^2$

## MATH TRIVIA 1-6

Do you remember what term is used instead of 2nd power?

Do you remember what term is used instead of 3rd power?

## PRACTICE THE SKILL 1-6

Express the following problems with exponents.

1. $2 \times 2 \times 2 \times 3 \times 3 =$ _____

2. $4 \times 4 \times 6 \times 6 \times 7 \times 7 =$ _____

3. $5 \times 5 \times 5 \times 5 \times 5 =$ _____

4. $3 \times 3 \times 2 \times 2 \times 7 \times 7 \times 7 =$ _____

5. $2 \times 3 \times 4 \times 4 \times 3 \times 2 \times 2 =$ _____

6. $7 \times 7 \times 7 \times 8 \times 8 \times 8 \times 8 =$ _____

7. $10 \times 10 \times 10 \times 12 \times 12 \times 12 =$ _____

8. $25 \times 25 \times 25 \times 30 \times 30 \times 30 =$ _____

9. $60 \times 60 \times 30 \times 30 \times 30 \times 10 \times 10 =$ _____

10. $6 \times 6 \times 6 \times 14 \times 14 \times 2 \times 2 =$ _____

## Positive and Negative Exponents

OBJECTIVE ④

Exponents can be either positive or negative numbers. As a reminder, any number that does not have an exponent is to the 1st power.

What happens when we have a negative exponent? It becomes the **reciprocal** of the indicated power of the number. Using the following example, we will go through a strategy for working with negative exponents.

*Example:*

$5^{-5}$

## STRATEGY 1-2

Disregard the negative symbol and find the answer to the exponent.

$$5^5 = 5 \times 5 \times 5 \times 5 \times 5 = 3,125$$

Now we need to address the negative symbol.

When we are working with a negative exponent, we must determine the reciprocal. The reciprocal of 3,125 is $\frac{1}{3,125}$.

In Chapter 3, we will be discussing fractions in detail. As a reminder, fractions are part of a whole number. Negative exponents will be moving the fraction closer to zero.

OBJECTIVE **4**

### Scientific Notation

Exponents are most commonly used when dealing with scientific notation.

Scientific notation is often used in the laboratory or in research when working with either a very large or a very small number. The use of an exponent decreases the chances of error. Scientific notation will be discussed in Chapter 10, but the following is an example of how exponents and scientific notation work.

Our number system and scientific notation are based on **powers of 10**. In scientific notation, we can change large numbers into numbers with exponents. Using exponents decreases the chance of computation errors or errors in the answer.

*Examples:*

$10^0 = 1$     $10^3 = 1,000$

$10^1 = 10$     $10^6 = 1,000,000$

$10^2 = 100$     $10^9 = 1,000,000,000$

*Examples:*

$10^{-1} = 0.1$

$10^{-2} = 0.01$

$10^{-3} = 0.001$

*Examples of writing scientific notation:*

$2,000 = 2 \times 10^3$

$400 = 4 \times 10^2$

$16,000 = 16 \times 10^3$

OBJECTIVE **4**

### Multiplication and Division of Exponents

When multiplying exponents with like bases, you add the exponents.

*Example:*

$3^3 \times 3^6 = 3^{3+6} = 3^9$ or $3 \times 3 \times 3 \times 3 \times 3 \times 3 \times 3 \times 3 \times 3 = 3^9$

If you are dividing exponents with like bases, you subtract the exponents.

*Example:*

$4^4 \div 4^2 = 4^{4-2} = 4^2$

But what would you do if you are multiplying or dividing exponents with unlike bases? You would compute the answer for each base separately and proceed to work the problem according to the operation.

## STRATEGY 1-3

*Example:*

$3^3 \times 4^2 =$

1. Compute the answer for $3^3$.
   27

2. Compute the answer for $4^2$.
   16

3. Insert the answers for steps 1 and 2 into the equation.
   $27 \times 16 =$

4. Solve the equation.
   $27 \times 16 = 432$

5. Your answer is **432**.

You would use the same strategy for division of exponents with unlike bases.

*Example:*

$10^3 \div 5^2 =$

1. Compute the answer for $10^3$
   $10 \times 10 \times 10 = 1000$

2. Compute the answer for $5^2$
   $5 \times 5 = 25$

3. Insert the answer from step 1 and 2 into the equation.
   $1000 \div 25 =$

   Solve the equation.
   $1000 \div 25 = 40$

   Your answer is **40**.

## MATH QUICK TIPS 1-3

To multiply powers of the same base, add their exponents.

## MATH QUICK TIPS 1-4

To divide powers of the same base, subtract the exponent of the divisor from the exponent of the dividend.

OBJECTIVE **4**

## PRACTICE THE SKILL 1-7

Perform the following exponent computations.

1. $4^3 \times 4^2 =$ _____

2. $5^6 \times 5^3 =$ _____

3. $10^2 \times 10^4 =$ _____

4. $8^3 \times 8^3 =$ _____

5. $6^3 \times 6^2 =$ _____

6. $6^2 \times 8^3 =$ _____

7. $4^3 \times 8^2 =$ _____

8. $5^5 \times 2^5 =$ _____

9. $3^2 \times 2^3 =$ _____

10. $10^1 \times 10^3 =$ _____

11. $5^2 \times 5^{-4} =$ _____

12. $2^{-4} \times 4^{-2} =$ _____

OBJECTIVE **4**

## PRACTICE THE SKILL 1-8

Perform the following exponent computations.

1. $24^3 \div 24^2 =$ _____

2. $35^5 \div 35^2 =$ _____

3. $49^8 \div 49^6 =$ _____

4. $63^3 \div 63^2 =$ _____

5. $150^{12} \div 150^2 =$ _____

6. $300^3 \div 50^2 =$ _____

7. $810^{10} \div 9^5 =$ _____

8. $450^9 \div 9^3 =$ _____

9. $320^4 \div 8^3 =$ _____

10. $121 \div 11^2 =$ _____

11. $25^{-2} \div 5^{-2} =$ _____

12. $3^{-4} \div 4^{-3} =$ _____

OBJECTIVE **5**

## PARENTHESES

Parentheses are used to distinguish specific numbers that are grouped together to determine a specific quantity. The grouping inside the parentheses is considered one quantity.

*Example:*

2(4) is the same as $2 \times 4 = 8$
4(5 + 6) is the same as $4 \times 11 = 44$
3(4 − 1) + 6(5 − 1) is the same as $3(3) + 6(4) = 9 + 24 = 33$

As a reminder, the **Associative Property of Multiplication** states that the product stays the same when the *grouping* of factors is changed.

*Examples:*

$(5 \times 3) \times 3 = 15 \times 3 = 45$
$5 \times (3 \times 3) = 5 \times 9 = 45$

## PRACTICE THE SKILL 1-9

Perform the following mathematical computations involving parentheses.

1. $2(4 + 5) =$ _____

2. $6(3 + 10) =$ _____

3. $15(2 + 3) =$ _____

4. $45(4 + 5) =$ _____

5. $12(6 + 6) =$ _____

6. $2(4 + 5) + 6(3 + 10) =$ _____

7. $15(2 + 3) + 45(4 + 5) =$ _____

8. $12(6 + 6) + 4(20 + 5) - 2(5 - 3) =$ _____

9. $2(3 + 4) + 5(6 + 7) - 8(9 - 1) - 10 =$ _____

10. $8(9 + 2) - 4(9 - 1) + 5(1 + 3) =$ _____

11. $5(20 + 37) \times 2(40 + 37) =$ _____

12. $6(20 + 7 + 2) \times 5(20 - 7 - 2) =$ _____

13. $8(41 + 40 + 1) \times 4(10 + 2 + 5) - 8(-6 - 4 + 2) =$ _____

14. $3(225 + 522) - 2(522 - 225) =$ _____

15. $2(9 + 8) + 3(7 - 6) + 4(6 + 5) =$ _____

16. $2(9 \times 8) + 3(7 \times 6) + 4(6 \times 5) =$ _____

17. $2(2 + 3) \div 5(3 - 2) =$ _____

18. $4(4 + 2) \div 3(4 - 2) =$ _____

19. $5(5 \times 4) \div 2(5 \times 4) =$ _____

20. $8(81 + 81) \div 3(9 + 9) =$ _____

21. $5(6 \div 3) + 3(10 \div 2) =$ _____

22. $9(27 \div 3) + 3(30 \div 2) =$ _____

23. $5(36 \div 3) + 8(10 \div 5) =$ _____

24. $5(16 \div 8) + 3(24 \div 2) =$ _____

25. $5(24 \div 3) + 2(12 \div 4) =$ _____

OBJECTIVE **5**    ## ORDER OF OPERATIONS

Please Excuse My Dear Aunt Sally is a great mnemonic for remembering the order of operations: Parentheses, Exponents, Multiplication, Division, Addition, and Subtraction. Think of it as directions for working a math problem. When solving math problems use the order of operations and work from left to right.

*Example:*

$5(6-2) + 5(6 \times 7) + 2(6^3) + 4 - 1 =$

## STRATEGY 1-4

1. Parentheses: $(6 - 2) = 4$   $(6 \times 7) = 42$
   *Problem rewritten:* $5(4) + 5(42) + 2(6^3) + 4 - 1 =$

2. Exponents: $6^3 = 6 \times 6 \times 6 = 216$
   *Problem rewritten:* $5(4) + 5(42) + 2(216) + 4 - 1 =$

3. Multiplication or division, whichever comes first from left to right:
   $5 \times 4 = 20$   $5 \times 42 = 210$   $2 \times 216 = 432$
   *Problem rewritten:* $20 + 210 + 432 + 4 - 1 =$

4. Addition or subtraction, whichever comes first from left to right:
   *Problem rewritten:* $20 + 210 + 432 + 4 - 1 = 665$

5. Your answer is **665**.

## PRACTICE THE SKILL 1-10

Using order of operations, perform the following mathematical computations.

1. $4(2 + 3) \times 6(4 - 3) \times 8(3 \times 3) \div 2 =$ _____

2. $5 + 7 + 9 + 4(50 - 17) - 3(45 - 17) =$ _____

3. $2(35 + 47)^2 - 3(47 - 35)^2 + 5 - 4 =$ _____

4. $5(6 + 4 - 3)^4 \times 3(5 + 6 - 2) + 4(6^4) =$ _____

5. $5 - 7 + 3 \times 6(4^2 - 2^3 + 7) \div 7 - 4 + 3(2^2 + 2^3) =$ _____

6. $6(45 + 9)^2 - 16(3 + 6)^2 - 4(60 \div 5) - 10 =$ _____

7. $9 + 7 - 5 + 3(50 - 62) - 4(48 \div 8)^2 =$ _____

*(Continued)*

## PRACTICE THE SKILL 1-10
*Continued from p. 18*

8. $5(225 \div 5)^3 - 3(3{,}636 \div 9)^2 =$ _____

9. $6(18 - 9 + 3) + 4(5)^3 - 8(34 - 6 + 4) - 15 =$ _____

10. $7(108 \div 12)^3 - 6(96 \div 8)^2 - (4^5 - 5^4 - 12^2) =$ _____

## FACTORING

OBJECTIVE **6**

There are very few strategies when it comes to factoring. Most of the time, factoring is trial and error. A **factor** is an integer that divides evenly into another. When does factoring come in handy?

- Converting fractions into their simplest form
- Determining greatest common factors of two or multiple numbers
- Determining if a number can divide evenly into another number

Many people learned to factor using the factor tree. This allows a visualization to make sure you have factored all the way to the prime numbers. **Prime numbers** are numbers whose only factors are 1 and that number.

*Examples of prime numbers:*
1, 2, 3, 5, 7, 11

*Example of a factor tree:*

```
   45
   ∧
 5    9
 |    ∧
 5  3  3
```
Therefore the *factors* of 45 in this factor tree are 3, 5, and 9.

If we wanted to check our answer, we would write the prime numbers in a multiplication sentence known as *prime factorization*.

*Example:*
Prime factorization for 45:   $3 \times 3 \times 5 = 45$

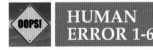

## HUMAN ERROR 1-6

*All solutions should be expressed in their simplest form.*

*Example of prime factorization for 45 in simplest form:*

$3^2 \times 5 = 45$

## MATH TRIVIA 1-7

Ten is a factor of any number that ends in a zero.

*Example:*
$10 \times 45 = 450$

*(Continued)*

## MATH TRIVIA 1-7
*Continued from p. 19*

Nine is a factor of any number if the digits add up to nine.

*Example:*
  81      $8 + 1 = 9$   9 is a factor of 81
126   $1 + 2 + 6 = 9$   $9 \times 14 = 126$

Five is a factor of any number that ends in a zero or five.

*Example:*
$5 \times 87 = 435$

Three is a factor if the sum of the numbers is divisible by three.

*Example:*
24      $2 + 4 = 6$   $3 \div 6 = 2$
3 is a factor of 24   $3 \times 8 = 24$

Two is a factor of any number that ends in an even number.

*Example:*
$24 = 2 \times 12$

Six is a factor of any number if the number satisfies the rule of two being a factor AND three being a factor.

*Example:*
$24 = 3 \times 8$   AND   $24 = 2 \times 12$   SO   $24 = 6 \times 4$
6 is a factor of 24.

## PRACTICE THE SKILL 1-11

Yes or No: Identify if the following is a prime number.

1. 2 _____     6. 49 _____

2. 13 _____     7. 61 _____

3. 15 _____     8. 79 _____

4. 29 _____     9. 83 _____

5. 35 _____     10. 99 _____

## PRACTICE THE SKILL 1-12

Write all of the factors for each of the following numbers.

1. 45 _____    6. 108 _____

2. 75 _____    7. 210 _____

3. 100 _____    8. 76 _____

4. 35 _____    9. 36 _____

5. 27 _____    10. 124 _____

## Greatest Common Factor

 OBJECTIVE 7

The **greatest common factor** (GCF) is the largest factor common to two or more numbers.

*Example:*
Find the GCF for 48 and 72.

## STRATEGY 1-5

1. Write out all the factors for 48: 1, 2, 3, 4, 6, 8, 12, 16, 24, 48

2. Write out all the factors for 72: 1, 2, 3, 4, 6, 8, 9, 12, 18, 24, 36, 72

3. Compare the numbers and determine the common factors: 1, 2, 3, 4, 6, 8, 12, 24

4. The GCF for both 48 and 72 is **24**.

## PRACTICE THE SKILL 1-13

Find the GCF for the following numbers.

1. 10, 15, 35 _____    9. 24, 48, 88 _____

2. 2, 3, 6 _____    10. 9, 81, 162 _____

3. 7, 21, 35 _____    11. 12, 144, 288 _____

4. 14, 49, 63 _____    12. 7, 49, 343 _____

5. 121, 44, 11 _____    13. 64, 108, 200 _____

6. 75, 150, 300 _____    14. 75, 525, 1125 _____

7. 124, 54, 32 _____    15. 332, 468, 839 _____

8. 66, 72, 138 _____

OBJECTIVE **7**

### Least Common Multiple

A multiple is the product of a whole number and any other whole number. The **least common multiple (LCM)** is the smallest multiple that is common to two or more numbers. Some of the functions of LCMs have to do with reducing, converting, and comparing fractions and mixed numbers. Fractions are discussed in detail throughout Chapter 3, but let's do a quick review of how to determine LCM.

*Example:*
Find the LCM for 6 and 18.
Multiples of 6 are: 6, 12, 18.
Multiples of 18 are: 18.          STOP! 18 is a multiple of both 6 and 18.

## PRACTICE THE SKILL 1-14

Find the least common multiple for the following numbers.

1. 4 and 8 _____     9. 13 and 2 _____

2. 4 and 6 _____    10. 11 and 121 _____

3. 20 and 60 _____   11. 15 and 75 _____

4. 5 and 8 _____    12. 150 and 750 _____

5. 12 and 5 _____   13. 64 and 72 _____

6. 30 and 3 _____   14. 9 and 378 _____

7. 40 and 20 _____   15. 8 and 120 _____

8. 8 and 9 _____

## BUILDING CONFIDENCE WITH THE SKILL 1-2

Complete the following operations.

*Find the LCM for the following numbers.*

1. 4 and 7 _____

2. 5 and 3 _____

3. 5 and 75 _____

4. 3 and 7 _____

5. 15 and 25 _____

*(Continued)*

## BUILDING CONFIDENCE WITH THE SKILL 1-2
*Continued from p. 22*

   **6.** 7 and 9 _____

   **7.** 144 and 12 _____

   **8.** 3 and 45 _____

   **9.** 7 and 6 _____

   **10.** 13 and 7 _____

   **11.** 32, 96, and 128 _____

   **12.** 45, 90, and 135 _____

   **13.** 60, 300, and 360 _____

   **14.** 100, 250, and 450 _____

   **15.** 8, 104, and 240 _____

*Find the GCF for the following numbers.*

   **16.** 49 and 84 _____

   **17.** 155 and 350 _____

   **18.** 4,104 and 81 _____

   **19.** 525 and 35 _____

   **20.** 81 and 63 and 108 _____

   **21.** 32, 96 and 128 _____

   **22.** 45, 90 and 135 _____

   **23.** 60, 300, and 360 _____

   **24.** 100, 250, and 450 _____

   **25.** 8, 104, and 240 _____

## MATH IN THE REAL WORLD 1-1

Word problems are discussed in detail in Chapter 4, but let's warm up with some practical application problems that include words. As you work through these problems, identify which operation you will use, write out your computations, and solve the problem.

*(Continued)*

## MATH IN THE REAL WORLD 1-1
*Continued from p. 23*

1. Gas prices are $3.98/gallon and your car holds 16 gallons. You have $40.00 to buy gas and to purchase a gallon of milk, which will cost $2.75 with tax.

   a. How much will it cost to completely fill your gas tank?

   b. If you completely fill your gas tank and purchase milk, will you have change or a negative balance?

   c. Figure out how much gas and milk you can purchase with your $40.00.

2. Your paycheck is $1,456.00 on payday. You are paid twice a month. Your bills include:
   Rent:         $700.00
   Utilities:      $176.80
   Phone:       $45.56
   Cable:        $25.50
   Food:         $476.00
   Car Payment: $504.00
   Gas:          $30.00/week
   Child Care:   $75.00/week

   a. What is your total income for the month?

   b. What are your total expenses for the month?

   c. Are you able to put $300.00 in your savings account each paycheck?

   d. If you save half of your remaining balance, how much would you have saved at the end of 1 year?

## CONCLUSION

I hope this walk down mathematical computation memory lane has built your confidence in your basic math skills. Many of these operations will appear in the same or slightly different formats in the following chapters. If you are still struggling with these concepts, talk to your instructor, find a classmate to study with, or speak with a counselor. Most people don't realize how much math health professionals encounter on a daily basis when performing their jobs. Math is needed for much more than just figuring out medication dosages; health care professionals use it when determining the weight of a patient, temperature variance, laboratory testing, patient and laboratory statistics, fluid balance, and the list goes on. Remember, there is more than one way to attack a math problem. Use the rules and strategies in the manner that works best for you.

## MASTER THE SKILL

Perform the following mathematical computations without the use of a calculator.

1. $15,690 + 368 =$ _____

2. $3,056 + 465 =$ _____

3. $435 + 350 =$ _____

4. $1,256 + 15,247 + 498 + 6,808 =$ _____

5. $5,025 + 4,995 =$ _____

6. $163 - 69 =$ _____

7. $3,655 - 29 =$ _____

8. $58 - 16 =$ _____

9. $1,002 - 103 - 65 =$ _____

10. $65,031 - 1,256 - 56 - 6 =$ _____

11. $256 \times 42 =$ _____

12. $256 \times 16 =$ _____

13. $65,031 \times 1,256 =$ _____

14. $65,508 \times 120 =$ _____

15. $410 \times 25 =$ _____

16. $105 \div 5 =$ _____

17. $840 \div 40 =$ _____

18. $296 \div 4 =$ _____

19. $1,125 \div 15 =$ _____

20. $162 \div 18 =$ _____

Perform the following calculations.

21. $(-24) + 43 =$ _____

22. $(-12) + (-4) =$ _____

23. $12 + (-56) =$ _____

*(Continued)*

## MASTER THE SKILL
*Continued from p. 25*

**24.** $5 - (-8) =$ _____

**25.** $7 - (-12) =$ _____

**26.** $9 \times (-2) =$ _____

**27.** $45 \div (-5) =$ _____

**28.** $8 \times (-4) =$ _____

**29.** $(-8) \div (-4) =$ _____

**30.** $(-3) \times (-12) =$ _____

Compute the following mathematical sentences.

**31.** $(65 \times 10^2) \times (39 \times 10^3) =$ _____

**32.** $(7 \times 2^5) - 4(4 \times 5^3) =$ _____

**33.** $77 \times 10^{-2} =$ _____

**34.** $6^6 \times 2(3 - 7^{-2}) =$ _____

**35.** $(35 \times 10^{-2}) - (57 \times 10^{-3}) =$ _____

**36.** $(45 \times 10^3) - (63 \times 10^{-3}) =$ _____

**37.** $4(23 + 17)^2 + 4(14 - 3)^3 + 50 - 44 =$ _____

**38.** $15(2^2 - 10) + (3^{-3} + 9) - 18 + 2 =$ _____

Write answer in the exponent form.

**39.** $5^5 \div 5^3 =$ _____

**40.** $14^{20} \times 14^{38} =$ _____

**41.** $100^{-4} \div 100^2 =$ _____

Write the following number sentences using exponents.

**42.** $2 \times 2 \times 2 \times 3 \times 4 \times 4 \times 4 \times 5 \times 3 =$ _____

**43.** $10 \times 10 \times 10 \times 50 \times 50 \times 35 \times 35 \times 35 \times 2 =$ _____

**44.** $7 \times 7 \times 7 \times 7 \times 7 \times 8 \times 8 \times 8 \times 8 \times 9 \times 9 \times 9 \times 6 \times 6 \times 5 =$ _____

*(Continued)*

## MASTER THE SKILL
*Continued from p. 26*

Complete the table.

| Numbers | GCF | LCM |
|---|---|---|
| **45.** 7 and 49 | _____ | _____ |
| **46.** 43 and 52 | _____ | _____ |
| **47.** 18 and 24 | _____ | _____ |
| **48.** 13 and 79 | _____ | _____ |
| **49.** 81 and 108 | _____ | _____ |
| **50.** 123 and 59 | _____ | _____ |
| **51.** 145 and 360 | _____ | _____ |
| **52.** 125 and 450 | _____ | _____ |
| **53.** 64 and 72 | _____ | _____ |
| **54.** 747 and 2,241 | _____ | _____ |
| **55.** 488 and 864 | _____ | _____ |

Solve the following problems.

**56.** $5(2 + 7^2) + 6^3 + 25(4 - 3) + 2^2 - 17 + 5 =$ _____

    a. What is the answer cubed? _____

**57.** $4 \times 6 - 4 \div 2 + (17 - 9) \times 2(14 + 8 - 2) \times 10 \div 5 =$ _____

    a. What is the answer squared? _____

**58.** Find the GCF for the following numbers: 108, 72, 63, 54, 45, 36, 27, and 18

**59.** Find the LCM for the following numbers: 24, 36, 48, 72, 90, 336, and 480

**60.** $3 - (-2) + (-4) + 15 - 7 + (-25) - (-35) + 14 - 2(3 + 6) + 5(-3 + 6) =$

_____

    a. What is the answer squared? _____

    b. What is the answer cubed? _____

    c. What is the answer to the 5th power? _____

*(Continued)*

## MASTER THE SKILL
*Continued from p. 27*

Identify the prime number(s) in each grouping:

**61.** 7, 21, 27, 35, 49, and 70 _____

**62.** 82, 97, 127, 149, and 166 _____

**63.** 89, 105, 144, 167, 184, and 193 _____

**64.** 185, 187, 193, 197, and 200 _____

**65.** 31, 35, 41, 45, 79, 97, and 108 _____

# Roman Numerals, Military Time, and Graphs

## CHAPTER OUTLINE

## LEARNING OBJECTIVES

*Upon completion of this chapter, the learner will be able to:*

1. Define the key terms that relate to Roman numerals, military time and graphs.

2. Demonstrate how to convert Arabic numerals into Roman numerals and vice versa.

3. Convert times from a 12-hour clock to a 24-hour clock and vice versa.

4. Demonstrate proper strategies for rounding numbers with 100% accuracy.

5. Discuss how graphs can be used in the health care fields.

6. Create line, bar, and circle graphs.

7. Transcribe information on the correct chart.

## KEY TERMS

OBJECTIVE 1

Bar Graph
Circle Graph (Pie Graph)
Graph
Hindu–Arabic Numerals
Intake and Output Graph
Measurement Graph
Military Time

Roman Numerals
Rounding Down
Rounding Numbers
Rounding Up
Traditional Time
Vital Sign Graph

This chapter discusses topics that I like to refer to as the brief concepts that are relevant in a variety of health occupations. In the health care careers, we encounter:

- Documentation using military time
- Roman numerals used in documentation
- Roman numerals used to identify laboratory testing

OBJECTIVE ②    **REVIEW OF ROMAN NUMERALS**

The Arabic, sometimes known as Hindu–Arabic, number system is the numbering system most of us have grown up with. It consists of numbers 0 to 9. All other numbers are made of a combination of those digits, and their value is determined by the place value of each digit.

Roman numbers are commonly written in upper-case letters, though lower-case letters are sometimes used, too. Putting the letters together in a specific order creates numbers. As the letters are put together, a different number is created (Table 2-1).

| TABLE 2-1 | *Roman Numerals Compared with Arabic Numerals* |
|---|---|
| Roman Numeral (Letter) Upper Case and Lower Case | Arabic Numeral |
| $\overline{ss}$ | ½ |
| I i | 1 |
| V v | 5 |
| X x | 10 |
| L l | 50 |
| C c | 100 |
| D d | 500 |
| M m | 1,000 |

*Data from Mulholland JM: The nurse, the math, the meds: Drug calculations using dimensional analysis, St. Louis, 2007, Mosby, and Fulcher RM, Fulcher EM: Math calculations for pharmacy technicians: A worktext, St. Louis, 2007, Saunders.*

## MATH TRIVIA 2-1

If you have problems remembering the sequence of the Roman numerals, try this mnemonic:

    <u>I</u> <u>V</u>alue <u>X</u>ylophones <u>L</u>ike <u>C</u>ats <u>D</u>rink <u>M</u>ilk

    I = 1, V = 5, X = 10, L = 50, C = 100, D = 500, M = 1000

## MATH QUICK TIP 2-1

Arabic numerals use commas to separate thousands. Roman numerals do not use commas.

## MATH QUICK TIP 2-2

Lower-case Roman numerals are used in the medical field.

## MATH TRIVIA 2-2

Do you remember what a period is in math?

*Answer:* A period is when larger numbers are grouped by three places. The number 564,321 has two periods in it—thousands period and ones period.

## Why Do We Use Roman Numerals?

Many factors influence when and where Roman numerals are used. Roman numerals are a part of the apothecary system of measurement, which has been used by physicians in the past for writing medication orders. It was common practice to use Roman numerals when writing medications in small dose increments. They were usually written in lower case with a line drawn over the numerals to prevent misinterpretation of the order. The implementation of the Joint Commission's current guidelines, however, has led to many changes in the way physicians write medication prescriptions to reduce the potential for error. One change has been the elimination of the apothecary system for writing medication orders. However, Roman numerals continue to be used to identify different clotting factors found in a person's blood.

*Example:*
iii [3]

*Example:*
v [5] or vii [7]

## How to Write Roman Numerals

Roman numerals have their own set of rules to ensure proper translation of these numeric symbols.

If the letter is repeated, the number of times the letter is written represents the Arabic numeral.

*Example:*
II = 2

Letters are never to be repeated more than three times.

## MATH QUICK TIP 2-3

Roman Numeral Rules
Addition Rule: If smaller values are placed to the right of larger values or if values are repeated, the values are to be added.

*(Continued)*

## MATH QUICK TIP 2-3
*Continued from p. 31*

*Examples:*

vi = 5 + 1 = 6

xi = 10 + 1 = 11

xxvi = 10 + 10 + 5 + 1 = 26

7 = vii (5 + 2)

18 = xviii (10 + 5 + 3)

65 = LXV (50 + 10 + 5)

## MATH QUICK TIP 2-4

Subtraction Rule: If smaller values are placed to the left of larger values, the smaller value is subtracted.

Only 1 smaller value can be placed to the left of a larger value
i can be deducted only from v or x
x may be deducted only from l or c
c may be deducted only from d or m

*Examples:*

iv = 1 − 5 = 4

xi = 50 − 10 = 40

cm = 1000 − 100 = 900

90 = xc    100 − 10 = 90

400 = dc   500 − 100 = 400

9 = ix     10 − 1 = 9

## MATH TRIVIA 2-3

v, l, d, m are not used for subtraction.

## MATH QUICK TIP 2-5

Subtraction Precedence: When a larger value is between two smaller values, the subtraction is done first; when a smaller value is between two larger values, the subtraction is done first.

*Examples:*

xxix = 10 + 10 + (10 − 1) = 29

cxc = 100 + (100 − 10) = 190

XLII = (50 − 10) + 2 = 42

## MATH TRIVIA 2-4

If it seems like there are two ways to write a Roman numeral, write the shorter version.

## PRACTICE THE SKILL 2-1

Express the following Arabic numerals as Roman numerals.

1. 7 _____
6. 42 _____

2. 5 _____
7. 65 _____

3. 8 _____
8. 100 _____

4. 11 _____
9. 2006 _____

5. 15 _____
10. 75 _____

Express the following Roman numerals as Arabic numerals.

11. IV _____
16. LXV _____

12. CC _____
17. VIII _____

13. XXX _____
18. XXXII _____

14. XIX _____
19. XVI _____

15. MVIII _____
20. III _____

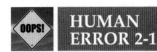

### HUMAN ERROR 2-1

*Be very careful when interpreting medication orders written with Roman numerals or written with both Roman numerals and Arabic numerals. Many errors occur when a V, which represents a 5, is confused with a U, which represents units. (For example, vii [seven] might be confused with 2 units.) This is why many facilities have discontinued the use of Roman numerals when writing medication orders.*

## MILITARY TIME

OBJECTIVE

Documentation in **military time** involves converting a traditional 12-hour clock into 24 hours. This eliminates the need to write "a.m." or "p.m." after a time entry, thereby avoiding confusion. Military time is always written with four digits. The first two digits represent the hour, and the last two digits represent the minutes. A 0 is used as a placeholder for recording time with only three digits.

## MATH QUICK TIP 2-6

Military time does not use a colon (:) or the abbreviations "a.m." or "p.m."

*Examples:*
1:00 a.m.　0100
2:15 a.m.　0215
3:30 a.m.　0330

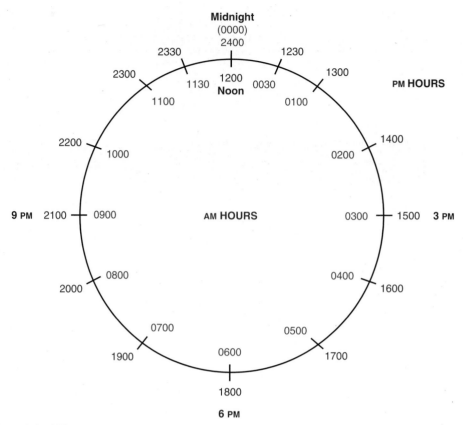

**Figure 2-1**  Military clock. (From Brown M, Mulholland JM: *Drug calculations: Process and problems for clinical practice*, ed 8, St. Louis, 2008, Mosby.)

At 10:00 a.m., a 0 is no longer needed as a placeholder. Simply write 1000 for 10:00 a.m. This method is used until 1:00 p.m.

*Examples:*
10:15 a.m.  1015
11:45 a.m.  1145
12:20 p.m.  1220

As stated before, military time is expressed by converting a 12-hour clock to a clock that counts 24 hours. The conversion begins when the time hits 1:00 p.m., which is referred to as 1300 hours. As you can see from Figure 2-1, each hour is counted from 1300 to 2359. Midnight (12 a.m.) can be documented in two different formats: 2400 or 0000. Your facility's policy will state which format you should use to document midnight.

A way to determine traditional afternoon times (p.m.) from military times is to subtract 12 from the number.

*Example:*
$14 - 12 = 2$
1400 is 2:00 p.m.

Remember this method only works on afternoon (p.m.) time.

*Examples:*
2:15 p.m.   1415
3:30 p.m.   1530
7:30 p.m.   1930
11:58 p.m.  2358

| BOX 2-1 | *Facilities Open 24 Hours a Day* |
|---|---|

- Hospital
- Nursing homes
- Rehabilitation centers
- Emergency rooms
- EMT/fire stations
- Pharmacy
- Home care
- Laboratory facilities

| BOX 2-2 | *Facilities Open Longer Than 8 Hours a Day* |
|---|---|

- Urgent care centers
- Same-day surgery centers
- Practices of large physician groups
- Phlebotomy/outpatient laboratory facilities
- Outpatient rehabilitation centers
- Adult day care
- Clinics

## Use of Military Time in Health Care

Why do health care facilities use military time in their documentation? Most health care facilities operate 24 hours a day, 7 days a week, and 365 days a year (Box 2-1). The use of military time reduces documentation errors, medication errors, and treatment errors. Facilities use a 24-hour clock to differentiate between an order written for a.m. versus p.m. administration. Many facilities are not open 24 hours a day but are open 12 to 15 hours a day (Box 2-2). Military time is used to identify when a patient has been seen, has been treated, has had medication dispensed, or when follow-up phone calls are made.

# MATH IN THE REAL WORLD 2-1

Where can you find Roman numerals in the real world?

- Super Bowl (e.g., Super Bowl XXVII)

- Movie credits (the year the movie was produced)

- Movie sequels (e.g., the *Rocky* series)

- Car styles (e.g., Speed Racer's Mach V)

- TV shows involving math as the plot

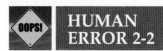

## HUMAN ERROR 2-2

*Did you remember to label your answers with a.m. or p.m.?*

## BUILDING CONFIDENCE WITH THE SKILL 2-1

Convert the following traditional times of day into military time.

1. 9:00 p.m. _____
2. 10:00 a.m. _____
3. 7:00 a.m. _____
4. 8:00 p.m. _____
5. 12 noon _____

6. 11:00 p.m. _____
7. 3:00 a.m. _____
8. 4:30 a.m. _____
9. 1:45 p.m. _____
10. 6:30 a.m. _____

Convert the following military times into 12-hour traditional time.

11. 0700 _____
12. 1530 _____
13. 2330 _____
14. 0015 _____
15. 0600 _____

16. 1800 _____
17. 2100 _____
18. 1015 _____
19. 1400 _____
20. 1830 _____

Convert the following Arabic numerals into Roman numerals.

21. 19 _____
22. 40 _____
23. 41 _____
24. 76 _____
25. 110 _____

26. 499 _____
27. 4 _____
28. 8 _____
29. 1965 _____
30. 1989 _____

Write the solutions to the following math problems in Roman numerals.

31.　27
　　 − 4

32.　14
　　 + 3

33.　56
　　 − 25

34.　2007
　　 − 450

35.　XXV
　　 + IV

36.　IX
　　 − IV

*(Continued)*

## BUILDING CONFIDENCE WITH THE SKILL 2-1
*Continued from p. 36*

37.  $\overline{\text{ii}}$ss
    $+ \overline{\text{iii}}$ss

38.  LV
    + XXI

39.  $\overline{\text{xxvi}}$
    $- \overline{\text{ix}}$ss

40.  XL
    + VII

## ROUNDING NUMBERS

OBJECTIVE **4**

Here are the rules for rounding numbers:

- Look one place to the right of the digit you want to round.
- If the digit is 5 or more, round the number to the next highest digit. This is known as **rounding up**.
- If the digit is less than 5, do not change the number at all. This is known as **rounding down**.

*Examples:*
Round to whole numbers:
347.987 would round to 348
23.43 would round to 23

Rounding with decimals (tenths):
243.12 would round to 243.1
896.712 would round to 896.7

### Whole and Decimal Place Value

| 5 | 3 | 1 | 4 | 2 | 8 | 9 | . | 8 | 2 | 4 | 1 | 3 | 5 |
|---|---|---|---|---|---|---|---|---|---|---|---|---|---|
| Million | Hundred-Thousand | Ten-Thousand | Thousand | Hundred | Ten | One | Decimal | Tenths | Hundredths | Thousandths | Ten-Thousandths | Hundred-Thousandths | Millionths |

## PRACTICE THE SKILL 2-2

Correctly write the following numbers, rounded to the thousandths place.

1. 32.56889 _____

2. 2.17421 _____

3. 1986.2007 _____

4. 0.875342 _____

5. 89.20491 _____

*(Continued)*

## PRACTICE THE SKILL 2-2
*Continued from p. 37*

Correctly write the following numbers, rounded to the hundredths place.

**6.** 765.3984 _____    **9.** 4476.568 _____

**7.** 210.1145 _____    **10.** 99.0678 _____

**8.** 2789.509 _____

Correctly write the following numbers, rounding to the tenths place.

**11.** 2.57985 _____    **14.** 56.83492 _____

**12.** 0.99742 _____    **15.** 0.10354 _____

**13.** 1.2430 _____

## BUILDING CONFIDENCE WITH THE SKILL 2-2

Complete the following chart by rounding numbers to the correct place.

| Problem | Ones | Thousandths | Tenths | Hundredths |
|---|---|---|---|---|
| **1.** 0.97341 | | | | |
| **2.** 6.37104 | | | | |
| **3.** 15.97523 | | | | |
| **4.** 0.601078 | | | | |
| **5.** 12.20914 | | | | |
| **6.** 1.25873 | | | | |
| **7.** 0.55645 | | | | |
| **8.** 0.46975 | | | | |
| **9.** 0.27743 | | | | |
| **10.** 2.35702 | | | | |

Match the following traditional times and military times.

**11.** 2057 _____    **a.** 6:37 p.m.

**12.** 0105 _____    **b.** 5:00 a.m.

*(Continued)*

## BUILDING CONFIDENCE WITH THE SKILL 2-2
*Continued from p. 38*

13. 0500 _____    c. 8:57 p.m.

14. 1837 _____    d. 1:05 a.m.

15. 1420 _____    e. 12:30 p.m.

16. 0830 _____    f. 12:15 a.m.

17. 1040 _____    g. 10:40 a.m.

18. 1230 _____    h. 8:30 a.m.

19. 2356 _____    i. 2:20 p.m.

20. 0015 _____    j. 11:56 p.m.

## GRAPHS

OBJECTIVE 5

**Graphs** are a visual way to express information regarding the relationship between two or more factors. Looking at a long page of numbers can be not only boring, but intimidating. After a while, the numbers blur together and misinterpretation of the information can occur. A graph can quickly convey information such as gross profit or loss, most profitable months, where most of the budget is used, and so on.

## MATH IN THE REAL WORLD 2-2
*Graphs in the Health Care Setting*

- Growth and development charts
- Vital sign charts
- Intake and output charts
- Budget charts
- Statistical information

In this chapter, we use different types of graphs and charts. You will learn how to create charts to reflect specific information. Depending on the availability of a computer, many of these exercises can be completed with the use of an electronic spreadsheet. Typically, working from an electronic spreadsheet will allow you to set up data sheets and create a graph. Once your graph is created, you can copy it to a word-processing document for reports.

A graph is a picture or diagram that reflects a relationship between two or more data sets. All graphs have a vertical axis and a horizontal axis. These scales are divided into increments that represent a ratio to the exact quantity. Once the variables for the axis have been established, the information is plotted. Line graphs are one of the most common types of graphs for plotting points from one or more data sets. Line graphs are commonly used to plot information that may have an increased chance for change. Once the information is plotted, a line is drawn from point to point. This gives a visual representation of the changes that occur in the data set or sets. If you are using more than one data set, each data set will be assigned a specific color to represent the information.

Graphs can be used to give a general description or illustration of the data set, trends, or the highs and lows of the information. To get actual information from a line graph, however, it helps to have the actual data set available for reference.

*Example:*
Number of people seen at Brightwood Hospital per year

| Year | Number of people seen |
|------|-----------------------|
| 1995 | 15,000 |
| 1996 | 22,000 |
| 1997 | 25,000 |
| 1998 | 23,500 |
| 1999 | 24,500 |
| 2000 | 26,500 |

Here is the same information plotted as a line graph.

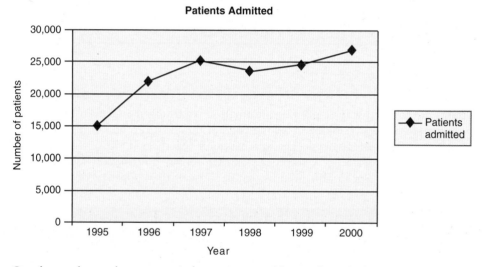

Graphs can be used to extract information quickly. Look at the line graph regarding the number of people seen at Brightwood Hospital per year (above) and answer the following questions:

1. In which year was the lowest number of patients seen? _____

2. In which year was there a decrease in the number of patients seen?

_____

3. In which year were the most patients seen? _____

OBJECTIVE ⑥        STRATEGY 2-1
*Creating a Line Graph Manually*

1. Identify the vertical (y) axis and the horizontal (x) axis with specific labels.

2. Determine the scale for each variable.

3. Plot each value for the data set. If you are comparing more than one data set, use different colors. Create a chart key and identify each data set in the chart key.

4. Using a ruler, connect the data set points to create a line.

Use the above strategies to plot the information from the following data set:

| Year | Patients seen in Emergency Room | Patients seen in outpatient surgery | Patients seen as inpatients |
|------|------|------|------|
| 2000 | 25,000 | 15,000 | 18,500 |
| 2001 | 25,500 | 16,500 | 20,000 |
| 2002 | 27,500 | 16,000 | 21,500 |
| 2003 | 26,500 | 15,500 | 22,000 |
| 2004 | 28,000 | 17,000 | 23,500 |
| 2005 | 27,500 | 18,000 | 23,000 |
| 2006 | 25,000 | 16,000 | 21,500 |

Here is what the line graph would look like:

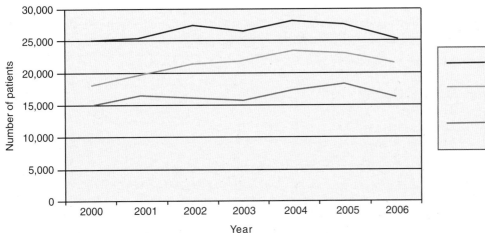

**Utilization of Specialty Areas**

STRATEGY 2-2
*Creating a Chart on the Computer*

OBJECTIVE 7

1. Open a spreadsheet program (e.g., Excel).

2. Input the data into the cells.

3. Highlight the cells you would like to include in the chart.

4. Click on the "Insert" tab and click on "Chart."

5. Follow the tutorial regarding the type of chart and labels.

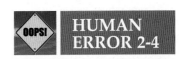

**HUMAN ERROR 2-3**

*When setting up your graph, allow enough space for accurate documentation of the data values.*

**HUMAN ERROR 2-4**

*If you are creating a graph by hand, remember that the x axis is the horizontal line and the y axis is the vertical line.*

# PRACTICE THE SKILL 2-3

1. Use graph paper or a computer to plot the following data to create a line graph.

| Year | Live infants born |
|------|-------------------|
| 2000 | 550 |
| 2001 | 475 |
| 2002 | 575 |
| 2003 | 600 |
| 2004 | 525 |
| 2005 | 500 |
| 2006 | 625 |

2. The following data set represents the number of patients seen in a physician's office per day for one month.

| | |
|---|---|
| Monday | 32 |
| Tuesday | 26 |
| Wednesday | 22 |
| Thursday | 28 |
| Friday | 32 |
| Saturday | 17 |

Based on the above data set, answer the following questions:

a. On which day(s) are the most patients seen?

_____

b. If you need to decrease the schedule by one day, which day would you consider eliminating? _____

3. The following data set represents the number of males and females ages 12 to 18 seen in the laboratory in the first half of the year. Create a chart to represent the data sets.

| | | |
|---|---|---|
| January | 150 males | 175 females |
| February | 112 males | 145 females |
| March | 125 males | 115 females |
| April | 100 males | 120 females |
| May | 90 males | 85 females |
| June | 75 males | 90 females |

*(Continued)*

**PRACTICE THE SKILL 2-3**
*Continued from p. 42*

**4.** Answer the following questions based on the graph below.

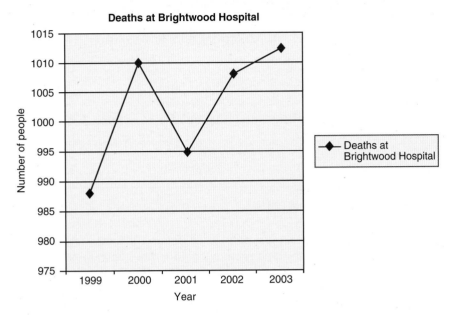

a. Which year had the lowest number of deaths at Brightwood Hospital?

_____

b. Which year had the greatest number of deaths at Brightwood Hospital?

_____

c. How many deaths occurred at Brightwood Hospital in 2002? _____

d. How many deaths occurred at Brightwood Hospital in 2001? _____

**5.** Answer the following questions based on the graph below.

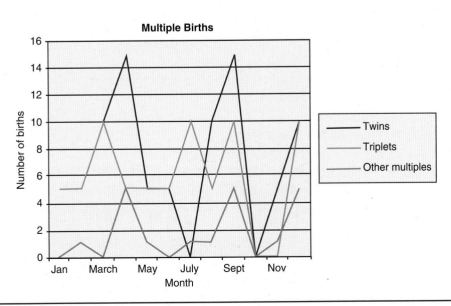

*(Continued)*

**PRACTICE THE SKILL 2-3**
*Continued from p. 43*

*Continued from p. 43*

a. Which month(s) had the greatest number multiple births other than twins and triplets? _____

b. In which month(s) were there no twins born at Brightwood Hospital? _____

c. In which month(s) were the most triplets born? _____

d. Which month(s) had the greatest total number of multiple births? _____

e. Which month(s) had the most twin births? _____

OBJECTIVE     **CIRCLE AND BAR GRAPHS**

**Circle graphs** are also known as **pie graphs**. Each data set is illustrated by a wedge or slice of the pie. This type of graph is commonly used to compare percentages of the total amount. The example below illustrates the number of people seen at Brightwood Hospital with two different circle graphs—one based on the total number of admissions and the second based on percentages. I used the strategies from Chapter 4 to determine the percentage for each value.

**Patients Admitted**

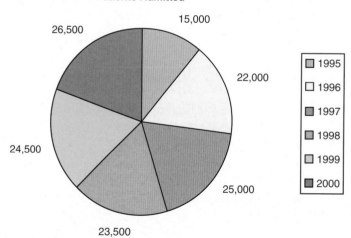

**Patients Admitted**

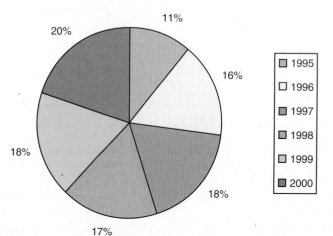

Bar graphs are commonly used to give a vertical or horizontal representation of data from different years or different sections of the facility. The following graph compares the total number of people seen in three different divisions of the hospital.

As the bar graph demonstrates, the emergency room (ER) has the greatest flow of patients each year. The graph also shows that the outpatient surgery center sees the fewest patients each year.

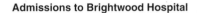

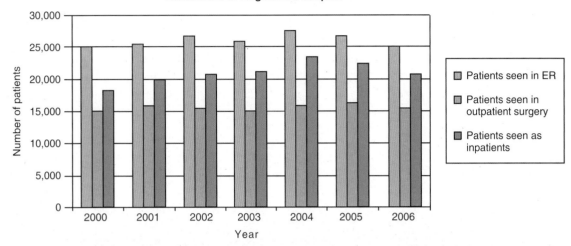

## BUILDING CONFIDENCE WITH THE SKILL 2-3

1. Using your computer, create a circle chart for each category.
   *Expenses per year*

   | Malpractice insurance | $32,000 |
   |---|---|
   | Retirement fund | $10,000 |
   | Casting supplies | $14,000 |
   | Medication supplies | $22,000 |
   | Salaries | $225,000 |
   | Software | $8,000 |

2. Using your computer, create a bar graph for the following data values.
   *Number of patients seen in a clinic each month for 3 years*

   |  | 2006 | 2007 | 2008 |
   |---|---|---|---|
   | January | 323 | 330 | 350 |
   | February | 275 | 310 | 330 |
   | March | 350 | 365 | 345 |
   | April | 275 | 290 | 280 |
   | May | 290 | 275 | 265 |
   | June | 200 | 150 | 200 |
   | July | 150 | 175 | 150 |
   | August | 225 | 200 | 180 |
   | September | 285 | 310 | 300 |
   | October | 305 | 325 | 340 |
   | November | 400 | 375 | 399 |
   | December | 325 | 280 | 300 |

3. Using your computer and the above data, create a line graph.

*(Continued)*

## BUILDING CONFIDENCE WITH THE SKILL 2-3
*Continued from p. 45*

4. Using your computer, create a bar graph and line graph to represent the data below.

|  | Respiratory diseases | Ear, nose, throat diseases | Gastric diseases |
|---|---|---|---|
| January | 25 | 80 | 36 |
| February | 23 | 74 | 22 |
| March | 32 | 66 | 18 |
| April | 14 | 56 | 29 |
| May | 22 | 55 | 42 |
| June | 10 | 40 | 7 |
| July | 9 | 27 | 11 |
| August | 11 | 32 | 26 |
| September | 25 | 88 | 34 |
| October | 32 | 78 | 41 |
| November | 45 | 69 | 32 |
| December | 76 | 75 | 24 |

5. Using your computer create 2 different charts that represent the data values listed below.

|  | Urinary diseases | Rashes | Pneumonia |
|---|---|---|---|
| January | 18 | 0 | 57 |
| February | 26 | 2 | 45 |
| March | 22 | 5 | 37 |
| April | 65 | 11 | 16 |
| May | 32 | 15 | 8 |
| June | 12 | 81 | 5 |
| July | 6 | 50 | 0 |
| August | 14 | 25 | 14 |
| September | 35 | 45 | 22 |
| October | 75 | 10 | 31 |
| November | 30 | 8 | 42 |
| December | 25 | 14 | 55 |

## MEASUREMENT GRAPHS

Many facilities have standardized graphic sheets. These sheets can be used to record vital signs (**vital sign graphs**) and fluid intake and output (**intake and output graphs**). Intake and output is discussed in Chapter 12. Because necessary information is recorded in one place on the graphic sheets, a reviewer can look at trends over a specified period. Please refer to the vital sign graphic sheet found in Chapter 12. As you see the top portion is designated for vital signs and the bottom portion is designated for intake and output values.

The purpose of this section is to introduce you to the use of different **measurement graphs** in the health care setting. To become familiar with the organization of the measurement graphs and how they can be used, in this section, you will be transferring information to the correct section of a graph. As you continue on your educational pathway in health care, you will receive detailed instruction on the use and values of measurement graphs. In addition, with the advancement of electronic health records, graphing of these values will be done by a computer program. However, it is important to understand the function or use of graphs when interpreting data of any type.

## Vital Sign Graphs

Look at Chapter 12, Figure 12-1. Which part of the chart is considered the vital sign graphic sheet? By viewing the graphic sheet, you can easily tell when the patient's temperature was above normal (98.6°F). With the increased use of electronic health records (EHR), as information is added the graph will automatically be updated.

## MATH IN THE REAL WORLD 2-3
### Vital Signs (T, P, R, and BP)

*Temperature (T):* Normal body temperature ranges from 97°F to 99°F.

*Pulse (P):* The pulse represents how quickly or slowly the heart is pumping. Normal pulse ranges from 60 to 100 beats per minute. Many things can influence a person's pulse, such as activity, age, disease, and illness.

*Respirations (R):* Respirations are measured to determine how quickly or slowly a person is breathing. Normal respirations are 12 to 20 breaths per minute. Respiration can be affected by age, smoking, activity, disease, and illness.

*Blood pressure (BP):* Blood pressure measures the pressure of the blood against the artery walls. Blood pressure is represented by two numbers written as a fraction. The systolic pressure is the highest pressure level that occurs when the heart is contracting. The systolic reading is written as the numerator. Diastolic pressure is the lowest pressure level when the heart is relaxed. Diastolic pressure is written as the denominator. Guidelines for the normal blood pressure range change periodically. Under current guidelines, the normal systolic reading is less than 120 and the normal diastolic pressure reading is less than 80. Thus, normal blood pressure should be less than $^{120}/_{80}$ millimeters of mercury (mm Hg).

## Height and Weight Graphs

Growth and development charts are completed at every well-baby and well-child check. There are different charts for infants to 36 months and for children and adolescents 2 to 20 years, as well as for boys (blue) and girls (pink) (Figures 2-2 and 2-3). These charts are used to record the child's height and weight. Based on this information, the physician can determine if the child is developing on the normal growth curve.

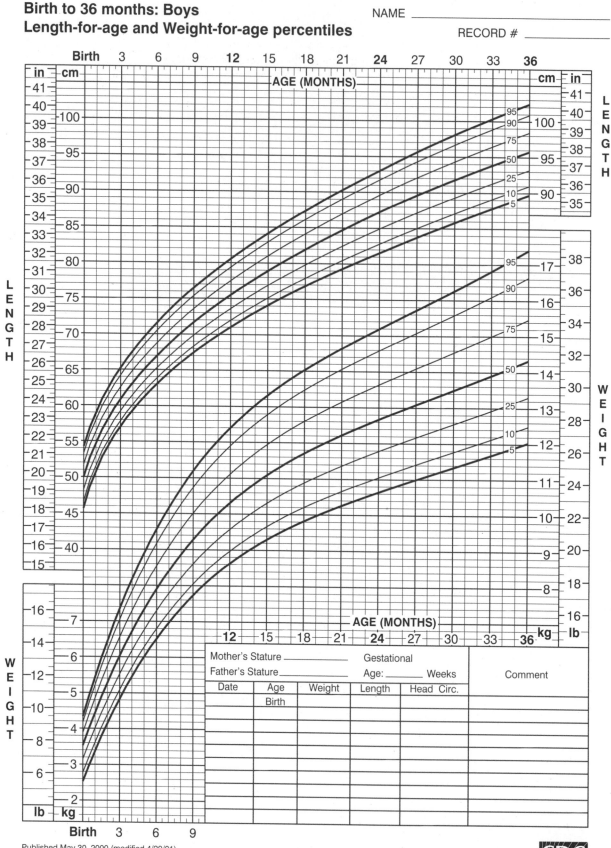

**Birth to 36 months: Boys**
**Length-for-age and Weight-for-age percentiles**

NAME _____

RECORD # _____

Published May 30, 2000 (modified 4/20/01).
SOURCE: Developed by the National Center for Health Statistics in collaboration with
the National Center for Chronic Disease Prevention and Health Promotion (2000).
http://www.cdc.gov/growthcharts

SAFER · HEALTHIER · PEOPLE™

**Figure 2-2**    Growth chart: Birth to 36 months: boys. Length-for-age and weight-for-age percentiles.
(Published May 30, 2000 [modified 4/20/01]. Developed by the National Center for Health Statistics in
collaboration with the National Center for Chronic Disease Prevention and Health Promotion [2000].
http://www.cdc.gov/growthcharts)

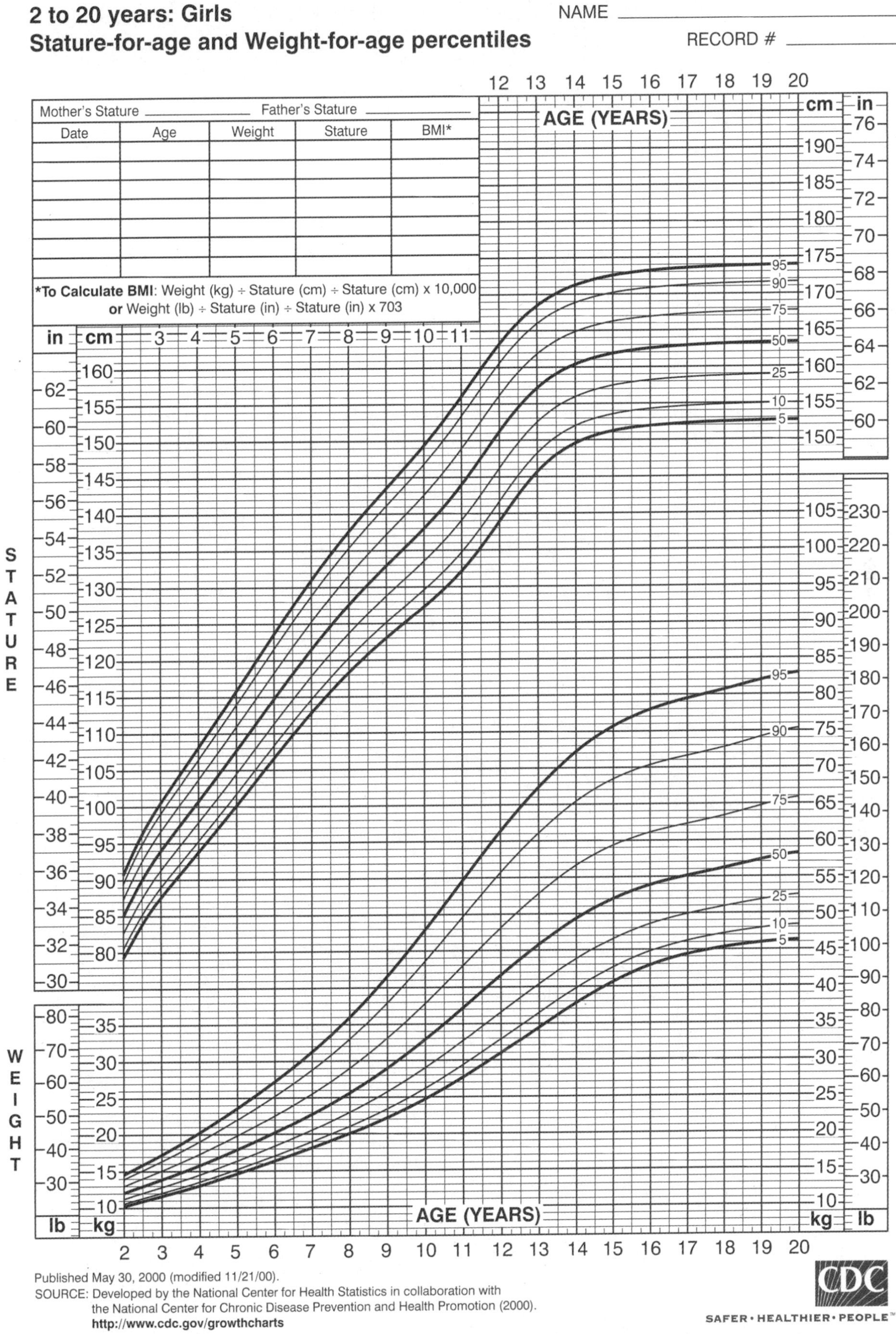

## 2 to 20 years: Girls
## Stature-for-age and Weight-for-age percentiles

NAME _____

RECORD # _____

| Date | Age | Weight | Stature | BMI* |
|------|-----|--------|---------|------|
| | | | | |
| | | | | |
| | | | | |
| | | | | |
| | | | | |

Mother's Stature _____ Father's Stature _____

**\*To Calculate BMI**: Weight (kg) ÷ Stature (cm) ÷ Stature (cm) x 10,000
**or** Weight (lb) ÷ Stature (in) ÷ Stature (in) x 703

Published May 30, 2000 (modified 11/21/00).
SOURCE: Developed by the National Center for Health Statistics in collaboration with
the National Center for Chronic Disease Prevention and Health Promotion (2000).
http://www.cdc.gov/growthcharts

CDC
SAFER • HEALTHIER • PEOPLE™

**Figure 2-3** Growth chart: 2 to 20 years: girls. Stature-for-age and weight-for-age percentiles. (Published May 30, 2000 [modified 11/21/00]. Developed by the National Center for Health Statistics in collaboration with the National Center for Chronic Disease Prevention and Health Promotion [2000]. http://www.cdc.gov/growthcharts.)

# PRACTICE THE SKILL 2-4

Using your computer, create a line graph for each set of values.

1. Write today's date.

2. Record the following vital signs:

|  | 6:00 a.m. | 8:00 a.m. | 12:00 p.m. | 2:00 p.m. | 4:00 p.m. | 6:00 p.m. | 8:00 p.m. | 11:00 p.m. |
|---|---|---|---|---|---|---|---|---|
| T | 99.7 | 99.1 | 98.8 | 99.1 | 100 | 100.8 | 101.2 | 100.6 |
| P | 80 | 82 | 82 | 88 | 90 | 88 | 88 | 84 |
| R | 18 | 18 | 20 | 18 | 20 | 20 | 20 | 20 |
| BP | $124/76$ | $132/78$ | $120/80$ | $134/76$ | $130/78$ | $128/76$ | $134/70$ | $128/80$ |

**Using a computer, create a graph chart to document values for height and weight.**

3. Baby boy Luke had the following height and weight measurements from birth through 3 years:

|  | Height | Weight |
|---|---|---|
| Birth | 19 inches | 8 lb 2 oz |
| 2 weeks | 19.5 inches | 8 lb 10 oz |
| 1 month | 20 inches | 9 lb 2 oz |
| 3 months | 22 inches | 9 lb 7 oz |
| 6 months | 23 inches | 11 lb |
| 9 months | 24 inches | 12 lb 2 oz |
| 1 year | 28 inches | 14 lb |
| 18 months | 31 inches | 17 lb 8 oz |
| 2 years | 34 inches | 22 lb 6 oz |
| 3 years | 36 inches | 28 lb |

# CONCLUSION

Confidence in your math skills is what allows you to solve problems. Accuracy with your computations is what keeps you from making errors. Both aspects are equally important in the world of health care professionals. For many of you, this chapter has been a review, but as with many skills you have learned, if you don't use it, you lose it. As you build on these skills, challenge yourself to think outside the box. As mentioned before, there is more than one way to attack a math problem. Share your strategies with your classmates. Remember, math can give you instant gratification. You work the problem and receive the correct answer—*success, confidence, and mastery of the skill.* If you work a problem and don't get the right answer, don't get discouraged! Discuss how you solved the problem and find out where you made your error. Most errors have to do with mistakes in computation or transposition of numbers.

Graphs and graphic charting are a visual way to compare information. A chart easily identifies any values that are not within normal limits. In addition, graphs are useful tools to illustrate the following:

Where money from the budget is spent
Frequency of patients or diseases
Frequency of orders for a test
Frequency of laboratory requisitions

## MASTER THE SKILL

Write the Arabic numeral that is equivalent to each of the following Roman numerals.

1. XV _____          6. XLI _____

2. xiv _____          7. LIX _____

3. XXII _____          8. CCC _____

4. viii _____          9. CD _____

5. iv _____          10. MMM _____

Write the Roman numeral that is equivalent to each of the following Arabic numerals. Write all answers in upper case letters.

11. 10 _____          16. 64 _____

12. 25 _____          17. 14 _____

13. 30 _____          18. 1903 _____

14. 49 _____          19. 2000 _____

15. 60 _____          20. 43 _____

Round the following numbers to the nearest tenth.

21. 0.34 _____          24. 1.92 _____

22. 1.27 _____          25. 0.06 _____

23. 0.788 _____

Round the following numbers to the nearest hundredth.

26. 0.6892 _____          29. 2.376 _____

27. 3.752 _____          30. 0.051 _____

28. 0.888 _____

Round the following numbers to the nearest thousandth.

31. 0.68923 _____          34. 2.37678 _____

32. 3.75243 _____          35. 0.05198 _____

33. 0.88824 _____

*(Continued)*

**MASTER THE SKILL**
*Continued from p. 51*

Round the following numbers to the nearest whole number.

**36.** 2.38 _____

**37.** 10.643 _____

**38.** 0.97423 _____

**39.** 1.5245 _____

**40.** 3.47 _____

OBJECTIVE **3**

Convert the following times from military time to 24-hour or traditional time.

**41.** 1436 _____

**42.** 0730 _____

**43.** 0001 _____

**44.** 1845 _____

**45.** 1120 _____

Write the following traditional times in military time for both a.m. and p.m.

| | *a.m.* | *p.m.* |
|---|---|---|
| **46.** 3:00 | _____ | _____ |
| **47.** 11:30 | _____ | _____ |
| **48.** 7:00 | _____ | _____ |
| **49.** 8:00 | _____ | _____ |
| **50.** 12:00 | _____ | _____ |

OBJECTIVES **6 7 8**

Answer questions 51 to 55 using the graph below.

**Number of TVs Sold in August**

Legend: Tom, Cindy, Amy

Y-axis: Number of TVs (0 to 40)
X-axis: Days of the week (Mon, Tue, Wed, Thur, Fri, Sat, Sun)

*(Continued)*

## MASTER THE SKILL
*Continued from p. 52*

**51.** On what day(s) of the week were the most TVs sold? _____

**52.** Which day of the week did Tom sell the most TVs? _____

**53.** Which day of the week did Cindy sell the fewest TVs? _____

**54.** Which day of the week did Amy sell the most TVs? _____

**55.** Which day of the week did everyone sell the same number of TVs?

_____

**Answer questions 56 to 58 using the data set below.**

|  | Tom |
|---|---|
| Monday | 12 |
| Tuesday | 20 |
| Wednesday | 32 |
| Thursday | 11 |
| Friday | 8 |
| Saturday | 35 |
| Sunday | 18 |

**56.** Create a circle chart based on percentages of TVs sold.

**57.** Create a line chart for the information provided in the data set above.

**58.** Create a bar chart for the information provided in the data set above.

**Answer questions 59 to 65 using the data set below.**

|  | X-ray | Laboratory values |
|---|---|---|
| 1991 | 5,657 | 8,976 |
| 1992 | 6,432 | 7,891 |
| 1993 | 7,864 | 7,254 |
| 1994 | 6,334 | 8,986 |
| 1995 | 8,136 | 10,001 |
| 1996 | 9,321 | 10,876 |
| 1997 | 9,558 | 11,225 |
| 1998 | 9,989 | 11,489 |
| 1999 | 10,025 | 10,445 |
| 2000 | 11,000 | 11,089 |

**59.** Create a pie chart representing x-ray values and percentage.

**60.** Create a pie chart representing laboratory values and percentage.

**61.** In what year was the highest percentage of laboratory specimens drawn?

_____

**62.** In what year was the lowest percentage of x-rays taken? _____

*(Continued)*

**MASTER THE SKILL**
*Continued from p. 53*

63. In what year were the most laboratory specimens drawn? _____

64. In what year were the most x-rays taken? _____

65. Of the three types of charts (bar, line, or circle), which one would provide the required information and be easiest to read? _____

Using your computer, create a line graph to represent each of the following vital sign values.

66. Write today's date.

67. Record the following vital signs:

|     | 6:00 a.m. | 8:00 a.m. | 12:00 p.m. | 2:00 p.m. | 4:00 p.m. | 6:00 p.m. | 8:00 p.m. | 11:00 p.m. |
|-----|-----------|-----------|------------|-----------|-----------|-----------|-----------|------------|
| T   | 98.7      | 98.1      | 97.8       | 98.1      | 98.6      | 99.0      | 100.2     | 101.6      |
| P   | 80        | 82        | 82         | 88        | 84        | 88        | 88        | 94         |
| R   | 18        | 18        | 20         | 18        | 20        | 18        | 20        | 22         |
| BP  | $124/76$  | $132/78$  | $120/80$   | $134/76$  | $130/78$  | $128/76$  | $134/70$  | $128/80$   |

Using the vital signs information above, answer the following questions.

68. What time did the patient have the highest temperature?

_____

69. What happened to the temperature throughout the day?

_____

70. What time did the patient have the highest blood pressure?

_____

71. What time did the patient have the lowest blood pressure?

_____

# Fractions

## CHAPTER OUTLINE

## LEARNING OBJECTIVES

*Upon completion of this chapter, the learner will be able to:*

1. Define the key terms that relate to fractions.

2. Identify situations where fractions would be used in real world situations and benefit the health care professional.

3. Manipulate fractions into a specified order of value.

4. Convert fractions from an improper fraction to a mixed number and from a mixed number to an improper fraction.

5. Perform mathematical operations involving fractions.

## KEY TERMS

OBJECTIVE 1

| | |
|---|---|
| Common Factor | Improper Fraction |
| Denominator | Least Common Denominator (LCD) |
| Equivalent Fraction | Mixed Number |
| Factor | Numerator |
| Fraction | Proper Fraction |
| Fractions with Common Denominators | Reduce or Simplify Fractions |
| Greatest Common Factor (GCF) | Whole Number |

OBJECTIVE 1

Health care professionals perform a variety of mathematical computations during the course of the day. Professionals involved in the clinical side of health care frequently encounter fractions while performing the following duties:

OBJECTIVE 2

- Medical assistant: preparing medications, measuring height and weight, measuring for the length of a cast or splint
- Pharmacy technician: assisting in the preparation of medication
- Physical therapy assistant: supervising rehabilitation exercises involving weights, documenting endurance in minutes or hours
- Nurse: administering medication, IV therapy, and blood transfusions

- Dietician: calculating dietary intake or calorie needs
- Paramedic: preparing medication doses based on weight, calculating length of time for transport from a scene

However, there is more to health care than just the clinical application. Many careers fall under the administrative aspects of health care. Anyone who deals with money, payroll, time sheets, or ordering of supplies will probably manipulate fractions or at least convert fractions into decimals.

Like most people, you have probably used fractions since grade school. However, your confidence in your ability to manipulate fractions may be weak. In this chapter, we will review fractions and provide strategies for properly manipulating fractions.

OBJECTIVE 2

OBJECTIVE 3

## UNDERSTANDING FRACTIONS

As a teacher, I am always surprised by the negative responses the word "fractions" evokes from students. Comments include:

"Fractions—I just don't understand them and never could."
"I can't do math because of fractions."
"I'm fine with math, except for fractions, but that doesn't matter because I never use them."

Do these statements sound familiar? Is this how you feel about fractions? Why do people become so anxious when they just hear the word *fractions*? People use fractions every day, whether they realize it or not. Here are a few examples:

"Who left ¼ of a tank of gas in the car?"
"About ¾ of the students in the class are girls."
"We have ½ an hour for lunch."
"You need to add ⅔ cup of sugar to the recipe."

See more examples in Box 3-1.

To understand fractions, we need to review their purpose. Let's get down to basics by answering the following questions:

1. What is a fraction?
2. Why do we use fractions?
3. Can fractions be equivalent?

I'm sure you know the answers. Now it is a matter of taking that knowledge and applying it in a different manner.

OBJECTIVE 1

### BOX 3-1    *Fractions in the Real World*

- Cooking: measuring ingredients
- Carpentry: measuring materials
- Plumbing: measuring the length and diameter of pipes
- Health care: measuring height, weight, and medications
- Science: establishing the amount of each chemical in a compound
- Payroll: determining the amount of pay for a fractional part of an hour
- Music: reading a time signature to find out what fraction of the beat in a measure each note is
- Interior design: figuring out wallpaper and fabric measurements

## What Is a Fraction?

A **fraction** is a mathematical way to describe a part or unit used in relation to the total quantity. The **numerator** represents the total number of units being used, and the **denominator** represents the total number of pieces.

*Example:*

Figure of a fraction    $\dfrac{2}{5}$ numerator  denominator

Many people learned fractions by visualizing a pizza pie. So, let's take what we know and apply it.

*Example:*

Three friends have ordered a pizza. The pizza comes in eight slices. Each friend has two slices (Figure 3-1).
Describe what fraction of the pizza has been eaten:

3 friends × 2 slices each = 6 slices of pizza eaten.
The pizza had a total of 8 slices.

The fraction ⁶⁄₈ represents how much of the pizza has been consumed. Did you automatically reduce ⁶⁄₈ to ¾ ? If so, great! If you are unsure how to reduce a fraction, that is all right because we will address this in the next few paragraphs.
What is the fractional expression for the amount of pizza that has *not* been consumed?

8 total slices − 6 slices already eaten = 2 slices left.
So, the fraction of the pizza that has not been consumed is ²⁄₈, or ¼.

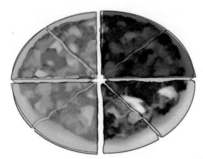

**Figure 3-1**    Example of fractions with pizza pie.

Now let's apply this concept to the work world. You work a 12-hour shift. You needed to leave 4 hours early. What fraction of the shift did you work? What fraction of the shift did you *not* work?
You worked 8 out of the 12 hours. The 8 hours you worked is the part or unit that you worked out of the total scheduled 12 hours. So, the fraction of the shift you did work is ⁸⁄₁₂ (or ⅔ if you automatically reduce the fraction).
You left 4 hours early; this represents the part or unit that you did not work out of the total scheduled 12 hours. Therefore, the fraction of the shift you did *not* work is ⁴⁄₁₂ (or ⅓ if you automatically reduce the fraction).

## How Do We Use Fractions?

OBJECTIVE ②

As we have learned, fractions are a descriptive way to identify a portion, either used or remaining, of the total. For the visual learners and kinesthetic learners of the world, however, fractions can be hard to visualize. If you are having problems in determining the size of a series of fractions, try drawing a box into the number of sections indicated in the denominator and then shading the sections indicated in the numerator (Figure 3-2).

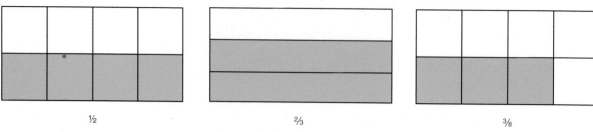

Figure 3-2   Comparison of fractions.

### STRATEGY 3-1

If you are having difficulty determining the order of a series of fractions, try this method:

1. Draw a rectangular box.

2. Divide the box into equal portions as determined by the denominator.

3. Shade the total portions used as determined by the numerator.

4. Finally, answer the question.

### PRACTICE THE SKILL 3-1

Circle the largest fraction in each series.

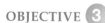

1. $5/11$            $3/8$            $2/3$

2. $1/15$            $1/10$           $1/6$

3. $1/4$             $1/3$            $1/2$

4. $2/3$             $3/5$            $5/7$

5. $1/10$            $1/100$          $1/50$

OBJECTIVE **3**

### Can Different Fractions Be Equivalent?

Yes, **equivalent fractions** are fractions that represent the same relationship of a part to the whole. The fractions are equal even though there are variations in the size of the pieces or parts of the total. Many times we refer to equivalent fractions when we reduce a fraction to its lowest form. When we **reduce or simplify fractions,** we are finding the lowest equivalent fraction by dividing the numerator and the denominator by the **greatest common factor (GCF).** Remember the example discussed above regarding the pizza pie: $6/8$ slices were eaten. We need to find the greatest **common factor** that can be divided into both 6 and 8. In other words, what is the highest number that can be divided into both 6 and 8? In this case, the GCF is 2.

$$\frac{6}{2} = 3$$

$$\frac{8}{2} = 4$$

Thus, $\frac{6}{8}$ is equivalent to $\frac{3}{4}$. The fractions involved have different denominators; however, they represent the same number of pieces.

Let's try another example. Are the following fractions equivalent?

$\frac{4}{8}$ and $\frac{4}{16}$

Reduce the fractions:

$\frac{4}{8}$ has the GCF of 4.

Dividing the numerator by 4 equals 1.

Dividing the denominator by 4 equals 2.

$$\frac{4}{8} = \frac{1}{2}$$

Using the steps stated above, $\frac{4}{16}$ has the GCF of 4.

Dividing the numerator by 4 equals 1.

Dividing the denominator by 4 equals 4.

$$\frac{4}{16} = \frac{1}{4}$$

Therefore $\frac{4}{8}$ and $\frac{4}{16}$ are **not** equivalent fractions.

### Why Does It Matter How We Express the Fraction?

Many people reduce fractions automatically either on paper or in their heads. Why? Because it is how they were taught: "Express your answer in its lowest form." Let's just say it is math etiquette.

Refer to the bulleted list of statements in the first section of this chapter. People describe fractions in their lowest form. People do not say $\frac{4}{16}$ gallon of gas was left in the tank. It sounds awkward. However, $\frac{4}{16}$ and $\frac{1}{4}$ are equivalent fractions. Your instructor will most likely deduct points from your test scores if you do not reduce answers to their lowest form.

Let's try another problem. Are the fractions $\frac{4}{20}$ and $\frac{5}{25}$ equivalent?

Step 1: Reduce your fractions:

$$\frac{4}{20} = \frac{1}{5}$$

$$\frac{5}{25} = \frac{1}{5}$$

Yes, these fractions are equivalent.

## MATH QUICK TIP 3-1

Express your answers in the lowest form.

## PRACTICE THE SKILL 3-2

Reduce the fraction to its lowest form.

1. $\frac{4}{12}$ _____

4. $\frac{5}{20}$ _____

2. $\frac{8}{48}$ _____

5. $\frac{10}{50}$ _____

3. $\frac{5}{15}$ _____

Are the following fractions equivalent? Answer "Yes" if they are equivalent and "No" if they are not equivalent.

6. $\frac{4}{12}$ and $\frac{5}{15}$ _____

9. $\frac{2}{3}$ and $\frac{12}{36}$ _____

7. $\frac{3}{9}$ and $\frac{6}{18}$ _____

10. $\frac{5}{8}$ and $\frac{3}{16}$ _____

8. $\frac{3}{4}$ and $\frac{7}{9}$ _____

## BUILDING CONFIDENCE WITH THE SKILL 3-1

Are the following series of fractions equivalent? Answer "Yes" if they are equivalent and "No" if they are not equivalent.

1. $\frac{1}{2}$, $\frac{25}{50}$, $\frac{50}{100}$ _____

6. $\frac{1}{18}$, $\frac{3}{18}$, $\frac{2}{9}$ _____

2. $\frac{1}{3}$, $\frac{3}{9}$, $\frac{2}{6}$ _____

7. $\frac{6}{12}$, $\frac{24}{48}$, $\frac{9}{81}$ _____

3. $\frac{1}{4}$, $\frac{4}{5}$, $\frac{3}{12}$ _____

8. $\frac{3}{18}$, $\frac{7}{10}$, $\frac{6}{43}$ _____

4. $\frac{1}{10}$, $\frac{8}{80}$, $\frac{9}{90}$ _____

9. $\frac{23}{46}$, $\frac{57}{114}$, $\frac{78}{156}$ _____

5. $\frac{1}{15}$, $\frac{6}{30}$, $\frac{9}{45}$ _____

10. $\frac{2}{3}$, $\frac{4}{6}$, $\frac{6}{9}$ _____

Reduce the following fractions.

11. $\frac{12}{24}$ _____

16. $\frac{5}{75}$ _____

12. $\frac{6}{18}$ _____

17. $\frac{12}{48}$ _____

13. $\frac{24}{36}$ _____

18. $\frac{7}{21}$ _____

14. $\frac{30}{48}$ _____

19. $\frac{72}{96}$ _____

15. $\frac{9}{15}$ _____

20. $\frac{15}{45}$ _____

*(Continued)*

# BUILDING CONFIDENCE WITH THE SKILL 3-1
*Continued from p. 60*

**Solve the following word problems.**

21. An RN and an LPN both are scheduled to work a 12-hour shift at the hospital. The RN receives a phone call and must leave the hospital after working only 3 hours. The LPN becomes ill after working 8 hours and must leave.

    a. What fraction of the work day did the RN work? _____

    b. What fraction of the work day did the LPN *not* work? _____

22. You are ordering pizza for everyone at the fire station. A large pizza has 12 slices. Your order includes one large supreme pizza, one large pepperoni pizza, and one large cheese pizza. The personnel consume the following:

    Paramedic #1 eats two slices of supreme and three slices of pepperoni.

    Paramedic #2 eats one slice of supreme and three slices of pepperoni.

    Firefighter #1 eats four slices of pepperoni and two slices of cheese.

    Firefighter #2 eats three slices of cheese.

    Captain eats six slices of supreme and two slices of pepperoni.

    a. What fraction of each type of pizza has been consumed? _____

    b. What fraction of each pizza remains? _____

## Different Types of Fractions

OBJECTIVE 4

In many occupations, it is acceptable to work with improper fractions; however, it is common practice for health care professionals to reduce fractions to their lowest form when recording results.

## MATH QUICK TIP 3-2

**Proper Fraction:** A fraction in which the denominator is greater than the numerator.
   *Examples:* $\frac{3}{5}$, $\frac{3}{4}$, $\frac{1}{8}$, $\frac{3}{10}$, $\frac{1}{2}$

**Improper Fraction:** A fraction in which the numerator is greater than the denominator.
   *Examples:* $\frac{12}{10}$, $\frac{9}{5}$, $\frac{15}{14}$, $\frac{27}{25}$

**Mixed Number:** Number expression that consists of a whole number and a fraction.
   *Examples:* $1\frac{1}{5}$, $1\frac{4}{5}$, $1\frac{1}{14}$, $1\frac{2}{25}$

**Whole Number:** Any fraction where the numerator is a multiple of the denominator can be rewritten as a whole number.
   *Examples:* $\frac{32}{32} = 1$, $\frac{3}{3} = 1$, $\frac{8}{4} = 2$, $\frac{9}{3} = 3$

Many mathematical operations involve converting an improper fraction to a mixed number or vice versa. To convert an improper fraction into a proper fraction, you must divide the denominator into the numerator. Sometimes this will result in a whole number.

*Example:*

$$\frac{6}{3}$$

6 divided by 3 = 2

## HUMAN ERROR 3-1

*Review GCF and LCM strategies in Chapter 1 to help reduce error with the concept of changing improper fractions into mixed numbers.*

Some improper fractions will not divide evenly to create a whole number. Some improper fractions will have a whole number and a fraction.

*Example:*

$$\frac{29}{7}$$

29 divided by 7 = 4 with a remainder of 1; the remainder is placed in the numerator and the denominator remains unchanged, so the answer is written as $4\frac{1}{7}$.

## MATH QUICK TIP 3-3

Mixed numbers must also be reduced to the lowest form.

## MATH QUICK TIP 3-4

An improper fraction is not changed to a mixed number when the fraction is being used in an operation involving multiplication or division.

Now that you remember how to reduce improper fractions, can you change a mixed number into an improper fraction?

*Example:*

$$3\frac{7}{10}$$

Multiply the denominator by the whole number: $10 \times 3 = 30$.
Then add the numerator: $30 + 7 = 37$.
The number 37 is your new numerator and will go over the existing denominator.
$\frac{37}{10}$ is your improper fraction.

## STRATEGY 3-2

((Denominator × Whole number) + Numerator)/Denominator = Improper fraction

*Example:* $5\frac{3}{5}$
Multiply the denominator by the whole number:
$5 \times 5 = 25$
Add the numerator to the above sum:
$25 + 3 = 28$
28 becomes the new numerator and will go over the existing denominator.
$\frac{28}{5}$ is your improper fraction.

## PRACTICE THE SKILL 3-3

Change the following improper fractions into mixed numbers. Record all answers in their lowest form.

1. $\frac{27}{4}$ _____

2. $\frac{35}{8}$ _____

3. $\frac{12}{10}$ _____

4. $\frac{47}{8}$ _____

5. $\frac{63}{6}$ _____

6. $\frac{25}{11}$ _____

7. $\frac{45}{7}$ _____

8. $\frac{56}{9}$ _____

9. $\frac{23}{2}$ _____

10. $\frac{81}{9}$ _____

## PRACTICE THE SKILL 3-4

Convert the following mixed numbers to improper fractions.

1. $3\frac{3}{4}$ _____

2. $8\frac{1}{6}$ _____

3. $5\frac{1}{2}$ _____

4. $7\frac{3}{4}$ _____

5. $11\frac{5}{8}$ _____

6. $9\frac{3}{16}$ _____

7. $12\frac{2}{3}$ _____

8. $15\frac{1}{2}$ _____

9. $4\frac{7}{8}$ _____

10. $9\frac{5}{9}$ _____

People use fractions every day. In this section, we have reviewed the different properties of fractions as well as how to manipulate fractions. In the following sections, we will build on these concepts to perform mathematical operations. As a reminder, all fractions should be stated in their lowest form.

## BUILDING CONFIDENCE WITH THE SKILL 3-2

In the following series, place the fractions in order from least to greatest.

1. $\frac{1}{12}$, $\frac{1}{16}$, $\frac{1}{24}$ _____

2. $\frac{2}{5}$, $\frac{7}{9}$, $\frac{3}{16}$ _____

3. $\frac{5}{24}$, $\frac{5}{36}$, $\frac{5}{15}$ _____

4. $\frac{1}{10}$, $\frac{2}{50}$, $\frac{75}{100}$ _____

5. $\frac{2}{3}$, $\frac{3}{4}$, $\frac{1}{8}$ _____

Convert the following improper fractions into either whole numbers or mixed numbers. Write all answers in their lowest form.

6. $\frac{18}{3}$ _____

7. $\frac{15}{4}$ _____

8. $\frac{24}{5}$ _____

9. $\frac{45}{36}$ _____

10. $\frac{23}{7}$ _____

Reduce the following fractions to their lowest form.

11. $\frac{7}{21}$ _____

12. $\frac{16}{32}$ _____

13. $\frac{24}{72}$ _____

14. $\frac{4}{24}$ _____

15. $\frac{6}{48}$ _____

Convert the mixed numbers into improper fractions.

16. $6\frac{5}{8}$ _____

17. $9\frac{3}{10}$ _____

18. $4\frac{7}{11}$ _____

19. $7\frac{9}{10}$ _____

20. $5\frac{1}{2}$ _____

*(Continued)*

## BUILDING CONFIDENCE WITH THE SKILL 3-2
*Continued from p. 64*

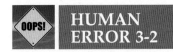

*Continued from p. 64*

### HUMAN ERROR 3-2

*Did you add correctly?
Did you subtract correctly?*

*Is your answer in its lowest form?*

*Does your answer make sense?*

**Match the fractions that are equivalent.**

21. $\frac{2}{3}$ _____ $\frac{12}{60}$

22. $\frac{1}{2}$ _____ $\frac{12}{18}$

23. $\frac{3}{4}$ _____ $\frac{16}{32}$

24. $\frac{1}{5}$ _____ $\frac{9}{48}$

25. $\frac{3}{16}$ _____ $\frac{15}{20}$

26. $\frac{12}{24}$ _____ $\frac{12}{60}$

27. $\frac{5}{25}$ _____ $\frac{16}{32}$

**Answer the following word problems.**

28. The patient drank $\frac{1}{2}$ cup of milk, $\frac{2}{3}$ cup of orange juice, and $\frac{3}{4}$ cup of coffee. Of which type of fluid did the patient drink the most?

_____

29. Due to a computer error, the following time sheet was submitted as improper fractions. Monday—$1\frac{1}{2}$ hours, Tuesday—$\frac{27}{4}$ hours, Wednesday—$\frac{15}{4}$ hours, Thursday—$1\frac{1}{2}$ hours, and Friday—$\frac{49}{7}$ hours. Based on the information, which day had the least amount of hours worked? _____ Which day had the most hours worked? _____

30. The prep instructions read: drink 2 oz of prep every hour starting at 6:00 p.m. and ending at 10:00 p.m. The patient should consume 6 oz at 10:00 p.m. The patient is given a 16 oz bottle of prep. What fraction of the prep will the patient consume?

## ADDITION AND SUBTRACTION OF FRACTIONS

OBJECTIVE 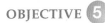 5

As much as we would like to just compare, reduce, and measure fractions, the most common operation performed with fractions is manipulation. In this section, we will refresh our knowledge of how to properly add and subtract with fractions.

*Example:*
Here is Ryan's time sheet for work:
Monday     $6\frac{1}{4}$ hours
Thursday   $4\frac{1}{4}$ hours
Saturday   5 hours

How many hours did Ryan work this week?
You may feel compelled to convert the mixed numbers into decimals before you add, and that is an acceptable way to figure this problem. However, fractions can be user friendly, so let's work this problem using the fractions.

When adding fractions, it is essential to have common denominators. In our example above, the common denominator is 4.

$6\frac{1}{4}$     Add the numerators.
$4\frac{1}{4}$     The denominators will remain the same because they are common.
$+\ 5$     Add the whole numbers.
$\overline{\ 15\frac{2}{4}}$

Once you have calculated the sum of the problem, you still need to reduce the fractions to the lowest form. In this case, $\frac{2}{4}$ can be reduced to $\frac{1}{2}$. So your final answer is $15\frac{1}{2}$ hours.

## MATH QUICK TIPS 3-5

As with whole numbers, addition and subtraction of fractions can be computed in either horizontal or vertical fashion. Either method is acceptable.

## PRACTICE THE SKILL 3-5

**Perform the following operations.**

1. $\dfrac{2}{5} + \dfrac{1}{5} =$ _____

2. $\dfrac{3}{16} + \dfrac{9}{16} =$ _____

3. $\dfrac{4}{13} + \dfrac{7}{13} =$ _____

4. $\dfrac{5}{24} + \dfrac{15}{24} =$ _____

5. $\dfrac{2}{3} + \dfrac{1}{3} =$ _____

6. $\dfrac{3}{8} + \dfrac{5}{8} =$ _____

7. $\dfrac{3}{14} + \dfrac{8}{14} =$ _____

8. $\dfrac{7}{8} + \dfrac{5}{8} =$ _____

9. $\dfrac{4}{35} + \dfrac{8}{35} =$ _____

10. $\dfrac{45}{60} + \dfrac{15}{60} =$ _____

Subtraction of fractions with like denominators is performed in the same manner as addition problems.

*Example:*

$$\frac{5}{8} - \frac{3}{8} =$$

Numerator: $5 - 3 = 2$

Because 8 is the common denominator, the answer is $\frac{2}{8}$. Or is it? Check yourself; do you need to reduce? If so, what is the correct answer?

## PRACTICE THE SKILL 3-6

Perform the following operations.

1. $\dfrac{7}{10} - \dfrac{4}{10} =$ _____

2. $\dfrac{7}{13} - \dfrac{6}{13} =$ _____

3. $\dfrac{4}{5} - \dfrac{1}{5} =$ _____

4. $\dfrac{22}{25} - \dfrac{14}{25} =$ _____

5. $\dfrac{14}{32} - \dfrac{10}{32} =$ _____

6. $\dfrac{45}{75} - \dfrac{32}{75} =$ _____

7. $\dfrac{58}{75} - \dfrac{32}{75} =$ _____

8. $\dfrac{8}{14} - \dfrac{6}{14} =$ _____

9. $\dfrac{42}{35} - \dfrac{7}{35} =$ _____

10. $\dfrac{81}{72} - \dfrac{56}{72} =$ _____

## Adding Fractions or Mixed Fractions with Uncommon Denominators

Unfortunately, most of the everyday math problems we encounter do not have common denominators. To work addition and subtraction problems with different denominators, we must find equivalent fractions with common denominators. Before performing this operation, we need to review the properties of the **least common denominator (LCD)** and **least common factor (LCF)**.

The LCD is the smallest common multiple that the denominators of two or more fractions have in common. To find the LCD, you must establish the LCF. If factoring is not your strongest skill, an easy way to determine a common denominator is to multiply the two denominators together.

*Example:*

$$\dfrac{1}{4} + \dfrac{3}{5} =$$

Multiplying denominators: $4 \times 5 = 20$

So a common denominator for 4 and 5 is 20. This might not be the LCD, but you have established a common denominator for the problem.

Next, you must convert your fractions to equivalent **fractions with common denominators.**

## STRATEGY 3-4

Finding common denominators.

1. Establish what multiples have both denominators as **factors**.

2. When in doubt, multiply both denominators together to establish a common denominator.

3. Once a common denominator has been established, multiply both the numerator and the denominator by the factor that produces the common denominator.

4. Complete the mathematical operation required to solve the problem.

$$\frac{1}{4} \rightarrow \frac{1 \times 5}{4 \times 5} \rightarrow \frac{5}{20}$$

$$+\frac{3}{5} \rightarrow \frac{3 \times 4}{5 \times 4} \rightarrow +\frac{12}{20}$$

*Answer:* $^{17}/_{20}$

To find the least common multiple, you can find the multiples of both denominators. Let's use the same example as above.

*Example:*

$$\frac{1}{4} + \frac{3}{5} =$$

$4 = 4, 8, 12, 16, 20, 24, 28, 32$

$5 = 5, 10, 15, 20, 25, 30, 35$

20 is the LCM of both 4 and 5. So, 20 is the least common denominator.

It would be to your advantage to find the least common multiple because the larger the number, the greater the chance of math error. In most cases, you can reduce fractions with large numbers before you work the calculation.

Let's try another example.

*Example:*

$$\frac{3}{7} + \frac{4}{5} =$$

$7 = 7, 14, 21, 28, 35$

$5 = 5, 10, 15, 20, 25, 30, 35$

The least common multiple of both 7 and 5 is 35.

**OR**

$7 \times 5 = 35$

$$\frac{3}{7} \rightarrow \frac{3 \times 5}{7 \times 5} \rightarrow \frac{15}{35}$$

$$+\frac{4}{5} \rightarrow \frac{4 \times 7}{5 \times 7} \rightarrow +\frac{28}{35}$$

*Answer:* $^{43}/_{35}$

Look at your answer. Is it in the correct, acceptable format? You should have recognized that the answer $^{43}/_{35}$ is an improper fraction. As stated before, it is common practice to convert an improper fraction into a mixed number. So what is your correct answer? If you determined that the answer is $1^{8}/_{35}$, you are correct.

 **MATH QUICK TIP 3-6**

If you multiply or divide the numerator, you must also multiply or divide the denominator by the same number.

## PRACTICE THE SKILL 3-7

Find the LCM for each series of numbers.

1. 2, 3, 6 _____          6. 6, 9, 12 _____

2. 3, 4, 6 _____          7. 5, 15, 30 _____

3. 5, 9, 45 _____         8. 15, 45, 60, 75 _____

4. 4, 6, 8 _____          9. 2, 3, 4 _____

5. 3, 6, 9 _____          10. 6, 8, 9 _____

## PRACTICE THE SKILL 3-8

Perform the following operations. Please write all answers in their lowest form.

1. $\begin{array}{r} \frac{1}{2} \\ +\frac{5}{7} \\ \hline \end{array}$

5. $\begin{array}{r} \frac{5}{12} \\ +\frac{11}{24} \\ \hline \end{array}$

9. $\begin{array}{r} \frac{7}{10} \\ +\frac{3}{4} \\ \hline \end{array}$

2. $\begin{array}{r} \frac{2}{3} \\ +\frac{5}{9} \\ \hline \end{array}$

6. $\begin{array}{r} \frac{3}{5} \\ +\frac{1}{6} \\ \hline \end{array}$

10. $\begin{array}{r} \frac{6}{7} \\ +\frac{5}{6} \\ \hline \end{array}$

3. $\begin{array}{r} \frac{3}{4} \\ +\frac{5}{16} \\ \hline \end{array}$

7. $\begin{array}{r} \frac{4}{9} \\ +\frac{4}{6} \\ \hline \end{array}$

4. $\begin{array}{r} \frac{1}{4} \\ +\frac{6}{9} \\ \hline \end{array}$

8. $\begin{array}{r} \frac{7}{8} \\ +\frac{8}{9} \\ \hline \end{array}$

Now that we know how to find common denominators, it is time to put the pieces together so we can successfully add fractions and mixed numbers. Don't forget—when adding and subtracting fractions, convert all improper fractions to a mixed number because this is common practice in health care.

OBJECTIVE 5

## STRATEGY 3-5

1. Find a common denominator. If the common denominator is not obvious, multiply the two denominators together to establish the LCD.

2. Establish an equivalent fraction using the common denominator.

3. Establish your new numerator by multiplying by the same factor that was used for the denominator.

4. Add the numerators together to find the sum.

5. Place the sum of your numerators over your established denominator.

6. Add any whole numbers together.

7. If you have an improper fraction, change it to a mixed number. Then, add the mixed number to your whole number.

8. Check your answer. Is it in its lowest form?

*Example:*

$$6\frac{4}{5}$$
$$+\,4\frac{2}{3}$$

Follow the strategy steps:

Step 1.    $LCD = 15$
Steps 2-3.   $4 \times 3 = 12$
             $5 \times 3 = 15$
             $2 \times 5 = 10$
             $3 \times 5 = 15$

*New Problem:*

Step 4.
$$6\frac{12}{15}$$
$$+\,4\frac{10}{15}$$

Steps 5-6.   $10\dfrac{22}{15}$

Step 7.    $\dfrac{22}{15} = 1\dfrac{7}{15}$

$$10 + 1\frac{7}{15} = 11\frac{7}{15}$$

*Answer:* $6\frac{4}{5} + 4\frac{2}{3} = 11\frac{7}{15}$

*Example:*

$$15\frac{3}{5}$$

$$+\ 2\frac{5}{6}$$

Follow the strategy steps:

Step 1.    LCD = 30
Steps 2-3.   $3 \times 6 = 18$
                $5 \times 6 = 30$
                $5 \times 5 = 25$
                $6 \times 5 = 30$

*New Problem:*

$$15\frac{18}{30}$$

Step 4.

$$+\ 2\frac{25}{30}$$

Step 5.   $17\frac{43}{30}$

Step 6.   $^{43}\!/_{30}$ can be changed to a mixed number: $1^{13}\!/_{30}$
Step 7.   Add your whole numbers: $17 + 1 = 18^{13}\!/_{30}$
Step 8.   Yes, the answer is in its lowest form.
*Answer:* $18^{13}\!/_{30}$

# PRACTICE THE SKILL 3-9

Perform the following operations.

1.  $\dfrac{4}{5}$
    $+\dfrac{2}{3}$

2.  $\dfrac{3}{4}$
    $+\dfrac{3}{16}$

3.  $\dfrac{5}{7}$
    $+\dfrac{5}{6}$

4.  $\dfrac{3}{8}$
    $+\dfrac{7}{12}$

5.  $\dfrac{8}{9}$
    $+\dfrac{3}{5}$

6.  $\dfrac{8}{15}$
    $+\dfrac{24}{45}$

7.  $\dfrac{23}{30}$
    $+\dfrac{15}{60}$

8.  $\dfrac{32}{42}$
    $+\dfrac{5}{7}$

9.  $\dfrac{7}{8}$
    $+\dfrac{5}{6}$

*(Continued)*

## PRACTICE THE SKILL 3-9
*Continued from p. 71*

10.
$$\frac{3}{13}$$
$$+\frac{5}{26}$$

11.
$$\frac{4}{32}$$
$$+\frac{8}{64}$$

12.
$$\frac{11}{22}$$
$$+\frac{22}{44}$$

## PRACTICE THE SKILL 3-10

Perform the following operations.

1. $3\frac{2}{3} + 4\frac{1}{4} =$ _____

2. $5\frac{9}{10} + 2\frac{1}{5} =$ _____

3. $14\frac{3}{8} + 6\frac{5}{6} =$ _____

4. $12\frac{5}{16} + 8\frac{1}{3} =$ _____

5. $33\frac{1}{2} + 11\frac{5}{11} =$ _____

6. $6\frac{6}{7} + 5\frac{3}{5} =$ _____

7. $15\frac{2}{3} + 1\frac{5}{9} =$ _____

8. $4\frac{4}{5} + 11\frac{6}{7} =$ _____

9. $12\frac{2}{3} + 6\frac{4}{5} =$ _____

10. $3\frac{3}{5} + 2\frac{4}{15} =$ _____

OBJECTIVE **5**    **Subtracting Fractions or Mixed Fractions with Uncommon Denominators**

Do you remember when you learned addition in elementary school? After you mastered that skill, what was the next skill you learned? Subtraction. Why was this the next logical skill to master? Because it has the opposite effect that addition has. When we are subtracting fractions and mixed numbers, we need to follow the same procedure, just substituting subtraction for addition.

What is one major skill that we had to learn for subtraction that is not performed in addition? Borrowing of numbers. This, of course, also occurs when subtracting fractions. When do we need to borrow? Borrowing occurs when we are trying to subtract a larger number from a smaller number and must "borrow" from a place value to the left to complete the operation. The same is true with fractions; however, when we borrow from the whole number, we must convert the whole number into a fraction and add it to the existing fraction.

*Example:*

$$3\frac{1}{3}$$
$$-2\frac{2}{3}$$

You need to borrow from the whole number 3 and regroup so that $\frac{2}{3}$ can be subtracted from $\frac{1}{3}$. If you borrow the whole number 1, that is the same as $\frac{3}{3}$ in fraction form. Once you add $\frac{3}{3} + \frac{1}{3} = \frac{4}{3}$,

$$3\frac{1}{3} \rightarrow 2\left(\frac{3}{3} + \frac{1}{3}\right) \rightarrow 2\frac{4}{3}$$

This changes the above problem to:

$$2\frac{4}{3}$$
$$-2\frac{2}{3}$$

*Answer:* $\frac{2}{3}$

## STRATEGY 3-6

1. Find a common denominator. If the common denominator is *not* obvious, multiply the two denominators together to establish a common denominator.

2. Establish an equivalent fraction using the common denominator.

3. Establish your new numerator by multiplying by the same factor that was used for the denominator.

4. Perform the appropriate subtraction computation with the numerators. If the computation requires you to borrow from the whole number, remember to write the borrowed number as a fraction using the denominator and adding the numerator and reduce the whole number by 1.

5. Place the difference of your numerators over your established denominator.

6. Perform the appropriate subtraction computation for the whole numbers.

7. Check your answer. Is it in the lowest form?

*Example:*

$$7\frac{5}{8}$$
$$-\,4\frac{7}{8}$$

It is necessary to borrow the whole number 1 and add it to the numerator. The whole number that is being borrowed must be represented as a fraction. In this case, the fraction is ⅜.

$$7\frac{5}{8} \rightarrow 6\left(\frac{5}{8}+\frac{8}{8}\right) \rightarrow \quad 6\frac{13}{8}$$
$$-\,4\frac{7}{8} \qquad\qquad\qquad\quad -\,4\frac{7}{8}$$
$$\qquad\qquad\qquad\qquad\quad 2\frac{6}{8} \quad \text{which in its lowest form is } 2\frac{3}{4}$$

## MATH QUICK TIP 3-7

Remember that when you are adding or subtracting fractions, you add or subtract only the numerators.

## PRACTICE THE SKILL 3-11

Perform the following operations.

1. $\dfrac{13}{18} - \dfrac{1}{2} =$ _____

2. $\dfrac{16}{7} - \dfrac{13}{21} =$ _____

3. $\dfrac{3}{5} - \dfrac{1}{4} =$ _____

4. $\dfrac{1}{4} - \dfrac{1}{7} =$ _____

5. $\dfrac{23}{24} - \dfrac{5}{12} =$ _____

6. $\dfrac{8}{42} - \dfrac{1}{7} =$ _____

7. $\dfrac{7}{8} - \dfrac{4}{5} =$ _____

8. $\dfrac{12}{24} - \dfrac{6}{12} =$ _____

*(Continued)*

## PRACTICE THE SKILL 3-11
### *Continued from p. 74*

9. $\dfrac{3}{4} - \dfrac{2}{3} =$ _____

10. $\dfrac{7}{8} - \dfrac{2}{6} =$ _____

## PRACTICE THE SKILL 3-12

Perform the following operations.

1.  $\begin{aligned} 17\tfrac{15}{45} \\ -\ 6\tfrac{1}{3} \end{aligned}$

5.  $\begin{aligned} 5\tfrac{9}{10} \\ -\ 2\tfrac{1}{5} \end{aligned}$

9.  $\begin{aligned} 9\tfrac{1}{2} \\ -\ 3\tfrac{1}{3} \end{aligned}$

2.  $\begin{aligned} 33\tfrac{1}{2} \\ -\ 11\tfrac{5}{11} \end{aligned}$

6.  $\begin{aligned} 4\tfrac{1}{4} \\ -\ 3\tfrac{2}{3} \end{aligned}$

10.  $\begin{aligned} 5\tfrac{3}{7} \\ -\ 3\tfrac{1}{3} \end{aligned}$

3.  $\begin{aligned} 12\tfrac{5}{16} \\ -\ 8\tfrac{1}{3} \end{aligned}$

7.  $\begin{aligned} 15\tfrac{3}{5} \\ -\ 12\tfrac{4}{5} \end{aligned}$

11.  $\begin{aligned} 15\tfrac{3}{4} \\ -\ 3\tfrac{7}{24} \end{aligned}$

4.  $\begin{aligned} 14\tfrac{3}{8} \\ -\ 6\tfrac{5}{6} \end{aligned}$

8.  $\begin{aligned} 45\tfrac{8}{15} \\ -\ 22\tfrac{11}{15} \end{aligned}$

12.  $\begin{aligned} 22\tfrac{1}{2} \\ -\ 14\tfrac{6}{8} \end{aligned}$

Many activities involve adding and subtracting fractions. If the measurements have the same denominator, the computation can be done quickly and accurately. Unfortunately, most computations involve uncommon denominators. Using the steps outlined in the Strategy boxes should help you gain confidence and accuracy with this form of computation. As a reminder, all answers should be stated in their lowest form and as mixed fractions.

# BUILDING CONFIDENCE WITH THE SKILL 3-3

Add the following fractions.

1. $\dfrac{8}{11} + \dfrac{10}{11} =$ _____

2. $\dfrac{9}{16} + \dfrac{4}{16} =$ _____

3. $\dfrac{2}{3} + \dfrac{3}{4} =$ _____

4. $\dfrac{5}{8} + \dfrac{1}{16} =$ _____

5. $\dfrac{9}{12} + \dfrac{32}{48} =$ _____

6. $\dfrac{7}{8} + \dfrac{12}{16} =$ _____

7. $\dfrac{12}{36} + \dfrac{5}{8} =$ _____

8. $\dfrac{14}{28} + \dfrac{3}{4} =$ _____

9. $\dfrac{5}{16} + \dfrac{3}{4} =$ _____

10. $\dfrac{42}{50} + \dfrac{23}{25} =$ _____

Subtract the following fractions.

11. $\dfrac{9}{11} - \dfrac{7}{11} =$ _____

12. $\dfrac{8}{23} - \dfrac{6}{23} =$ _____

13. $\dfrac{5}{16} - \dfrac{1}{8} =$ _____

14. $\dfrac{18}{21} - \dfrac{6}{7} =$ _____

15. $\dfrac{4}{5} - \dfrac{1}{20} =$ _____

16. $\dfrac{13}{16} - \dfrac{1}{8} =$ _____

17. $\dfrac{3}{4} - \dfrac{1}{2} =$ _____

18. $\dfrac{1}{8} - \dfrac{1}{24} =$ _____

19. $\dfrac{3}{33} - \dfrac{2}{22} =$ _____

*(Continued)*

## BUILDING CONFIDENCE WITH THE SKILL 3-3
*Continued from p. 76*

20. $\frac{4}{5} - \frac{1}{3} =$ _____

Add the following mixed numbers.

21. $2\frac{3}{8} + 7\frac{1}{2} =$ _____

22. $4\frac{9}{10} + 8\frac{2}{3} =$ _____

23. $9\frac{6}{16} + 12\frac{1}{32} =$ _____

24. $2\frac{2}{3} + 12\frac{1}{4} =$ _____

25. $9\frac{1}{2} + 7\frac{3}{16} =$ _____

26. $6\frac{4}{5} + 5\frac{2}{3} =$ _____

27. $14\frac{4}{5} + 16\frac{7}{11} =$ _____

Subtract the following mixed numbers.

28.  $\begin{array}{r} 2\frac{3}{8} \\ -1\frac{1}{4} \\ \hline \end{array}$

30.  $\begin{array}{r} 4\frac{15}{16} \\ -3\frac{1}{16} \\ \hline \end{array}$

32.  $\begin{array}{r} 15 \\ -6\frac{7}{8} \\ \hline \end{array}$

29.  $\begin{array}{r} 9\frac{1}{3} \\ -6\frac{1}{2} \\ \hline \end{array}$

31.  $\begin{array}{r} 2\frac{1}{2} \\ -1\frac{1}{2} \\ \hline \end{array}$

Answer the following word problems.

33. The patient was instructed to drink 4½ cups of x-ray prep for a test. The patient was only able to drink 3¾ cups of prep. How much of the prep was not consumed? _____

34. On Monday, the toddler's weight was 22¾ lb. When the toddler returned on Wednesday, her weight was 21½ lb. What is the weight difference between the two visits? _____

35. The physician ate ⅔ cup of meat, ½ cup of vegetables, and 1 cup of dessert. What was the total amount of food consumed by the physician? _____

## HUMAN ERROR 3-3

*Did you use common denominators?*

*Did you reduce your answer to its lowest form?*

*When you subtracted, did you need to borrow?*

*Does your answer make sense?*

OBJECTIVE 5    **MULTIPLICATION AND DIVISION OF FRACTIONS**

One difference between the multiplication operation and the addition operation for fractions is that multiplication does not require fractions to have common denominators.

Multiplication of fractions has two different formats. Calculating the same problem with either format will result in the same answer. The following examples demonstrate the horizontal multiplication method and the canceling method to calculate the appropriate answer. You can decide which method works best for you. We begin with the horizontal multiplication method.

*Example:*

$$\frac{3}{5} \times \frac{2}{3} =$$

$3 \times 2 = 6$       Multiply the numerators.
$5 \times 3 = 15$      Multiply the denominators.
*Answer:* $\frac{6}{15}$      Is this answer in lowest form? No.
The correct answer is $\frac{2}{5}$ because it is expressed in the lowest form.

The same computation can be completed by another method called *canceling*. The canceling method is used when any numerator or denominator is divisible by a common factor. What is the advantage to using the canceling method? When you are working with larger numbers, canceling will help reduce fractions to a smaller form.

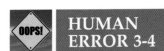

**HUMAN ERROR 3-4**

*Before multiplying or dividing, make sure your fractions are reduced to their lowest form.*

*Example:*

$$\frac{3}{5} \times \frac{2}{3} =$$

The 3 in the numerator will cancel the 3 in the denominator.

This changes the problem to: $\frac{1}{5} \times \frac{2}{1}$

We then multiply across as we did above: $\frac{1}{5} \times \frac{2}{1} = \frac{2}{5}$

This is the same product as in the problem above.

**MATH QUICK TIP 3-8**

Unlike addition and subtraction with fractions, when multiplying and dividing with fractions, perform the math function to both the numerator *and* the denominator.

**MATH IN THE REAL WORLD 3-1**

Math computations can be performed with the aid of many basic and scientific calculators. However, a calculator is only as smart as the person programming the information. With practice and confidence, you will be able to figure out fraction problems on paper as fast as it would take you to input the information into the calculator.

# PRACTICE THE SKILL 3-13

Compute the following problems. Write your answers in the lowest form.

1. $\dfrac{4}{5} \times \dfrac{7}{8} =$ _____

2. $\dfrac{5}{8} \times \dfrac{1}{3} =$ _____

3. $\dfrac{13}{26} \times \dfrac{1}{2} =$ _____

4. $\dfrac{15}{25} \times \dfrac{1}{4} =$ _____

5. $\dfrac{6}{7} \times \dfrac{4}{9} =$ _____

6. $\dfrac{3}{14} \times \dfrac{6}{7} =$ _____

7. $\dfrac{1}{8} \times \dfrac{5}{12} =$ _____

8. $\dfrac{2}{15} \times \dfrac{4}{5} =$ _____

9. $\dfrac{7}{10} \times \dfrac{4}{5} =$ _____

10. $\dfrac{6}{7} \times \dfrac{1}{3} =$ _____

## Multiplying Mixed-Number Fractions

When you are multiplying a mixed number, the first step of the computation is to convert the mixed number into an improper fraction. The next step involves multiplying as we did above.

If your calculations involve an improper fraction multiplied by a whole number, you can convert the whole number into a fraction by placing the whole number in the numerator and a 1 in the denominator.

*Example:*

$2\dfrac{3}{5} \times 4\dfrac{2}{3} =$

$5 \times 2 + 3 = 13 \quad 3 \times 4 + 2 = 14$

$\dfrac{13}{5} \times \dfrac{14}{3} = \dfrac{182}{15}$

*Answer:* $12\dfrac{2}{15}$

OBJECTIVE 5

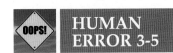

## HUMAN ERROR 3-5

*Converting a mixed number to an improper fraction:*

((Denominator × Whole Number) + Numerator)/ Denominator

*Example with a whole number:*

$$4\frac{2}{3} \times 5 =$$

$$3 \times 4 + 2 = 14$$

To make the whole number 5 a fraction, put a 1 in the denominator.

$$\frac{14}{3} \times \frac{5}{1} = \frac{70}{3}$$

*Answer:* 23⅓

## PRACTICE THE SKILL 3-14

Compute the following problems.

1. $2\frac{3}{4} \times 5\frac{1}{6} =$ _____

2. $7\frac{1}{9} \times 6\frac{1}{3} =$ _____

3. $10\frac{1}{2} \times 5\frac{1}{4} =$ _____

4. $6\frac{2}{3} \times 5\frac{3}{5} =$ _____

5. $11\frac{1}{2} \times 3\frac{1}{9} =$ _____

6. $15\frac{2}{3} \times 14\frac{3}{7} =$ _____

7. $4\frac{2}{3} \times 6\frac{5}{8} =$ _____

8. $11\frac{2}{3} \times 15\frac{1}{5} =$ _____

9. $14\frac{1}{2} \times 6\frac{3}{4} =$ _____

10. $5\frac{2}{3} \times 7\frac{1}{2} =$ _____

OBJECTIVE 5    ## Dividing Fractions

Division of fractions is a two-step problem that involves inverting the second fraction and making the computation into a multiplication problem. Once the computation has been made into a multiplication problem, we follow the same steps outlined above.

## STRATEGY 3-7

1. Make sure the fractions are in lowest form.

2. Invert the second fraction by putting the numerator in the denominator place and the denominator in the numerator place.

3. Change the division symbol to a multiplication symbol.

4. Multiply the numerators.

5. Multiply the denominators.

6. Reduce the answer from an improper fraction to a mixed number.

7. Make sure the answer is expressed in the lowest form.

*Examples:*

$$\frac{5}{8} \div \frac{2}{3} =$$

$$\frac{5}{8} \times \frac{3}{2} = \frac{15}{16}$$

$$5 \div \frac{1}{2} =$$

$$\frac{5}{1} \times \frac{2}{1} = 10$$

## PRACTICE THE SKILL 3-15

Compute the following problems.

1. $\frac{2}{3} \div \frac{1}{4} =$ _____

2. $\frac{2}{5} \div \frac{1}{8} =$ _____

3. $\frac{5}{7} \div \frac{1}{6} =$ _____

4. $\frac{2}{15} \div \frac{1}{8} =$ _____

5. $\frac{3}{16} \div \frac{4}{9} =$ _____

6. $\frac{5}{12} \div \frac{7}{10} =$ _____

*(Continued)*

## PRACTICE THE SKILL 3-15
*Continued from p. 81*

7. $\dfrac{4}{5} \div \dfrac{2}{3} =$ _____

8. $\dfrac{7}{8} \div \dfrac{3}{4} =$ _____

9. $\dfrac{5}{16} \div \dfrac{1}{8} =$ _____

10. $\dfrac{1}{4} \div \dfrac{1}{2} =$ _____

**OBJECTIVE 5**

### Dividing Fractions with Mixed Numbers

Just as when multiplying fractions, when dividing mixed number fractions, you must first convert the mixed number into an improper fraction. Once the fractions are in an improper format, proceed to work the problem the same as you would any other division of fraction computation.

## STRATEGY 3-8

1. Convert the mixed numbers into improper fractions.

2. Make sure the fractions are in lowest form.

3. Invert the second fraction by putting the numerator in the denominator place and the denominator in the numerator place.

4. Change the division symbol to a multiplication symbol.

5. Multiply the numerators.

6. Multiply the denominators.

7. Reduce the answer from an improper fraction to a mixed number.

8. Make sure the answer is expressed in the lowest form.

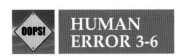

### HUMAN ERROR 3-6

*Before starting computations with fractions, always check to see that the fractions are in their lowest form. This will decrease the chance of error.*

*Example:*

$4\dfrac{3}{4} \div 5\dfrac{1}{5} =$

First New Numerator: $4 \times 4 + 3 = 19$
Second New Numerator: $5 \times 5 + 1 = 26$

$\dfrac{19}{4} \div \dfrac{26}{5} =$

$$\frac{19}{4} \times \frac{5}{26} = \frac{95}{104}$$

*Answer:* $^{95}\!/_{104}$

## PRACTICE THE SKILL 3-16

Compute the following problems.

1. $3\dfrac{1}{3} \div 2\dfrac{1}{2} =$ _____

2. $6\dfrac{3}{4} \div 5\dfrac{3}{5} =$ _____

3. $8\dfrac{2}{3} \div 6\dfrac{3}{5} =$ _____

4. $15\dfrac{1}{3} \div 12\dfrac{1}{8} =$ _____

5. $18\dfrac{3}{6} \div 12\dfrac{3}{4} =$ _____

6. $9\dfrac{7}{8} \div \dfrac{1}{3} =$ _____

7. $4\dfrac{4}{5} \div 2\dfrac{1}{2} =$ _____

8. $7\dfrac{8}{9} \div 4\dfrac{1}{3} =$ _____

9. $7\dfrac{2}{3} \div 6\dfrac{1}{4} =$ _____

10. $20\dfrac{1}{2} \div 14\dfrac{1}{3} =$ _____

## BUILDING CONFIDENCE WITH THE SKILL 3-4

Multiply the following fractions.

1. $\dfrac{2}{3} \times \dfrac{4}{5} =$ _____

2. $\dfrac{7}{28} \times \dfrac{4}{21} =$ _____

3. $\dfrac{5}{9} \times \dfrac{6}{7} =$ _____

4. $\dfrac{11}{15} \times \dfrac{5}{22} =$ _____

*(Continued)*

**BUILDING CONFIDENCE WITH THE SKILL 3-4**
*Continued from p. 83*

5. $\dfrac{8}{9} \times \dfrac{2}{3} =$ _____

6. $\dfrac{5}{6} \times \dfrac{4}{5} =$ _____

7. $\dfrac{5}{9} \times \dfrac{7}{8} =$ _____

8. $\dfrac{3}{5} \times \dfrac{2}{3} =$ _____

9. $\dfrac{2}{11} \times \dfrac{1}{2} =$ _____

10. $\dfrac{4}{7} \times \dfrac{6}{28} =$ _____

Divide the following fractions.

11. $\dfrac{6}{9} \div \dfrac{3}{5} =$ _____

12. $\dfrac{4}{7} \div \dfrac{5}{12} =$ _____

13. $\dfrac{18}{21} \div \dfrac{16}{24} =$ _____

14. $\dfrac{2}{3} \div \dfrac{1}{2} =$ _____

15. $\dfrac{7}{8} \div \dfrac{4}{5} =$ _____

16. $\dfrac{4}{5} \div \dfrac{2}{3} =$ _____

17. $\dfrac{5}{12} \div \dfrac{7}{8} =$ _____

Multiply the following mixed numbers.

18. $2\dfrac{1}{2} \times 3\dfrac{1}{3} =$ _____

19. $4\dfrac{1}{3} \times 5\dfrac{8}{9} =$ _____

20. $6\dfrac{3}{4} \times 1\dfrac{1}{16} =$ _____

21. $10\dfrac{1}{2} \times 12\dfrac{1}{2} =$ _____

22. $7\dfrac{7}{8} \times \dfrac{5}{9} =$ _____

*(Continued)*

## BUILDING CONFIDENCE WITH THE SKILL 3-4
*Continued from p. 84*

Divide the following mixed numbers.

23. $4\dfrac{1}{3} \div 5\dfrac{1}{8} =$ _____

24. $6\dfrac{1}{2} \div 3\dfrac{1}{3} =$ _____

25. $9\dfrac{7}{10} \div 11\dfrac{1}{14} =$ _____

26. $5\dfrac{1}{2} \div 3\dfrac{1}{16} =$ _____

27. $7\dfrac{7}{8} \div \dfrac{5}{9} =$ _____

Answer the following word problems.

28. The physician has instructed the parent of a patient to give the patient $1\frac{1}{2}$ tsp of medicine three times a day. What is the total amount of medicine the patient will receive in a 24-hour period? _____

29. The health care worker is scheduled to work 37 hours/week. Assuming she/he works the same number of hours each day. How many hours a day would she/he need to work in a 5-day work week?

_____

30. The patient has been instructed to take $\frac{1}{2}$ tablet of heart medication daily. The pharmacist is filling a 120-day prescription. How many tablets will be needed to complete this order? _____

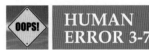

## HUMAN ERROR 3-7

*Did you perform the proper operation?*

*Did you reduce your answer to the lowest form?*

*Does your answer make sense?*

## CONCLUSION

I hope that you are starting to feel more comfortable with fractions. You may have noticed how often fractions sneak into our conversations and the workplace. The best way to feel confident with fractions is to keep working with them. The more calculations you perform successfully, the stronger your confidence in your knowledge will be. Most careers involve fractions in some way or another. Fractions can be tools for a career.

OBJECTIVES   **MASTER THE SKILL**

Complete the following problems.

1. $\dfrac{4}{9} + \dfrac{7}{9} =$ _____

2. $\dfrac{7}{9} - \dfrac{4}{9} =$ _____

3. $\dfrac{2}{3} + \dfrac{4}{5} =$ _____

4. $\dfrac{1}{3} - \dfrac{1}{6} =$ _____

5. $\begin{array}{r} 2\frac{4}{7} \\ + 6\frac{9}{10} \\ \hline \end{array}$

8. $\begin{array}{r} 16\frac{4}{5} \\ + 5\frac{1}{8} \\ \hline \end{array}$

11. $\begin{array}{r} 15\frac{7}{8} \\ - 5\frac{1}{3} \\ \hline \end{array}$

6. $\begin{array}{r} 15\frac{2}{3} \\ + 9\frac{1}{2} \\ \hline \end{array}$

9. $\begin{array}{r} 3\frac{1}{2} \\ - 1\frac{1}{13} \\ \hline \end{array}$

12. $\begin{array}{r} 24\frac{7}{18} \\ + 9\frac{8}{9} \\ \hline \end{array}$

7. $\begin{array}{r} 4\frac{5}{9} \\ + 17\frac{9}{8} \\ \hline \end{array}$

10. $\begin{array}{r} 6\frac{1}{8} \\ - 4\frac{1}{2} \\ \hline \end{array}$

13. $\dfrac{4}{5} \times \dfrac{7}{8} =$ _____

14. $\dfrac{2}{3} \times \dfrac{3}{4} =$ _____

15. $\dfrac{8}{16} \times \dfrac{9}{12} =$ _____

16. $2\dfrac{1}{2} \times 4\dfrac{7}{8} =$ _____

17. $5\dfrac{3}{5} \times 15\dfrac{1}{3} =$ _____

18. $10\dfrac{3}{4} \times 8\dfrac{1}{3} =$ _____

19. $\dfrac{45}{9} \times \dfrac{6}{36} =$ _____

*(Continued)*

## MASTER THE SKILL
*Continued from p. 86*

20. $\dfrac{4}{5} \div \dfrac{2}{3} =$ _____

21. $\dfrac{1}{8} \div \dfrac{1}{16} =$ _____

22. $\dfrac{3}{4} \div \dfrac{5}{7} =$ _____

23. $12\dfrac{1}{2} \div 3\dfrac{1}{4} =$ _____

24. $\dfrac{7}{21} \div \dfrac{9}{2} =$ _____

25. $\dfrac{9}{45} \div \dfrac{15}{3} =$ _____

26. $6\dfrac{2}{3} \div 3\dfrac{1}{2} =$ _____

27. The physician has ordered to weigh the patient daily for 3 days. The patient's weight on Monday was $197\frac{1}{2}$ lbs. The patient gained $\frac{3}{4}$ lb on Tuesday, and on Wednesday she/he lost $3\frac{3}{4}$ lbs. How much does the patient weigh at the end of 3 days? _____

28. The patient drank $1\frac{1}{2}$ cups of milk, $\frac{3}{4}$ cup of orange juice, and 2 cups of coffee every day. What is her daily fluid consumption? What is her total weekly fluid consumption? _____

29. The patient was instructed to drink the following prep for her x-ray:

    $2\frac{1}{2}$ oz every 15 minutes for 2 hours

    4 oz every 30 minutes for 2 hours

    $6\frac{1}{2}$ oz every hour for 2 hours

    What is the total quantity of prep that the pharmacist will need to dispense to the patient? _____

30. The employee works 40 hours per 5-day work week. She works the same number of hours per day and is only permitted to check her personal e-mail during a 30-minute lunch break. How much time does this person spend working each day? _____

# Word Problems, Percentages, and Decimals

## CHAPTER OUTLINE

## LEARNING OBJECTIVES

*Upon completion of this chapter, the learner will be able to:*

1. Define the key terms that relate to word problems, percentages, and decimals.

2. Identify key terms within a word problem and compute the problem.

3. Identify situations that benefit from using percentages and decimals in health care professions.

4. Manipulate decimal computations.

5. Manipulate percentage computations.

6. Convert numbers between their fraction, decimal, and percentage forms.

OBJECTIVE **1**

## KEY TERMS

| | |
|---|---|
| Decimal | Decimal Point |
| Decimal Fraction | Percentage or Percent |

OBJECTIVE **1**

Math plays a vital role in the delivery of services in a health care environment. Sometimes the math appears in an obvious, straightforward statement, but some orders are more complicated because of the available form of medication, fluids, or treatment modality that has been prescribed. One thing is certain—most mathematical problems appear in the form of a word problem.

How many of you just groaned? I am sure it was quite a few of you. For some reason, most people are not comfortable with solving word problems. They give such reasons as "I'm not sure if I performed the proper operation," "My answers never seem to make sense," and "I was never good with word problems in school." Yet, when I ask a student to estimate how much it will cost to fill up his or her 20-gallon gas tank at $3.00 per gallon, the student can quickly come up with the answer of $60.00. Students frequently state that this is not a word problem or not really math, just a factor of everyday life.

We perform mathematical calculations throughout every day. Many are in the form of word problems, and the most common word problems in health care have to do with medication calculations. Why is this? Because many medications do not come in the exact dosage that the physician has prescribed, or the dose is based on the person's weight.

Take a moment to write down a statement or two regarding how you feel about word problems. Are you comfortable solving them? Or do you feel uncertain about your skills? The first step in working through math anxiety is to identify the cause of the anxiety.

## MATH IN THE REAL WORLD 4-1
*Word Problems of Everyday Life*

- How much tip should you add to the bill?

- How much will it cost to fill up your gas tank?

- Did you collect the 20% coinsurance from the patient?

- Do you have enough to cover the cost of groceries if the bill is $275.00?

- Did you receive the correct change?

- Do you have enough time to run an errand while your child attends a 30-minute music lesson?

## UNDERSTANDING WORD PROBLEMS

OBJECTIVE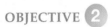

What is it about word problems that gives people the most difficulty? When I ask this question in class, the most common answer is, "I'm so worried about the numbers that I miss the key words in the problems." Most of the time, we do not communicate by writing math problems. We use words to describe the relationship between the numbers and the information we are trying to obtain (Boxes 4-1 and 4-2 and Table 4-1).

| BOX 4-1 | Key Terms for Addition and Subtraction Word Problems |
|---------|-----------------------------------------------------|

| Addition problems | Subtraction problems |
|-------------------|---------------------|
| Increase | Decrease |
| Plus | Minus |
| Additional | Difference |
| More | Fewer |
| Total | Remainder |
| Sum | Less |
| | Reduced |

| BOX 4-2 | Key Terms for Multiplication and Division Word Problems |
|---------|--------------------------------------------------------|

| Multiplication problems | Division problems |
|-------------------------|-------------------|
| Of | Ratio |
| Twice | Half |
| Product | Quotient |
| Times | Divided by |
| At | Divided into |
| Total | |

| TABLE 4-1 | Key Phrases for One or More Computations |
| --- | --- |

| Key Phrase | Operation |
| --- | --- |
| What is the total? | Addition and Multiplication |
| What is the average? | Addition and division |
| What is the total cost? | Addition |
| What is the discount? | Multiplication |
| What are the hidden charges? | Depending on how the problem is worded, involves addition and subtraction |
| What is the total discount? | Depending on how the problem is worded, involves multiplication, addition, or subtraction |

OBJECTIVE **2**

## HOW TO SOLVE A WORD PROBLEM

Depending on what the question is asking, many of us can solve simple or straightforward word problems in our heads. The difficulty occurs when a fellow student or coworker asks you to explain how you came up with your answer. Many of us find it hard to explain the steps we performed to obtain the correct answer because, to us, the answer is obvious. For example, *your lunch is $12.50 with tip. You give the waiter a $20.00 bill. How much is the change?* Without writing anything down, many of you came up with the answer $7.50. *How* did you come up with the answer?

The first step in solving any word problem is to read the problem completely. Circle key terms that will help, identify the operation you must perform to obtain the answer, and check to make sure your answer satisfies the question. Does the answer make sense?

## STRATEGY 4-1
*Solving Word Problems*

1. Read the question.

2. Identify what you are trying to find. Some students find it helpful to underline what the question is asking.

3. Pull out important information in the problem.

4. Identify the mathematical operation necessary to answer the question.

5. Perform the mathematical calculation accurately.

6. Label the answer.

7. Check to make sure the answer satisfies the question that was asked in the problem.

8. Ensure that the answer makes sense.

# MATH TRIVIA 4-1

When dealing with zeros remember the saying: Zeros ALWAYS lead but NEVER follow.

*Example:*
0.5 the zero is critical element for the problem.
5.0 the zero is not needed to solve the problem.

Use the steps in the box Strategy 4-1 to solve the following word problem: *Kevin spends a total of $30.00 for lunch during a 5-day workweek. What is the average amount he spends on lunch each day?*
Solution for the example question:

1. Read the question.
   *Did you read the entire question? If not, go back and reread the question.*
2. Underline what the question is asking.
   *What is the average amount Kevin spends on lunch each day?*
3. Identify what you are trying to find.
   *What is the average amount Kevin spends on lunch each day?*
4. Pull out important information in the problem.
   a. *Kevin spends a total of $30.00 for lunch in a 5-day workweek.*
   b. *What is the average amount Kevin spends on lunch each day?*
5. Identify the mathematical operation necessary to answer the question.
   *To find the average, divide the total amount spent by the number of days in the workweek (30 ÷ 5).*
6. Perform the mathematical calculation accurately.
   *30 ÷ 5 = 6*
7. Label the answer.
   *$6.00*
8. Check to make sure the answer satisfies the question that was asked in the problem.
   *Kevin spends on average $6.00 a day for lunch.*
9. Ensure that the answer makes sense.
   *Yes, the answer makes sense.*

Let's try one more example: *Amy is ordering supplies for the physician's office. Figure out the total cost of supplies based on the information given:*

| | | |
|---|---|---|
| Gloves | $3.50/box | Need 3 boxes |
| Gauze | $4.00/box | Need 2 boxes |
| Needles | $14.00/box | Need 3 boxes |

Solution for the example question:

1. Read the question.
   *Did you read the entire question? If not, go back and reread the question.*
2. Underline what the question is asking.
   *What is the total cost of the supplies Amy needs to order?*
3. Identify what you are trying to find.
   *What is the total cost of the supplies Amy needs to order?*

4. Pull out important information in the problem.
   *(1) Identify the quantity of supplies needed and (2) cost of each supply.*
5. Identify the mathematical operation necessary to answer the question.
   a. *Use multiplication to determine the total cost of each supply.*
   b. *Add the total cost of each supply to obtain the grand total of the order.*
6. Perform the mathematical calculation accurately.

   | | | |
   |---|---|---|
   | *Gloves* | *$3.50/box* | *Need 3 boxes* |

   *$3.50 × 3 = $10.50*

   | | | |
   |---|---|---|
   | *Gauze* | *$4.00/box* | *Need 2 boxes* |

   *$4.00 × 2 = $8.00*

   | | | |
   |---|---|---|
   | *Needles* | *$14.00/box* | *Need 3 boxes* |

   *$14.00 × 3 = $42.00*
   *Add the sums to obtain the total cost: $10.50 + $8.00 + $42.00 =*
   *$60.50*

7. Label the answer.
   *$60.50*
8. Check to make sure the answer satisfies the question that was asked in the problem.
   *The total cost of Amy's supplies is $60.50.*
9. Ensure that the answer makes sense.
   *Yes, the answer makes sense.*

As with any skill, start out slowly. Take your time when identifying the key words. If necessary, you could write the symbol for the operation that the word represents. Furthermore, you could rewrite the word problem into a mathematical expression and then solve it. If your problem has a fraction or decimal in it, round to a whole number to estimate the answer, and then perform the necessary calculations to determine the actual answer to the problem. As your confidence builds with word problems, so will your ability to perform "mental math" calculations. What is mental math? Mental math involves being able to solve math problems (in any format) in your head and produce the correct answer.

## MATH TRIVIA 4-2

1 cc (cubic centimeter) is equivalent to 1 mL (milliliter).
   1 cc = 1 mL

OBJECTIVE **2**

## PRACTICE THE SKILL 4-1

Perform the proper function to solve each word problem.

1. A man drove 12 miles to the grocery store, 8 miles to the dry cleaners, 30 miles to work, and 14 miles to an appointment at the clinic. How many miles did he drive? _____

2. The physician wrote the following Intravenous orders for the patient: Ancef 150 cc, 250 cc of blood, and 3000 cc of 0.9 normal saline. What is the total amount of fluids the patient will receive? _____

*(Continued)*

## PRACTICE THE SKILL 4-1
*Continued from p. 92*

3. The patient has been instructed to take 500 mg of medication 3 times a day for 10 days. What is the total amount of medication the patient will have taken when he completes the prescription? _____

4. Four people have tickets to today's baseball game. Based on the following information, how much will they spend during the baseball game?

_____

| | |
|---|---|
| Tickets | $15.00 each |
| Hot dogs | $2.50 each and everyone has two hot dogs |
| Soda | $4.00 each and everyone has two sodas |
| Ice cream | $3.50 each and everyone has one ice cream |

5. A physician orders 1000 cc of intravenous fluids for a dehydrated patient. The IV is running at 150 cc/hour. How long will it take to infuse 1000 cc?

_____

6. A woman spends $32.50 at the pharmacy. She gives the cashier a $50.00 bill. How much change will she receive? _____

7. The medication bottle contains 100 cc. The first prescription requires 66 cc, and the second prescription takes 17 cc. How much remains in the medication bottle? _____

8. The pharmacy stocked the medication cabinet with 35 vials of hepatitis B vaccine. The health care worker removes three vials at 9:00 a.m., two vials at 10:30 a.m., and four vials at 12:00 noon. The physician removes two vials at 12:30 p.m. and one vial at 2:00 p.m. The nurse removes three vials at 2:30 p.m. How many vials remain? _____

9. The patient has been instructed to wear the oral headgear equipment for a total of 12 hours/day (after school and at bed time). The patient wears it 7.5 hours while sleeping. How many additional hours will the patient need to wear the headgear equipment after school? _____

10. Gas prices are $3.89/gallon. You have a 14-gallon tank in your car. How much will it cost to fill your completely empty gas tank? _____

## DECIMALS                                          OBJECTIVES

"Decimals—something I feel comfortable with when it comes to math." I have heard this phrase many times during my teaching career. Most students say they feel at ease with decimals because they can associate them with money. In the medical field, decimals are used to describe

- Laboratory values
- Fluid concentrations
- Measurement of incisions and wounds
- Currency amounts for payment of services

As a reminder, when you are reading and writing **decimals**, whole numbers are written to the left of the **decimal point** and numbers on both sides of the decimal point are located in "place values." The part on the right of the decimal is the "fractional part."

The same strategy used for rounding whole numbers can be used for rounding decimals. Refer to the box Strategy 4-2 when completing the Practice the Skill problems that follow it.

Thousands Hundreds Tens Ones

## 1,234.56789

Tenths Hundredths Thousandths Ten thousandths Hundred thousandths

## STRATEGY 4-2
*Rounding Decimals*

1. Identify the place value to which you are rounding.

2. Look to the immediate right (one place value) to determine how to round.

3. If this number is 5 or greater, round the place value up by one digit and drop all the remaining numbers to the right.

4. If the number is 4 or less, leave the number alone and drop all the numbers to the right.

*Example 1:*
Round 3.4267 to the nearest hundredth.

1. Identify the place value to which you are rounding.
   *Identify the hundredths place: 3.4267.*

2. Look to the immediate right (one place value) of the place value you are rounding.
   *Look at the number 6, which is the number immediately to the right of the place value you are rounding.*

3. If this number is 5 or greater, round the place value up by one digit and drop all the remaining numbers to the right.
   *Since the number 6 is greater than 2, it is necessary to raise the 2 (found in the hundredths place) to a 3 and drop the remaining numbers to the right.*

Thus, your answer is 3.43.

*Example 2:*
Round 2.47315 to the nearest thousandth.

**1.** Identify the place value to which you are rounding.
   *Identify the thousandths place: 2.47315.*

**2.** Look to the immediate right (one place value) of the place value you are rounding.
   *Look at the number 1, which is the number immediately to the right of the place value you are rounding.*

**3.** If this number is 5 or greater, round the place value up by one digit and drop all the remaining numbers to the right.
   *Since the number 1 is less than 5, you would drop the remaining numbers to the right.*

Therefore, your answer is 2.473.

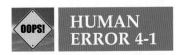

**HUMAN ERROR 4-1**

*To avoid confusion, place a 0 before the decimal point to show that there is not a whole number in front of it. Example: 0.5 or 0.05.*

## PRACTICE THE SKILL 4-2

OBJECTIVES **3** **4**

Round the following decimals to the nearest thousandth.

1. 2.3579 _____

4. 0.972354 _____

2. 15.153246 _____

5. 7.13244 _____

3. 12.9723 _____

Round the following decimals to the nearest hundredth.

6. 97.5326 _____

9. 14.3275 _____

7. 12.3673 _____

10. 0.252643 _____

8. 0.981423 _____

Round the following decimals to the nearest tenth.

11. 13.462 _____

14. 2.2534 _____

12. 75.631 _____

15. 109.8736 _____

13. 0.98263 _____

Round the following decimals to the nearest whole number.

16. 2.254 _____

19. 1.025 _____

17. 89.45 _____

20. 0.654 _____

18. 97.78 _____

If you are having difficulties with this section, review the concept of rounding numbers in Chapter 2 (p. 37).

## Addition and Subtraction of Decimals

Do you remember the strategy for adding and subtracting decimals? Always line your decimals up in a vertical manner. If you have uneven numbers, you can add zeros to the end. Once your math problem is formatted, all you need to do to solve the problem is perform the requested operation. The way your answer will be used determines whether you should round the number to a whole number, tenths, hundredths, or thousandths place value.

### STRATEGY 4-3
*Addition and Subtraction of Decimals*

1. Write the problem in a vertical format.

2. Line the decimals up vertically.

3. Add zeros to fill in any uneven place values.

4. Perform the required mathematical operation.

*Example 1:*

$45.679 + 2.35 + 0.2431 =$

1. Write the problem in a vertical format and line the decimals up vertically.
```
   45.679
    2.35
+   0.2431
```

2. Add zeros to fill in any uneven place values.
```
   45.6790
    2.3500
+   0.2431
```

3. Perform the required mathematical operation.
```
   45.6790
    2.3500
+   0.2431
   48.2721
```

*Example 2:*

$32.098 + 8.93 + 10.325 =$

1. Write the problem in a vertical format.
```
   32.098
    8.93
+  10.325
```

2. Line the decimals up vertically.
```
   32.098
    8.93
+  10.325
```

**3.** Add zeros to fill in any uneven place values.

```
    32.098
     8.930
+   10.325
```

**4.** Perform the required mathematical operation.

```
    32.098
     8.930
+   10.325
   ───────
    51.353
```

*Example 3:*

Step 1:
```
    127.18
+    13.9
```

Step 2:
```
    127.18
+    13.9
```

Step 3:
```
    127.18
+    13.90
```

Step 4:
```
    127.18
+    13.90
   ───────
    141.08
```

## PRACTICE THE SKILL 4-3

OBJECTIVES  3 4

Add the following decimals. Do not round your answers.

1.
```
    35.679
+   67.875
```

2.
```
    0.5632
+   0.235
```

3.
```
    15.782
+    4.444
```

4.
```
    10.45
    35.47
+   22.67
```

5.
```
    119.32
     19.32
      9.32
+     0.32
```

6.
```
     2.53
      .67
     8.942
+   12.2
```

7.
```
     5.75
     3
+    6.4231
```

8.
```
     8.9
    14.7
+   31.9
```

9.
```
    0.45
    0.55
+   0.89
```

10.
```
    0.125
    2.5
    0.25
+   1.025
```

*(Continued)*

## PRACTICE THE SKILL 4-3
*Continued from p. 97*

Subtract the following decimals.

**11.** 55 – 42.5 = _____

**12.** 275.45 – 75.45 = _____

**13.** 12.5 – 7.5 = _____

**14.** 35.89 – 14.50 = _____

**15.** 457.32 – 57.32 = _____

**16.** 3.5 – 1.2 = _____

**17.** 945.321 – 223.45 = _____

**18.** 67.45 – 23.31 = _____

**19.** 0.9534 – 0.0214 = _____

**20.** 0.4572 – 0.225 = _____

## Multiplication and Division of Decimals

Many students find multiplying decimals to be the easiest of all the mathematical computations because it involves only three steps to solve the problem:

1. Perform the multiplication problem.
2. Count the number of digits to the right of the decimal point in the multiplier and multiplicand.
3. Look at the answer. Starting from the last digit to the right, count to the left the number of decimal places determined in step 2. Place your decimal point before that digit.

*Example:*
$7.02 \times 5.17 =$

**1.** Perform the multiplication problem.

$$
\begin{array}{r}
7.02 \\
\times\, 5.17 \\
\hline
4914 \\
7020 \\
+\, 351000 \\
\hline
362934
\end{array}
$$

**2.** Count the number of digits to the right of the decimal point in the multiplier and multiplicand.

$$
\begin{array}{r}
7.02 \\
\times\, 5.17 \\
\hline
\end{array}
$$

*There are a total of four digits to the right of the decimals.*

**3.** Look at the answer. Starting from the last digit to the right, count to the left the number of decimal places determined in step 2. Place your decimal point before that digit.
*Answer:* 36.2934

## PRACTICE THE SKILL 4-4

OBJECTIVE 4

Multiply the following decimals.

**1.** $4.57 \times 5.3 =$ _____

**2.** $45.76 \times 3 =$ _____

**3.** $789.10 \times 10 =$ _____

**4.** $2.5 \times 3 =$ _____

**5.** $5.25 \times 12 =$ _____

**6.** $90.25 \times .25 =$ _____

**7.** $1.007 \times 5.0 =$ _____

**8.** $0.125 \times 2.5 \times 0.03 =$ _____

**9.** $2.5 \times 4 \times 10 =$ _____

**10.** $50 \times .8 \times 12.5 =$ _____

Do you remember how to divide numbers with decimals? If you have a whole number in the divisor and a decimal in the dividend, (a / b = c) perform the division operation and place a decimal point in the same location as the decimal in the dividend.

*Example:*
$3.4 \div 2 =$
*Answer:* 1.7

If you have a decimal in the divisor and a whole number in the dividend, however, you must move the divisor decimal until it becomes a whole number. Remember, whatever you do to the divisor, you must perform the same operation to the dividend. So move your decimal in the dividend the same number of positions the decimal was moved in the divisor (add 0 if needed to obtain the proper place value).

*Example:*
$3 \div 2.5 =$
Move the decimal to the right and create the whole number 25.
Add a decimal and 0 after the 3. Then move the decimal to create a whole number of 30.
Solve the math problem.
*Answer:* 1.2

What should you do if there is a decimal in both the divisor and the dividend? Move the decimal to the right until the divisor becomes a whole number. Again, remember to move the decimal in the dividend the same number of places as it was moved in the divisor.

*Example:*
$2.5 \div 7.5 =$

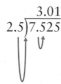

$$2.5 \overline{)7.525} \quad \overset{3.01}{}$$

1. Move the decimal to the right (the same number of places) for the divisor and the dividend.

$$25 \overline{)75.25} \quad \overset{3.01}{} \\ \underline{75}$$

2. Perform the mathematical operation.
   Reminder: Use a zero to demonstrate that the divisor cannot be divided into the dividend.

$$\begin{array}{r} 0\,2\,5 \\ \underline{2\,5} \\ 0 \end{array}$$

3. Place the decimal in the proper place value in the answer.

*Answer: 3.01*   4. Record your answer.

OBJECTIVE ④

# PRACTICE THE SKILL 4-5

Divide the following decimals.

1. $682.4 \div 4 =$ _____

2. $125 \div 0.25 =$ _____

3. $1.5 \div 0.3 =$ _____

4. $25.55 \div 10.5 =$ _____

5. $39.03 \div 0.03 =$ _____

6. $15.72 \div 0.9 =$ _____

7. $450 \div 1.5 =$ _____

8. $75.00 \div 24.50 =$ _____

9. $21.35 \div 7.33 =$ _____

10. $100 \div 50.25 =$ _____

## BUILDING CONFIDENCE WITH THE SKILL 4-1

OBJECTIVES

Perform the correct operation to solve the following problems. Round your answer to the hundredths place.

1.  4.678
    2.35
    + 3.1

2.  15.5 mg
    2.25 mg
    +  5    mg

3.  $14.79
    $37.89
    + $42.35

4.  2.75 ml
    4.25 ml
    +  15.20 ml

5.  $1457.90
    $235.46
    +  $987.34

6.  $42.35
    −  $6.78

7.  55 ml
    23 ml
    − 10 ml

8.  0.546
    −  .336

9.  18.3
    −  4.672

10.  1.354
    −  0.987

11.  2.5
    ×  5.8

12.  4.5
    ×  3.456

13.  15.2
    ×  .89

14.  2.25
    ×  .125

15.  32.7
    ×  .33

16.  33.30
    ÷  0.03

17.  150
    ÷  0.25

18.  15.66
    ÷  .20

19.  $25.81
    ÷  $0.90

20.  $720.00
    ÷   1.20

21. The prescription reads the following: Amoxil 500 mg every 4 hours times ten days. What is the total amount of medication needed to fill the prescription? _____

22. To fill a prescription, the pharmacy supplies 45 tablets. Each tablet has 1.25 mg of medication. What is the total amount of medication in the bottle? _____

23. The physician writes the following IV order: Normal Saline 1000 cc to be infused over 6 hours. How many milliliters will be infused each hour?

_____

24. The patient must keep track of their fluid intake for a 24-hour period. The patient records the following fluid intake in the provided diary:

| 8:00 a.m.   | 360 cc    | breakfast |
| 10:00 a.m.  | 45.25 cc  | snack     |
| 12:00 noon  | 450.75 cc | lunch     |
| 2:00 p.m.   | 180 cc    | snack     |
| 5:00 p.m.   | 345.50 cc | dinner    |
| 8:00 p.m.   | 245.45 cc | snack     |
| 11:00 p.m.  | 90 cc     | snack     |

*(Continued)*

## BUILDING CONFIDENCE WITH THE SKILL 4-1
*Continued from p. 101*

What is the total amount of fluids consumed in a 24-hour period?

_____

25. The health care consumer has a bill for $457.89. The patient would like to make payments over a 3-month period.

    a. How much will the patient pay each month? _____

    b. Were the installment payments equal over the 3-month period? Yes or No?

OBJECTIVES

## PERCENTAGES

**Percentage**, or **percent**, means a specified number of parts out of 100 pieces. To convert a percentage into a fraction, simply remove the percent sign and write the fraction with 100 in the denominator, then reduce the fraction to its lowest form. When converting a percentage to a decimal, remember to perform the proper mathematical computation and watch the placement of your decimal point.

## MATH QUICK TIP 4-1

The percentage 20% can be written as the fraction $^{20}\!/_{100}$ and reduced to $^1\!/_5$. The percentage 20% written as a decimal is 0.2.

*Example:* 235%
1. How to convert a percentage to a fraction. Place the number in the numerator and 100 in the denominator.
   $^{235}\!/_{100}$

2. Reduce the fraction
   $^{47}\!/_{20}$

3. Write your answer as an improper fraction or a mixed number.
   $^{47}\!/_{20}$ or $2^7\!/_{20}$

*Example:* $^4\!/_5$ is what percent?
1. Divide the denominator by the numerator.
   $^5\!/_4 = 0.80$

2. Multiple the decimal by 100 to obtain the percent.
   $0.80 \times 100 = 80\%$

3. *Answer:* $^4\!/_5 = 80\%$

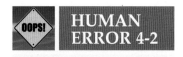

**HUMAN ERROR 4-2**

*Did you remember that all percentages are based on a part of 100?*

# PRACTICE THE SKILL 4-6

Convert the following percentages to fractions. Reduce fractions as appropriate.

1. 15% _____        6. 80% _____

2. 33% _____        7. 45% _____

3. 75% _____        8. 60% _____

4. 20% _____        9. 12% _____

5. 66% _____        10. 125% _____

Convert the following fractions into percentages.

11. ¾ _____%        16. 6½ _____%

12. ¹⁄₂₀ _____%      17. 5¼ _____%

13. ⅕ _____%         18. ²⁵⁄₇₅ _____%

14. ⅛ _____%         19. 1⅔ _____%

15. ¼ _____%         20. ⁴⁵⁄₉₀ _____%

## Finding the Percentage of a Number

Percentages are most commonly used in the sale of merchandise. Whether it be purchasing a new car, clothing, or furniture, consumers look for bargains. How much is 40% off the original price? Percentages are also involved when calculating interest rates and determining profit/loss values. Most percentage problems can be solved by multiplication or division operations.

Finding the percentage of a number is usually expressed as a word problem (review Box 4-2). The word *of* means that you will multiply. Finding the percentage of a number involves converting the percentage and the number into fractions and then multiplying. Another way to solve this type of problem is to change the percentage into a decimal then multiply.

*Example:*

30% of 900 =

$$\frac{30}{100} \times \frac{900}{1} = \frac{27000}{100}$$

Reduced to 270

*Answer:* 30% of 900 is 270

Or another way to solve this example problem is as follows:

Change 30% into a decimal: 0.3

Multiply 0.3 × 900 = 270

*Answer:* 30% of 900 is 270

You must determine which methods are logical and accurate for you. If you prefer to write the problem as a proportion, use that method for all problems.

If you prefer decimals, that's fine. Just remain consistent as you work through the practice problems.

When you are determining percentage, use this formula: divide the first number by the second number and multiply by 100.

**Example:**
10 is what percentage of 50?
$$\frac{10}{50} = \frac{1}{5} = .20$$
$.20 \times 100 = 20\%$

How do we solve a problem when we know that a specific number is a percentage of an unknown figure?

**Example:**
10 is 20% of what number?
Divide the number by the percentage.
$10/20\% =$
$10/0.2 =$
*Answer: 50*

**Example 3:**
3 is 75% of what?
$3/75\% =$
$3/.75 =$
*Answer: 4*

As mentioned in previous chapters, there can be more than one way to solve a math problem. Let's try a different strategy with this next example problem.

 **STRATEGY 4-4**

1. Write the problem in an algebraic format.

2. Perform the proper operation on both sides of the equation. (Refer to "Order of Operations" in Chapter 1 if you have difficulty.)

3. Solve the problem.

**Example:**
12 is 50% of what number?
$$\frac{12}{.5} =$$
*Answer: 24*
12 is 50% of the number 24.

This problem can also be written as a basic algebraic expression. The letter "X" is commonly used to identify the unknown value. Using the example question above, the problem can be written as follows:

$12 = 50\%$ of $X$

Divide both sides by 0.5 to have X (unknown) by itself.

$$\frac{12}{0.5} = \frac{0.5\,X}{0.5}$$

$$\frac{12}{0.5} = X$$

$$24 = X$$

Now check your answer by substituting your answer of 24 for X.

$12 = 50\%$ of 24

$12 = 0.5 \times 24$

$12 = 12$

If you are rusty on algebra, don't be concerned. We will be discussing ratios and proportions in the next chapter.

## MATH TRIVIA 4-3

% of a number means change to decimal and multiply by that number. That's how 50% of X turns into 0.5 X.

## PRACTICE THE SKILL 4-7

Find the solutions to the following problems.

1. What is 25% of $75.00? _____

2. What is 80% of $345.00? _____

3. What is 25% of $19.35? _____

4. What is 5% of 35.50? _____

5. What is 125% of 300? _____

6. 150 is what percentage of 450? _____

7. 35 is what percentage of 105? _____

8. 20 is what percentage of 85? _____

9. 15 is what percentage of 175? _____

10. 5 is what percentage of 20? _____

Solve the following word problems.

11. The health care consumer must pay 35% of all physician bills. The most recent bill is for $365.00. What is the consumer's responsibility toward the bill? _____

*(Continued)*

## PRACTICE THE SKILL 4-7
*Continued from p. 105*

**12.** The patient was able to drink only 85% of the 1000 mL bottle of x-ray prep. How much was consumed by the patient? _____

**13.** Hospital employees receive a 25% discount on all prescriptions. What will the employee pay for purchases that cost a total of $185.25? _____

**14.** Your gas tank holds 23 gallons of gas. How many gallons remain if your tank is 65% empty? _____

**15.** The patient's insurance policy will pay 90% of all ER charges. How much will the insurance policy pay for a bill of $678.35? _____

OBJECTIVE 6

## CONVERSION BETWEEN FRACTIONS, PERCENTAGES, AND DECIMALS

**Decimal fractions** are fractions whose denominator is a multiple of 10. Conversion from the fraction to a decimal can be done quickly and accurately by dropping the denominator and placing the decimal point in the proper place value represented by the denominator.

*Example:*
$^{25}/_{100}$
Drop the denominator.
Place your decimal point to represent the hundredths place value.
*Answer:* 0.25

Common fractions can be changed into decimals by simply dividing the numerator by the denominator. The answer is expressed as a decimal.

*Example:*
Format the fraction in vertical manner and show how to solve the problem.
$$\frac{32}{125} =$$
*Answer:* 0.256

Converting a percentage to a decimal involves removing the percent sign and moving the decimal point two places to the left. If necessary, add a 0 to create the proper place value. Reverse the process to change a decimal to a percentage.

*Example:*
6.5% = what decimal?
Drop the % to create the number 6.5.
Move the decimal two places to the left. You must add one 0 in order to create the hundredths place value.
*Answer:* 0.065

How do we convert a percentage to a fraction? We divide the percent by 100 and reduce the fraction into lowest terms.

*Example:*
9%   $^9/_{100}$

*Example:*
5%   $^5/_{100}$ reduced to $^1/_{20}$

*Example:*
$5^3/_4$ = _____%
Convert mixed number to an improper fraction.
$(4 \times 5) + 3 = 23/4$
Multiply the improper fraction by 100
$23/4 \times 100 = 2300/4$
Divide the numerator by the denominator to obtain the proper percentage.
*Answer: 575%*

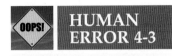

**HUMAN ERROR 4-3**

*Before converting a fraction into a decimal, make sure the fraction is reduced to its lowest form.*

Based on the above information, you should be able to convert decimals to percentages or fractions or any combination.

# PRACTICE THE SKILL 4-8

Convert the following fractions and mixed numbers into percentages.

1. $^3/_4$ = _____ %
2. $^4/_5$ = _____ %
3. $^1/_8$ = _____ %
4. $2^2/_3$ = _____ %
5. $4^5/_8$ = _____ %

6. $10^1/_3$ = _____ %
7. $^1/_5$ = _____ %
8. $^1/_6$ = _____ %
9. $^1/_4$ = _____ %
10. $12^3/_5$ = _____ %

Convert the following fractions and mixed numbers into decimals.

11. $^1/_6$ = _____
12. $2^1/_5$ = _____
13. $^3/_8$ = _____
14. $4^4/_5$ = _____
15. $^3/_4$ = _____

16. $10^1/_3$ = _____
17. $^5/_{12}$ = _____
18. $6^1/_3$ = _____
19. $^5/_7$ = _____
20. $3^1/_6$ = _____

OBJECTIVES  4 5 6

# BUILDING CONFIDENCE WITH THE SKILL 4-2

Complete the table by converting fractions, percentages, and decimals.

| Problem Number | Fraction | Percentage | Decimal |
|---|---|---|---|
| 1. | ½ | | |
| 2. | | 33% | |
| 3. | | | .45 |
| 4. | ¹⁄₂₀ | | |
| 5. | ¾ | | |
| 6. | | 10% | |
| 7. | | | .66 |
| 8. | ⅕ | | |
| 9. | | 60% | |
| 10. | | | .25 |
| 11. | ⅔ | | |
| 12. | | 75% | |
| 13. | | | .80 |
| 14. | ⅛ | | |
| 15. | | 40% | |

## Solve the following word problems.

16. A patient is seen at an urgent care facility. The following charges are applied to his bill: office visit, $60.00; urine test, $15.00; and antibiotic injection, $68.50. The patient is responsible for 20% of the total bill. How much would you collect from the patient? _____

17. The insurance company is billed $865.42 for an emergency room visit. The insurance company will pay 80% of the total bill. How much will the insurance company pay? How much is the patient responsible for?

_____

18. The physician orders 4.25 mg of medication to be taken three times a day for 10 days. What is the total amount of the medication the patient will be taking? _____

19. The pharmacist has a stock bottle of medication that contains 15.5 mL. The pharmacist needs to divide the medication into five equal parts. How many milliliters will be in each of the prescribed medication doses?

_____

20. During an emergency call, the paramedics must keep track of the mileage from the time they leave the fire station until they return. The following mileage was recorded during the previous call:

    Fire station to patient's home: 17.25 miles

    Patient's home to emergency department: 22.6 miles

    Emergency department to fire station: 19.6 miles

    a. What was the total mileage for this run? _____

    b. If the insurance agency will reimburse the fire station 41.5 cents/mile for this call, what would be the total reimbursement to the fire station?

    _____

## CONCLUSION

Health care professionals can expect to encounter percentages and decimals in many aspects of the work environment. Information regarding laboratory values, medication doses, patient billing, budgets, and use of equipment can be expressed as either a decimal or a percentage. As in our everyday world, in the health care environment you will be asked to work math problems in the form of straight computations or as word problems. As you continue your work within this text, you will encounter more word problems. Solving them will help increase your confidence in performing math in a clinical setting.

## MASTER THE SKILL

OBJECTIVES  3 4 5 6

Solve the following problems.

1.  14.567
    37.890
    4.576
    2.3
    + 3.0

2.  45.67
    2.389
    11.54
    + 7.980

3.  0.973521
    0.7854
    + 0.14237

4.  0.180
    5.0
    5.757
    0.75
    + 7.5

5.  14.32
    35.46
    148.75
    + 98.35

6.  57.895
    − 7.895

7.  14.95
    − 12.50

8.  35.70
    12.76
    − 5.50

9.  0.98421
    − 0.68315

10.  4689.03641
    − 322.67852

11.  4.6
    × 1.57

12.  2.85
    × 3.75

13.  14.68
    × 7.35

14.  2.50
    × 3

15.  987.035
    × 0.025

16.  12
    ÷ 36.60

17.  1025
    ÷ 1.25

18.  475
    ÷ 50

19.  37.50
    ÷ 2.5

20.  783.25
    ÷ 6

21.  16% of 125 = _____

22.  6.5% of 189 = _____

*(Continued)*

## MASTER THE SKILL
*Continued from p. 109*

23. 20% of 12,478.43 = _____

24. 80% of 12,478.43 = _____

25. 0.9% of 1000 = _____

26. 45% of 90 = _____

27. 12.5% of 184.5 = _____

28. 6.5% of 202.56 = _____

29. 1.5% of 5 = _____

30. 13% of 1365 = _____

31. 65 is what percentage of 517? _____

32. 45 is what percentage of 430? _____

33. 2.5 is what percentage of 12? _____

34. 0.33 is what percentage of 90? _____

35. 0.20 is what percentage of 89.50? _____

36. A consumer is being seen for an urgent medical issue. The insurance
    company will pay 50% for all ER visits and 70% of all urgent care visits.
    The total bill for the urgent care visit is $187.45. How much will the
    insurance company pay for this visit? _____

37. Hospital employees receive a 25% discount at the local health club.
    The health club charges a monthly membership fee of $65.80. What is
    the discounted monthly rate for hospital employees? _____

38. Customers receive a 35% discount on all purchases over $1000.00.
    A consumer orders $1365.00 in supplies.

    a. What is the discounted amount? _____

    b. How much will a consumer pay for the supplies? _____

39. Your patient has a 2500 cc bag of irrigation solution hanging, and 750 cc
    of fluid has been infused. What percentage of irrigation solution has been
    infused? _____

40. The physician orders 1500 flu injections. There were 300 shots given in
    September, 450 shots given in October, and 665 shots given in November.

    a. What percentage of flu vaccine has been given? _____

    b. What percentage of flu vaccine remains? _____

# Ratios and Proportions

## CHAPTER OUTLINE

## LEARNING OBJECTIVES

*Upon completion of this chapter, the learner will be able to:*

1. Define the key terms that relate to the chapter.

2. Identify the proper way to set up ratios.

3. Demonstrate how to set up a proportion.

4. Solve for *X*.

5. Solve word problems for *X*.

## KEY TERMS

OBJECTIVE ❶

Algebra

Cross Multiplication

Extremes

Means

Proportion

Ratio

I n this chapter, we will discuss different ways to set up and solve ratio and
proportion problems. I hope you will find a strategy that reinforces your
knowledge and allows you to be confident in these **algebra** equations.

## RATIO

OBJECTIVES ❷ ❸

By nature, human beings love to compare objects. Take a minute and list different
activities in your daily life that involve comparisons.

## MATH IN THE REAL WORLD 5-1
*Comparisons from Daily Living*

- Job descriptions

- Work hours

- Store prices

- Cars

- Homework

- Schools

When you think about it, a **ratio** is simply a comparison between two objects or amounts.

Health care uses ratios in determining medication dosage, IV additives, normal/abnormal lab values, disease statistics, and profit/loss margins. Once a ratio has been identified, it is easy to write a proportion to find a solution or the answer to a question.

Ratios can be written either as a fraction or with a colon to separate the items being compared. In word problems, you will commonly see the word *to* between the two items of comparison.

OBJECTIVE 2

*Example:*
The shelter houses 15 dogs to every 7 cats.

$15:7$, $\dfrac{15}{7}$, or 15 to 7

*Example:*
There are 7 boys and 12 girls in the class.

$7:12$, $\dfrac{7}{12}$, or 7 to 12

Look at the medication labels in Figures 5-1, 5-2, and 5-3. What are the examples in these three figures comparing?

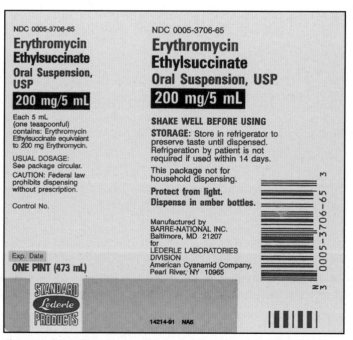

**Figure 5-1**    Erythromycin label. (From Fulcher RM, Fulcher EM: *Math calculations for pharmacy technicians: A worktext*, St. Louis, 2007, Saunders.)

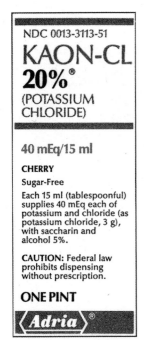

**Figure 5-2**   KAON-CL label.
(From Fulcher RM, Fulcher EM: *Math calculations for pharmacy technicians: A worktext*, St. Louis, 2007, Saunders.)

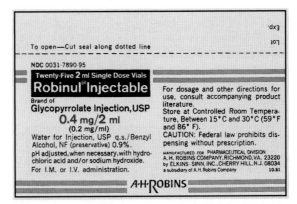

**Figure 5-3**   Robinul Injectable label. (From Fulcher RM, Fulcher EM: *Math calculations for pharmacy technicians: A worktext*, St. Louis, 2007, Saunders.)

If you said medication per milliliter, you are correct. Each of the labels compares the medication dose to a specified amount of liquid, expressed in milliliters (mL).

Now look at the labels of medications that are dispensed as tablets (Figures 5-4, 5-5, and 5-6).

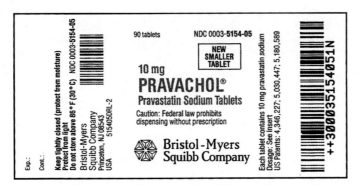

**Figure 5-4**   Pravachol label. (From Fulcher RM, Fulcher EM: *Math calculations for pharmacy technicians: A worktext*, St. Louis, 2007, Saunders.)

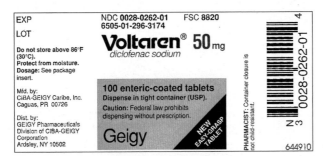

**Figure 5-5**   Voltaren label. (From Fulcher RM, Fulcher EM: *Math calculations for pharmacy technicians: A worktext*, St. Louis, 2007, Saunders.)

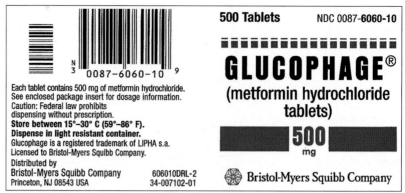

**Figure 5-6** Glucophage label. (From Fulcher RM, Fulcher EM: *Math calculations for pharmacy technicians: A worktext*, St. Louis, 2007, Saunders.)

The labels express the dosage per tablet.

## MATH QUICK TIP 5-1

When dealing with ratios, always reduce fractions to their lowest form before multiplying. This will reduce computation errors.

## PRACTICE THE SKILL 5-1

Write the ratio for the medication amounts shown in Figures 5-1, 5-2, 5-3, 5-4, 5-5, and 5-6.

1. _____     4. _____

2. _____     5. _____

3. _____     6. _____

Write a ratio for each of the following word problems that deal with everyday life.

7. The bouquet had two roses for every three carnations. _____

8. Add two scoops of coffee for every three cups of water. _____

9. The student to teacher ratio is twenty-five to one. _____

10. There are two bathrooms for every four bedrooms. _____

*(Continued)*

## PRACTICE THE SKILL 5-1
*Continued from p. 114*

11. Televisions run 2 minutes of commercials for every 17 minutes of programming. _____

12. Class runs 48 minutes out of every hour. _____

**Write a ratio for each of the following word problems that deal with use of ratios in health care.**

13. There is 25 mg of medication in every 5 cc of liquid.

_____

14. The injection has 75 mg of medication for every 1 mL.

_____

15. The IV has 20 milliequivalents of potassium for every 1000 cc of fluid.

_____

16. The patient's pulse was 72 beats per minute. _____

17. Autism affects 1 out of 158 children. _____

18. The medicated paste has 25 mg per 1/2 inch. _____

19. In 150 mL there is 50 mg of medication. _____

20. There is 5% glucose in 1000 mL of 0.45% normal saline solution.

_____

## PROPORTION

OBJECTIVE ③

A **proportion** is a mathematical equation that compares two equal ratios. Proportions can be written as fractions with an equal sign (=) between the two ratios or can be expressed by the use of double colons (::) between the ratios.

*Examples:*

$$\frac{1}{2} = \frac{3}{6} \quad \text{or} \quad 1{:}2 :: 3{:}6$$

The key to solving a proportion problem is how you set up your problem. Refer to the box Strategy 5-1 for steps in setting up a proportion.

## STRATEGY 5-1
*Writing Proportions*

1. Read the problem.

2. Identify the known information.

3. Write the proportion so that the same units appear in the same location for each proportion.

4. Solve the problem using **cross multiplication** if your proportion is written as a fraction. If the problem is written in linear fashion, multiply the **means** ("inside" numbers) together and the **extremes** ("outside" numbers) together.

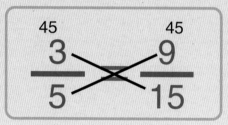

Example of cross multiplication.

*Example:*

In the second grade class in room 200 there is one boy for every two girls. In the second grade class in room 202 there are six girls for every three boys. Are these proportions equal?

1. Read the problem.

   *In the second grade class in room 200 there is one boy for every two girls. In the second grade class in room 202 there are six girls for every three boys. Are these proportions equal?*

2. Identify the known information.

   *In the second grade class in room 200 there is **one boy** for every **two girls**. In the second grade class in room 202 there are **six girls** for every **three boys**.*

3. Write the proportion so that the same units appear in the same location for each proportion.

   $$\frac{1 \text{ boy}}{2 \text{ girls}} = \frac{3 \text{ boys}}{6 \text{ girls}} \qquad 1 \text{ boy} : 2 \text{ girls} :: 3 \text{ boys} : 6 \text{ girls}$$

4. Solve the problem using cross multiplication if your proportion is written as a fraction. If your problem is written in linear fashion, multiply the means together and the extremes together.

   $$\frac{1}{2} = \frac{3}{6}$$
   $1 \times 6 = 2 \times 3$
   $6 = 6$
   *Yes, these proportions are equal.*

   $1:2 :: 3:6$
   $1 \times 6 :: 2 \times 3$
   $6 :: 6$
   *Yes, these proportions are equal.*

Is there a different way to solve this problem? You might think it would have been easier and just as accurate to reduce your fractions before multiplying. As previously stated, there is more than one way to solve a math problem. Yes, you would have come up with the same answer if you had reduced $\frac{3}{6}$ to $\frac{1}{2}$; then your answer would have been ½ = ½. Again, the answer to the problem would be, "Yes, these proportions are equal."

## Solving for *X*

OBJECTIVE 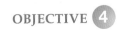 4

In the real world, we encounter proportion problems when we try to compare similar measurements but do not have all the information. The key to solving these problems is to set up the problem so the same measurements are in the same location on both sides of the equation. It is common to use the letter *X* to represent the unknown.

---

## STRATEGY 5-2
*Writing Proportions as a Fraction*

1. Read the problem.

2. Identify the known information.

3. Write the known information on the left side of the equation.

4. Identify the unknown information.

5. Represent the unknown information with the letter X.

6. Write the unknown information on the right side of the equation. Make sure you have the same measurements in identical positions for each portion.

7. Reduce any fractions before performing computations.

8. Solve the problem using cross multiplication. If you have forgotten how to cross multiply, refer to the box Strategy 5-3.

9. Check your answer by substituting your answer for X. You should obtain equal results for this to be a true proportion.

10. Label your answer.

---

## STRATEGY 5-3
*Cross Multiplication*

*Example:*

$\frac{2}{3} = \frac{X}{4}$

1. Multiply the numerator from the left side of the equation with the denominator of the right side of the equation.
$2 \times 4$

2. Multiply the numerator from the right side of the equation with the denominator of the left side of the equation.
$3 \times X$

*(Continued)*

**HUMAN ERROR 5-1**

*Many times, errors occur because we have entered the sequence of numbers incorrectly into the calculator. With division, enter in the dividend first, select the division button, then enter the divisor, and press the equal button to obtain your answer.*

 **STRATEGY 5-3**
*Continued from p. 117*

3. To isolate $X$, you must divide both sides of the equation by the number being multiplied to the $X$.

$$3 \times X = 2 \times 4$$

$$\frac{3X}{3} = \frac{8}{3}$$

$$X = \frac{8}{3}$$

$X = 2\frac{1}{3}$ or 2.666666666666, which rounded to the nearest tenth is 2.7.

4. Label your answer.

 **STRATEGY 5-4**
*Checking Your Work*

1. Insert your answer to replace the $X$ in the proportion.

2. Perform the mathematical calculations.

3. Your answer is correct if the solutions of both proportions are equal.

*Example:* using information from strategy box 5-2, 5-3, 5-4.
The physician orders 15 mg of medication for every 10 pounds of a person's weight. How much medication would be given for a person who weighs 120 pounds?

1. Read the problem.
   *The physician orders 15 mg of medication for every 10 pounds of a person's weight. How much medication would be given for a person who weighs 120 pounds?*

2. Identify the known information.
   *Known: 15 mg of medication for every 10 pounds of weight*
   *Known: person weighs 120 pounds*

3. Write the known information on the left side of the equation.
   $$\frac{15 \text{ mg}}{10 \text{ pounds}}$$

4. Identify the unknown information.
   *How much medication to give a person who weighs 120 pounds*

5. Represent the unknown information with the letter $X$.
   $X$ mg

6. Write the unknown information on the right side of the equation. Make sure you have the same measurements in identical positions for each portion.
   $$\frac{15 \text{ mg}}{10 \text{ pounds}} = \frac{X \text{ mg}}{120 \text{ pounds}}$$

7. Reduce any fractions before performing computations. 5 is a common factor of both 15 and 10.
   $$\text{Reduce } \frac{15 \text{ mg}}{10 \text{ pounds}} \text{ to } \frac{3 \text{ mg}}{2 \text{ pounds}}$$

8. Solve the problem using cross multiplication.

$$\frac{3 \text{ mg}}{2 \text{ pounds}} = \frac{X \text{ mg}}{120 \text{ pounds}}$$

$3 \times 120 = 2 \times X$

$$\frac{360}{2} = \frac{2X}{2} \quad \textit{Isolate the X by dividing both sides by 2}$$

$180 = X$

9. Check your answer by substituting your answer for X. You should obtain equal results for this to be a true proportion.

$$\frac{3 \text{ mg}}{2 \text{ pounds}} = \frac{180 \text{ mg}}{120 \text{ pounds}} \left( \textit{you can reduce to } \frac{3}{2} \right)$$

$3 \times 2 = 2 \times 3$

$6 = 6$

$3 \times 120 = 2 \times 180$

$360 = 360$

***Your answer is correct.***

10. Label your answer in order to answer the question.
*Answer: You would give 180 mg of medication to a person whose weight is 120 pounds.*

Take a few minutes to solve the following problems. Refer to the Strategy boxes if you forget what step comes next. Use the fraction method for these problems.

*Problem 1:* Your car gets 26 miles to the gallon. How many gallons of gas would you need to travel 250 miles?
*Answer: 9.62 gallons*

*Problem 2:* The store is selling beef roast at $2.56 per pound. You need 12 pounds of roast for a dinner party on Friday evening. How much do you expect to spend on the beef roast?
*Answer: $30.72, which would could be rounded to $31.*

Some students prefer to write proportions in a linear fashion rather than as fractions. Instead of cross multiplication, you would multiply the means and the extremes. As with cross multiplication, you need to isolate your unknown X by dividing both sides of the equation by the number being multiplied by X. Ensure that your answer not only makes sense, but also is labeled.

## STRATEGY 5-5
*Writing a Proportion with Linear Format*

1. Read the problem.

2. Identify the known information.

3. Write the known information on the left side of the equation.

4. Identify the unknown information.

5. Represent the unknown information with the letter X.

*(Continued)*

## STRATEGY 5-5
*Continued from p. 119*

6. Write the unknown information on the right side of the equation. Make sure you have the same measurements in identical positions for each portion.

7. Solve the problem by multiplying the means and the extremes.

8. Isolate *X* by dividing both sides of the equation with the number that is being multiplied by *X*.

9. Check your answer.

10. Label your answer.

*Example:*
The physician orders 40 mg of medication in every 5 mL of liquid. How much liquid is required to administer 120 mg of medication?

1. Read the problem.
   *The physician orders 40 mg of medication in every 5 mL of liquid. How much liquid is required to administer 120 mg of medication?*

2. Identify the known information.
   *There is 40 mg of medication in every 5 mL of liquid.*

3. Write your known information on the left side of the equation.
   *40 mg : 5 mL*

4. Identify the unknown information.
   *How many milliliters will be needed to administer 120 mg of medication?*

5. Represent the unknown information with the letter *X*.
   *120 mg : X*

6. Write the unknown information on the right side of the equation. Make sure you have the same measurements in identical positions for each portion.
   *40 mg : 5 mL :: 120 mg : X*

7. Solve the problem by multiplying the means and the extremes.
   *Means:* $5 \times 120 = 600$
   *Extremes:* $40 \times X = 40\,X$
   $$\frac{600 :: 40X}{40 :: 40}$$ *Divide both sides by 40*
   *15 :: X*

8. Check your answer.
   $5 \times 120 :: 40 \times 15$
   *600 :: 600*
   **Your answer is correct.**

9. Label your answer.
   *You need 15 mL of liquid for 120 mg of medication.*

Here are additional problems to work in the linear method.

*Problem 3:* There are 15 boys for every 20 girls in your college class. If there are 360 girls in the class, how many boys are in the class?
*Answer:* 270 boys

*Problem 4:* The patient weighs 210 pounds. The doctor orders 50 mg of medication for every 10 pounds. How much medication would you give?
*Answer:* 1050 mg of medication

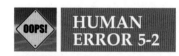

## HUMAN ERROR 5-2

*Incorrect setup is the most common error with proportion problems. Double-check your work. Do you have the same units of measure in the same location on both sides of the problem?*

*The second most common error is incorrectly performing the mathematical calculations. Take your time and check your work.*

# PRACTICE THE SKILL 5-2

Solve the following problems to determine the value of X.

1. $X : 25 :: 16 : 100$ _____

2. $\dfrac{6}{18} = \dfrac{X}{12}$ _____

3. $72 : 3 :: X : 7$ _____

4. $\dfrac{76}{26} = \dfrac{X}{2}$ _____

5. $X : 16 :: 16 : 32$ _____

6. $\dfrac{X}{92} = \dfrac{36}{24}$ _____

7. $3 : X :: 90 : 6$ _____

8. $\dfrac{16}{X} = \dfrac{9}{27}$ _____

9. $X : 8 :: 11 : 2$ _____

10. $\dfrac{X}{10} = \dfrac{11}{11}$ _____

11. $5 : 9 :: X : 40$ _____

12. $\dfrac{1}{2} = \dfrac{X}{65}$ _____

13. $9 : 16 :: 4 : X$ _____

14. $\dfrac{21}{30} = \dfrac{7}{X}$ _____

15. $3 : 4 :: 25 : X$ _____

16. $\dfrac{2}{3} = \dfrac{30}{X}$ _____

17. $1 : 3 :: 15 : X$ _____

18. $\dfrac{27}{50} = \dfrac{X}{16}$ _____

19. $61 : 108 :: X : 3$ _____

20. $\dfrac{20}{8} = \dfrac{X}{6}$ _____

*(Continued)*

## PRACTICE THE SKILL 5-2
*Continued from p. 121*

**21.** $\dfrac{20}{16} = \dfrac{3}{X}$ _____

**22.** $5 : 20 :: 25 : X$ _____

**23.** $5 : 6 :: 30 : X$ _____

**24.** $\dfrac{1}{5} = \dfrac{X}{1000}$ _____

**25.** $15 : 3 :: X : 7$ _____

OBJECTIVES ④ ⑤

## BUILDING CONFIDENCE WITH THE SKILL 5-1

Solve the following proportions. Round answers to the nearest tenth.

**1.** $\dfrac{3}{8} = \dfrac{X}{32}$ _____

**2.** $\dfrac{X}{15} = \dfrac{30}{150}$ _____

**3.** $\dfrac{13}{42} = \dfrac{7}{X}$ _____

**4.** $\dfrac{50}{X} = \dfrac{200}{1000}$ _____

**5.** $\dfrac{15}{70} = \dfrac{X}{14}$ _____

**6.** $\dfrac{500}{2} = \dfrac{750}{X}$ _____

**7.** $\dfrac{X}{32} = \dfrac{7}{56}$ _____

**8.** $\dfrac{40}{X} = \dfrac{14}{96}$ _____

**9.** $\dfrac{9}{15} = \dfrac{3}{X}$ _____

**10.** $\dfrac{5}{9} = \dfrac{X}{18}$ _____

**11.** $X : 25 :: 16 : 100$ _____

**12.** $6 : 18 :: X : 12$ _____

**13.** $72 : 3 :: X : 7$ _____

*(Continued)*

## BUILDING CONFIDENCE WITH THE SKILL 5-1
*Continued from p. 122*

**14.** 76 : 26 :: X : 2 _____

**15.** X : 16 :: 16 : 32 _____

**16.** X : 92 :: 36 : 24 _____

**17.** 3 : X :: 90 : 6 _____

**18.** 16 : X :: 9 : 27 _____

**19.** X : 8 :: 11 : 2 _____

**20.** X : 10 :: 11 : 11 _____

**Set up the following word problems as proportions. Solve the problems.**

**21.** A bouquet has two roses for every three carnations. There are 12 roses in the bouquet. How many carnations are in the bouquet? _____

**22.** Add two scoops of coffee for every three cups of water. How much coffee is added for 24 cups of water? _____

**23.** The student to teacher ratio is 25 to one. How many teachers are needed for a class of 48 students? _____

**24.** There are two bathrooms for every four bedrooms. The mansion has 12 bedrooms. How many bathrooms do you expect to find? _____

**25.** Televisions run 2 minutes of commercials for every 17 minutes of programming. How many minutes of commercials would be run for 85 minutes of programming? _____

**26.** Gas prices are $3.95 per gallon. Your car has a 14-gallon tank. What is the cost to fill your tank with gas? _____

**27.** Autism affects 1 out of 158 children. If there are 1,896 children in the preschool program, how many do you expect to be diagnosed with autism?

_____

**28.** A recipe for pudding requires 2 cups of milk for every four servings. How many cups of milk do you need for 12 servings of pudding? _____

**29.** When the cookie recipe is doubled, it yields 72 cookies. Based on that ratio, how many cookies will you have if you triple the recipe? _____

**30.** The baby formula calls for two scoops of powder for every four ounces of water. How many scoops do you need for 24 ounces of water? _____

**31.** The car wash takes 14 minutes to vacuum, wash, and dry a 4-door sedan. How many sedans can be cleaned in 98 minutes? _____

*(Continued)*

## BUILDING CONFIDENCE WITH THE SKILL 5-1
*Continued from p. 123*

32. The cashier spends 3.75 minutes per customer. How many customers are served in 120 minutes? _____

33. A trip to Washington, D.C., is 625 miles one way from your starting point. Your car can travel 450 miles on 18 gallons of gas. How many gallons of gas will it take from your starting point to Washington, D.C.? _____

34. Cleaning solution is to be diluted at a two cups to eight gallons of water ratio. How many gallons are needed for six cups of solution? _____

35. The farmer's yield from three apple trees is seven bushels of apples. How many bushels will 45 trees yield? _____

36. The lawnmower requires 2 ounces of oil for every 16 ounces of gas. How much oil is needed for 80 ounces of gas? _____

37. The raffle tickets are $2.50 for seven tickets. How many tickets can be bought with $20.00? _____

38. A salt-water fish tank requires 3 ounces of salt for every 5 gallons of water. How many ounces of salt are needed for a 75-gallon tank? _____

39. A cyclist rides 3 miles every 30 minutes. The bike trail is 45 miles long. How long will it take the cyclist to ride the trail without a break? _____

40. The tour boat can hold 95 people per trip. The boat runs 45 fully loaded trips per day. How many people ride the boat every day? _____

OBJECTIVES  ## Medication Proportions

In this chapter, we have been working on solving proportion problems and solving for *X*. In future chapters, we will be converting different measurements from metric to household equivalents. At this time, I would like to share common formulas that are used when calculating medication problems. Remember, the most common mistake when calculating medication dosage occurs when setting up the proportion. The proportion must have the same units in the same location.

## STRATEGY 5-6
*Different Medication Calculation Formulas*

$$\frac{\text{Dosage ordered}}{\text{Dosage available}} \times \text{Known dosage form} = \text{Amount to give}$$

$$\frac{\text{Known dosage available}}{\text{Known dosage form}} = \frac{\text{Dosage ordered}}{\text{Amount to be given}}$$

Students who have taken a prenursing pharmacology class may be aware of another formula that is commonly used:

$$\frac{\text{D(desire)}}{\text{H(have)}} \times \text{Q(quantity)} = \text{Amount}$$

This formula is further discussed in Chapter 7, where you are asked to solve different and more complex problems using metric and apothecary (household) measurements.

Each of the above formulas answers the same question, just in a different format. The following examples demonstrate the same problem using each of the different formulas.

*Example:*
The physician orders 300 mg of antibiotic. The antibiotic comes as 150 mg per capsule.

1. $\dfrac{300 \text{ mg}}{150 \text{ mg}} \times 1 \text{ capsule} = 2 \text{ capsules}$

2. $\dfrac{150 \text{ mg}}{1 \text{ capsule}} = \dfrac{300 \text{ mg}}{X \text{ capsule}}$   or   $150 : 1 :: 300 : X$

   $\dfrac{300}{150} = \dfrac{150 \, X}{150}$     or     $\dfrac{300}{150} :: \dfrac{150 \, X}{150}$

   $2 = X$       or     $2 :: X$

3. What do you know? $= \dfrac{\text{What do you want?}}{\text{What do you need?}}$

As you can see, all the above formulas produce the same answer. It is up to you to decide which formula works best for your learning style. Once you have decided, stay consistent—do not keep switching back and forth. We do our best work when we feel confident in our methodology.

# PRACTICE THE SKILL 5-3

OBJECTIVES  4 5

Solve the following problems. Round your answer to the nearest tenth.

1. There is 25 mg of medication in every 5 mL of liquid. The doctor orders 75 mg of medication. How many milliliters of liquid will you give?

_____

2. The injection has 75 mg of medication for every 1 mL. How many milliliters do you give for 225 mg of medication? _____

3. The IV has 20 milliequivalents (mEq) of potassium for every 1000 mL of fluid. How much fluid must be infused to obtain 70 mEq of potassium?

_____

4. The doctor orders an injection of 6 mg of medication. The medication is supplied as 2 mg per 1.5 mL. How many milliliters (ml) would you give?

_____

5. The IV contains 300 mg of medication in 150 mL of fluid. How many milliliters (mL) would you give for the patient to receive 750 mg of medication? _____

6. The vial holds 25 mg in 10 mL. How many milligrams (mg) are in each 1 mL dose? _____

*(Continued)*

**PRACTICE THE SKILL 5-3**
*Continued from p. 125*

7. The medication is supplied in 40 mg tablets. How many tablets should be given if the doctor orders 100 mg? _____

8. The medication is supplied as 40 mg for every 15 mL of fluid. How many milligrams will be given in 45 mL of fluid? _____

9. The doctor orders 2.5 mg for every 10 pounds the patient weighs. The patient's weight is 160 pounds. How many milligrams (mg) should you give? _____

10. Pain medication comes as 75 mg/mL. The physician orders 150 mg of medication. How many milliliters would you give? _____

11. A vial holds 0.5 mg of medication in every 1/2 mL. The physician orders 0.75 mg of medication to be given. How many mL do you need to give?

_____

12. The physician orders 2 grams of medication. The vial states 1 gram per 1.5 mL. How many milliliters would you give? _____

## CONCLUSION

There are many activities in which we use ratios and proportions without a conscious thought process. We do not realize how we came up with the answer; we just know what it is, especially when it comes to medication dosages. However, problems should be written out and computations double-checked to prevent errors. Just like carpentry: measure twice, cut once. Work carefully when performing any type of mathematical computation. Errors may occur if you become rushed or distracted. Calculators can perform these computations quickly and accurately, but only if the person entering the data understands the concepts. Just setting up your proportion incorrectly may cause an error. Take your time and enjoy your success in mastering the skills presented in this chapter.

OBJECTIVES

**MASTER THE SKILL**

Solve the following proportions. Round answers to the nearest tenth.

1. $\dfrac{740}{X} = \dfrac{35}{20}$ _____

2. $125 : X :: 15 : 10$ _____

3. $\dfrac{40}{X} = \dfrac{28}{14}$ _____

4. $X : 87 :: 110 : 122$ _____

*(Continued)*

## MASTER THE SKILL
*Continued from p. 126*

5.  $\dfrac{52}{X} = \dfrac{12}{3}$  _____

6.  $\dfrac{39}{40} = \dfrac{92}{X}$  _____

7.  23 : 46 :: X : 50  _____

8.  $\dfrac{11}{113} = \dfrac{15}{X}$  _____

9.  13 : 52 :: X : 90  _____

10.  $\dfrac{X}{7} = \dfrac{8}{200}$  _____

11.  7 : 30 :: X : 15  _____

12.  9 : 45 :: 3 : X  _____

13.  $\dfrac{1}{23} = \dfrac{14}{X}$  _____

14.  $\dfrac{55}{X} = \dfrac{65}{195}$  _____

15.  $\dfrac{8}{11} = \dfrac{64}{X}$  _____

**Round the answers to the nearest tenth.**

16.  The physician orders 40 mg of medication by mouth. The medication is supplied as 20 mg per tablet. How many tablets would you give? _____

17.  The doctor orders a 500 mL bolus of fluids. The IV comes in 125 mL bags. How many bags would you give? _____

18.  The patient takes Lasix 40 mg/tablet twice a day. How many tablets would she need for a 6-month (180-day) supply?

_____

19.  The doctor orders 75 mg of Demerol. Your facility has Demerol 25 mg/0.5 mL. How many milliliters (mL) should you give? _____

20.  The physician orders 0.25 mg of medication. The medication is available in 0.125 mg tablets. How many tablets would you give? _____

21.  The pharmacy receives an order for 350 mg of medication. The medication is available as 175 mg tablets. How many tablets would they supply?

_____

*(Continued)*

## MASTER THE SKILL
*Continued from p. 127*

22. You need to give 0.4 mg of medication. The medication comes as 0.2 mg/0.5 mL. How many milliliters (mL) would you give? _____

23. The doctor orders Keflex 125 mg/5 mL. You need to administer 175 mg. How many milliliters (mL) would you give? _____

24. The laboratory test requires 10 mL of blood. Each blood tube holds 2.5 mL of blood. How many tubes of blood do you need to run the test?

_____

25. The medication is supplied as 30 mg for every 3 mL. How many milligrams are in 18 mL of medication? _____

26. The orthopedic technician uses 14 inches of casting material for every short arm cast. Today, 13 short arm casts were applied. How much casting material was used? _____

27. Each suture repair kit holds six gauze pads. How many gauze pads are needed to complete 65 suture repair kits? _____

28. The dietary department serves 4 ounces of meat to every patient. Today, 80 ounces of meat were served. How many patients were served? _____

29. The blood bank takes 500 mL of blood from each donor. How many donors are needed to obtain 2500 mL of blood? _____

30. Patients are turned in their beds every 2 hours. How many times would you turn a patient in a 12-hour shift? _____

# General Accounting

## CHAPTER OUTLINE

## LEARNING OBJECTIVES

*Upon completion of this chapter, the learner will be able to:*

1. Define the key terms that relate to the chapter.

2. Calculate insurance deductibles and copayments.

3. Compute and analyze balances of day sheets and ledger cards with 100% accuracy.

4. Calculate and record petty cash transactions.

5. Utilize tax information to determine gross and net pay.

6. Complete purchase order forms.

## KEY TERMS

OBJECTIVE 1

| | |
|---|---|
| Coinsurance | Ledger Card |
| Copayment | Net Income |
| Day Sheet | Net Loss |
| Deductible | Net Profit |
| Encounter Form | Purchase Order |
| Gross Income | Solvent |

OBJECTIVE 1

Health care can be a double-edged sword. On one side is the art of assisting the community in maintaining healthy lifestyles. On the other is the business of health care. Although most people do not view health care as a business, it is one of the fastest growing industries in the United States. If facilities are not paid for services, they in turn cannot buy equipment or pay the salaries of the workers. In this chapter, we discuss accounting (fiscal health, or the business side of health care).

## MATH IN THE REAL WORLD 6-1
*Real World Expressions: Common Phrases Used to Discuss Finances*

- In the red
- Break even
- In the black
- **Net loss**
- **Solvent**
- Net profit
- Sinking
- Treading water
- Heads above water

OBJECTIVES **1** **2**

# INSURANCE

The number one source of income in health care is insurance reimbursement. Insurance can come in the form of private coverage, health maintenance plans, Medicare, Medicaid, military insurance, or disability plans. There are many types of insurance plans, and even if two companies receive insurance from the same provider, their plans could be very different. When it comes to insurance, there is *no* one-size-fits-all plan. This is why the following careers are in such demand:

- Medical insurance specialists
- Medical billers
- Medical coders
- Health information managers

Think about the last time you visited a physician's office, an urgent care facility, or an emergency room. How much did you have to pay for the visit? Your payment was based on whether your insurance policy had a **deductible, coinsurance,** or **copayment.** If you were not covered by an insurance plan, you might have had to pay the balance in full that day. Was your payment collected before you saw the physician? If so, that may mean that your insurance requires a copayment. If you paid for services after being seen by the physician, you probably have a deductible or coinsurance. If that is not confusing enough, insurance companies have benefits for hospitalization that may be different from the benefits for outpatient services.

There are many pieces to the insurance puzzle. Although management of a patient's insurance data is part of the growing field of health information management, it is important that all members of the health care team have basic insurance knowledge.

## MATH IN THE REAL WORLD 6-2

What mathematical tools are used when dealing with money? Addition, subtraction, multiplication, division, and percentages. This chapter will strengthen your skills by using these concepts in multistep problems.

In general, managed care policies (HMO, PPO, and EPO) require that a copayment be paid at the time of service. The copayment amount may vary based on the location and type of service. Copayments are paid each time the person sees the physician or therapist or receives any other service that falls under the insurance plan's copayment requirement. Copay IS deducted from the total bill, but does NOT count toward deductible.

Traditional insurance plans and Medicare typically have both a deductible that must be met before insurance coverage begins and coinsurance. Coinsurance amounts are determined by the insurance company. If the insurance policy is 70/30, this means the insurance will pay 70% of the usual and customary charges and the patient is responsible for 30%. Coinsurance varies from policy to policy; however, the insurer's responsibility and the patient's responsibility always add up to 100%. Payments toward deductibles and coinsurance are subtracted from the total bill for the visit.

You may encounter patients who have coverage from more than one insurance company. Many people carry secondary insurance to reduce their out-of-pocket expenses. Should you collect the deductible, and if so, how much? Should you collect the copayment from both insurance policies? Or only from the primary insurance policy? Or should you collect the highest copayment amount? Each facility has its own policy for handling primary and secondary insurance payments. The information to remember is that claims are submitted to the secondary insurance company to cover the cost of the visit not covered by primary insurance.

*Example:*
Mr. Ford has insurance from his employer (primary), and he is also covered under his wife's policy (secondary). When Mr. Ford is seen by the physician, the primary insurance company will pay 90% for the usual and customary services. Then, instead of Mr. Ford paying the remaining 10%, it is submitted to his wife's insurance company for payment.

## MATH QUICK TIP 6-1

When you are determining coinsurance responsibility, the total amount must always add up to 100%.

Accurate documentation regarding the collection of copayment, deductibles, and coinsurance amounts must be communicated to the insurance specialist. These amounts must be reported to the insurance company for accurate determination of benefits. This information directly affects the reimbursement amount to the physician. If the health care facility does not collect copayment, deductibles, and coinsurance, the result is a decrease in cash flow to the facility. A significant decrease or a failure to be fiscally sound may affect the services offered, which could affect your job.

## PRACTICE THE SKILL 6-1

**Identify whether coinsurance, copayment, or a deductible would be collected based on the question.**

1. A patient's insurance policy requires a payment of $25.00 for each visit to the physician's office. This is called a _____.

2. The patient has an appointment on January 5, 20XX. The patient has Medicare Part B insurance, which requires that a payment of $135.00 is paid by the patient at the beginning of each year before the insurance coverage begins. This is an example of a _____.

3. A patient has private insurance through Blue Cross/Blue Shield. The policy states that the patient is required to pay 20% of all charges that occur when seeing the physician. This is an example of _____.

4. A patient has a managed care insurance plan that covers emergency room expenses. According to the insurance card, the patient must pay a $150.00 at the time of the visit, and pay 35% of all emergency room charges. The $150.00 is an example of _____ and the 35% is an example of _____.

5. A _____, if required, is usually collected before the patient sees the physician.

6. _____ is commonly collected at the end of the visit.

7. Medicare Part B states that a patient will pay 80% of the usual and customary charges after the _____ has been met.

8. A patient has a doctor's appointment on January 13th. Based on the patient's insurance coverage, the patient must pay the yearly _____ before the insurance company will provide coverage.

9. Private insurance traditionally requires both a _____ and a _____.

10. Managed care plans require a _____ to be paid at the time of each visit.

**OBJECTIVES ② ③**

### Collecting Copayment, Deductibles, and Coinsurance

Depending on your job description, you may be required to collect copayments, deductibles, or coinsurance at the beginning or end of a visit. When working with copayments or coinsurance, you might easily find the collectable amount by looking at the insurance card or accessing the account through a secure website. It may be necessary, however, to contact the insurance company to determine what amount of the deductible has been satisfied. Correctly documenting the type of payment is important so that claims personnel can report this information to the insurance company when a claim has been filed.

## STRATEGY 6-1
*Determining Copayment Amounts*

1. Look at the insurance card in Figure 6-1.

2. Determine if the insurance plan has a copayment amount (copay).

3. Collect the copayment amount.

4. Record collection of fees as described later in the chapter. *Remember: this amount is deducted from the total amount of the bill.*

5. Copayments are collected every time the patient is seen by the physician; this includes follow-up visits.

---

**ABC** Health

Plan: **2468**
**POS**

Member name: **Sally L. Smith**          PCP: **James S. Jones**
Member number: **333-WTRTV-445522**
Group number: **987654**

COPAYMENT: Office Visit: **$15**
Emergency Room: **$75**
Urgent Care Facility: **$50**

*Member inquires: Call 800-555-1357*

**Figure 6-1**   Sample insurance card.

---

## PRACTICE THE SKILL 6-2

Refer to Figure 6-1 and answer the following questions.

1. Does the card indicate that the patient has hospital coverage? _____

2. Does the card indicate that the patient has a primary care physician? _____

3. Is there a different copayment amount for urgent care or emergency room visits? _____

4. What is the copayment amount for the emergency room, if indicated? _____

5. What is the copayment amount for an office visit, if indicated? _____

6. What is the copayment amount for an urgent care visit, if indicated? _____

## STRATEGY 6-2
*Determining Deductible Amounts*

1. Contact the insurance company or the designated secure website to determine if a deductible has been paid in full. If not, what portion of the deductible has been met?

2. Depending on the policy of the facility, you may be required to collect a portion of the deductible before the patient sees the physician. *Alternatively*, the deductible may be collected at the end of the visit once the total amount of the bill has been determined.

3. Properly document how much of the deductible was collected. This information must be turned in to the insurance company to determine when coverage will begin.

4. Subtract the amount of the deductible from the total bill to determine the billable amount.

5. Record collection of fees as described later in the chapter.

*Example:*

The patient's insurance policy has a $250.00 per year deductible. On January 13, 20XX, the patient is seen in the physician's office. The total bill is $185.00. This is the first time the patient has used his health insurance this year. Answer the following questions based on this scenario.

1. What is the total amount of Mr. Ryan's yearly deductible? _____

2. How much has been met this year toward the deductible?

   _____

3. How much should you collect from Mr. Ryan toward his deductible?

   _____

4. Has Mr. Ryan met his deductible for the year? _____
   If not, how much will he need to pay before his insurance becomes active?

   _____

## STRATEGY 6-3
*Determining Coinsurance Amounts*

1. Contact the insurance company, either by phone or on a secure website, to determine if the patient has coinsurance.

2. Find out whether there is a deductible and how much has been met. (Remember: the deductible must be met before insurance coverage begins.)

3. Verify the insurance company's responsibility for the bill and the patient's responsibility for the bill. (The total amount cannot equal more than 100%.)

*(Continued)*

## STRATEGY 6-3
*Continued from p. 134*

4. Once the total bill has been established, determine the patient's responsibility. (If you have forgotten how to determine percentage, refer to Chapter 4.)

5. Collect the amount for which the patient is responsible at the end of the visit.

6. Subtract the amount of the coinsurance from the total bill to determine the billable amount.

7. Record collection of fees as described later in the chapter.

## PRACTICE THE SKILL 6-3

**Determine the patient's responsibility in each of the following problems.**

1. The administrative assistant has verified that the insurance company's responsibility is 65%.

   a. What is the patient's responsibility? _____

   b. If the total bill for this visit is $65.40, how much will be collected from the patient? _____

   c. How much will the insurance company be billed? _____

2. The administrative assistant has verified that the patient's responsibility is 20%.

   a. What is the insurance company's responsibility? _____

   b. The total bill for this visit is $285.00. How much should you collect from the patient? _____

   c. What is the billable amount that the insurance company is responsible for? If there is a deductible, find out how much has been met?

   _____

3. The medical assistant has verified from the insurance company that the patient is responsible for 45% of the medical bill. The total bill is $314.75.

   a. What percentage of the bill will the insurance company pay? _____

   b. What is the billable amount that the insurance company is responsible for? _____

   c. How much should the medical assistant collect from the patient? _____

## STRATEGY 6-4
*Determining Deductibles and Coinsurance*

1. Contact the insurance company either by phone or on a secure website to determine if the patient has a yearly deductible and the coinsurance amount.

2. Find out whether there is a deductible and how much has been met.
   *$150.00 outstanding balance*

3. Verify the insurance company's responsibility for the bill and the patient's responsibility for the bill.
   *80/20          80% Insurance/20% Patient*

4. Determine the total amount of the bill.
   *$425.00*

5. First, subtract the outstanding deductible from the total bill to determine the billable amount.
   *$425.00 – $150.00 = $275.00 billable amount*

6. Next, determine what percentage of the billable amount is the patient's responsibility.
   *$275.00 × 20% = $55.00 is the patient's responsibility*

7. Determine the total amount that will be collected from the patient.
   *$150.00 + $55.00 = $ 205.00 will be collected from the patient*

8. If there is a deductible, find out how much has been met.
   $425.00 – $205.00 = $220.00 will be collected from the insurance company.

9. Record collection of fees as described later in this chapter.

## STRATEGY 6-5
*Copayment and Coinsurance Combination*

Some insurance plans require a copayment, which covers the office visit to the healthcare provider, and coinsurance for such services as radiology, laboratory, and durable medical equipment (crutches, cast, sling, etc.).

1. Check the insurance card to determine whether there is a copayment and the amount. Contact the insurance company either by phone or on a secure website to find out whether the patient has coinsurance for radiology, laboratory, or durable medical equipment (DME).
   *Copayment: $35.00*
   *Coinsurance: 25%*

2. Depending on the policy of the facility, collect the copayment before the patient sees the physician. If x-rays, laboratory work, or DME is a possibility, your facility might have you collect the total amount at the end of the visit.

*(Continued)*

## STRATEGY 6-5
*Continued from p. 136*

3. At the end of the visit, determine whether the coinsurance would apply toward any procedures.

   *Total bill for the visit: $230.00.*     *Lab fee: $15.00; x-ray fee: $92.00*
   *Doctor Fee: $123.00*                    *Total coinsurance amount: $107.00*

4. Determine the patient's coinsurance responsibility.
   $$\$107.00 \times 25\% = \$26.75$$

5. Subtract the coinsurance amount from the total bill to determine the billable amount.
   *Total bill $230.00 – $26.75 = $203.25*

6. Determine the total amount that will be collected from the patient.
   *Copayment + Coinsurance = Total amount that will be collected from the patient $35.00 + $26.75 = $61.75*

7. Record collection of fees as described later in this chapter.

## MATH IN THE REAL WORLD 6-3

You may encounter patients who have two or more insurance policies. The first step is to determine which insurance is primary. The patient must satisfy the conditions of the primary insurance before the secondary insurer pays its portion of the bill. Many facilities apply only the conditions of the primary insurance (collect copayment, coinsurance, or deductible) and submit this information to the primary insurer. Once coordination of benefits has been established, they submit the remaining balance to the secondary insurer. The patient may still be responsible for some part of the bill, which may be collected later.

## PRACTICE THE SKILL 6-4

Answer the following questions based on the information provided in the word problems.

1. The patient has Medicare Part B insurance. Medicare has a $134.00 yearly deductible. Once the deductible has been met, the coinsurance coverage is 80/20. The patient will be seeing the physician, for their first visit in the new year, on January 4th. His total bill is $95.00.

   a. What is the total amount of the yearly deductible? _____

   b. How much should the receptionist collect from the patient? _____

   c. Has this patient met their yearly deductible? If not, what is the remaining balance after this visit? _____

*(Continued)*

## PRACTICE THE SKILL 6-4
*Continued from p. 137*

The patient returns 2 weeks later to see the doctor for a follow-up visit. The total bill for this visit is $95.00. The patient has not seen any other physician since their last visit. Based on the answers to the previous questions, determine the answers to the following questions.

d. How much of the office visit charges will be applied to the patient's yearly deductible? _____

e. Will the patient have to pay coinsurance? If so, how much?

_____

f. What is the total amount that the medical assistant will need to collect from this patient? _____

g. What is the total billable amount for this visit? _____

2. The patient has scheduled an appointment for a complete physical. The patient has the following insurance:

MetLife PPO                     Deductible: $0.00
                                Copayment: $25.00
                                Coinsurance: 10% for radiology,
                                   laboratory, and DME
The patient's physical includes: Office visit: $350.00
                                X-ray: $95.00
                                Blood test: $15.00

The patient has scheduled an appointment in 10 days to review the test results.

a. What is the copayment amount? _____

b. Is the patient responsible for an additional coverage? If so, how much would the receptionist collect? _____

c. How much will you collect when the visit is over? _____

The patient returns 10 days later for test results. The patient states he or she has not had any change in insurance coverage. The patient see the physician to review the test results and discuss a new treatment plan.

d. How much should you collect for this visit? _____

e. When will you typically collect this fee? _____

## BUILDING CONFIDENCE WITH THE SKILL 6-1

1. The patient is being seen for a follow-up visit for her asthma. The patient is covered by a PPO insurance plan with a $25.00 copayment. The total charge for today's visit is $65.00. How much would the receptionist collect from the patient? _____

2. The patient arrives at the emergency room after a fall from a ladder at home. The intake specialist verifies that the patient's insurance coinsurance coverage is 85%. The patient is diagnosed with a fractured tibia. The cost of the visit is $1015.00. How much would the intake specialist collect from the patient? _____

3. Medicare Part B has a yearly deductible of $124.00 and coinsurance of 80/20. A patient is being seen in the clinic today. The receptionist has verified that the patient has paid $72.50 toward the yearly deductible. Today's bill is for $135.00.

   a. How much would the receptionist collect from the patient? _____

   b. What is the billable amount to Medicare? _____

4. The patient's managed care plan has a $35.00 copayment for all office visits and the insurance will pay 75% of all radiographic and laboratory procedures. The patient is being seen for a dislocated shoulder. The patient will be charged the following fees:
   Office visit: $135.00 and X-Ray: $112.00.

   a. How much should be collected from the patient? _____

   b. What is the billable amount to the insurance company? _____

5. The patient being seen has dual insurance, Medicare is primary and MetLife is secondary. Medicare has a $134.00 yearly deductible and the patient has paid 90.80 toward this amount. After the deductible has been paid, the patient is responsible for 20% of the bill. MetLife will not cover any of the expenses until the Medicare deductible amount has been satisfied, at which time they will pay 15% of any fees not covered by Medicare. The patient's charges for today's visit include:

   Office visit     $95.00
   EKG     $45.00
   Laboratory test    $35.00

   a. How much will you collect from Mr. Stephen? _____

   b. How much will you bill Medicare? _____

   c. How much will you bill MetLife? _____

6. Your physical therapy visit cost $168.00. The insurance will cover 75% of the bill. How much will you need to pay? _____

*(Continued)*

## BUILDING CONFIDENCE WITH THE SKILL 6-1
*Continued from p. 139*

7. The patient's insurance coverage has a 1500.00 deductible and coinsurance where the patient is responsible for 30% of the remaining expenses. So far the patient has paid 995.00 toward the deductible. The patient is having outpatient surgery with the estimated cost of $18,250.00. The patient must pay their portion of the bill prior to surgery.

   a. The outstanding amount for the deductible is? _____

   b. What amount will the patient pay toward the surgery?

   _____

   c. What amount will be collected from the patient prior to the surgery?

   _____

   d. What is the anticipated amount that the insurance company will pay for the surgery? _____

8. Your employer requires you to get a physical. This is not a benefit covered by your insurance carrier. The physical costs $65.00, which includes the office visits. According to your insurance card, you have a $30.00 copayment for all office visits. How much would you expect to pay for the physical? _____

9. The patient has dual insurance. Coordination of benefits agreement has established that the primary insurance will pay 75% of the medical expenses and the secondary insurance will cover the remaining amount. The following charges occur in todays visit:

   Office Visit: $115.00
   Lab Fees: $105.00
   Testing Fees: $95.00
   Medication: $65.00

   a. Determine the billable amount for the primary insurance company.

   _____

   b. What is the secondary insurance responsibility toward the bill?

   _____

   c. How much do you expect MetLife to pay? _____

10. The patient's insurance will pay 60% of all medical equipment. The patient was diagnosed with a dislocated patella. The patient will be charged $105.00 for a knee immobilizer and $27.50 for a set of crutches.

   a. What amount do you expect the insurance to pay?

   _____

   b. What amount will the patient be expected to pay? _____

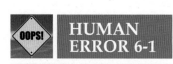

## HUMAN ERROR 6-1

*Look over your answers. Do they make sense? Most errors occur because of inaccurate math computations.*

## CASH DRAWER, DAY SHEETS, LEDGER CARDS, AND PETTY CASH

OBJECTIVES **3** **4**

Have you ever held a job in which you were responsible for the exchange of money? If so, you are ahead of the game. Just like grocery stores, medical offices exchange money with each transaction. Accurate documentation of the amount of charges, cash received, and other transactions is necessary to balance your cash drawer at the end of the day. Even in the hospital setting, money is exchanged for services rendered. This may be done at registration, upon discharge, or by individuals making payments on their accounts.

In this section, you will learn how to balance the cash drawer and **day sheets**. In addition, we will discuss the use of petty cash and the recording of transactions on ledger cards. Depending on the size of your facility, these tasks will be accomplished either electronically or by hand.

## MATH IN THE REAL WORLD 6-4

With the advancement in Electronic Health Records (EHR), patient financial and health records can be tabulated in real-time.

### Cash Drawer

Many facilities use a cash drawer worksheet. The purpose of this worksheet is to accurately document all *currency* transactions involving the cash drawer throughout the day. It is essential to have documentation of the beginning balance of your cash drawer at the start of each day.

In addition to cash, transactions can occur in other formats. To establish the total daily revenue, you must take into account payments made by check, credit and debit cards, and in some cases gift cards or promotional discounts.

## MATH QUICK TIP 6-2

In today's society, the computer performs many of the tasks described in this chapter electronically. However, it is important to know how to perform these tasks manually.

Use the charts provided in the text (or create your own) and see if you can create or find a template to perform the problems electronically.

The true test of skill mastery is when you can come up with the correct answer in a manual and electronic format.

## STRATEGY 6-6
*Balancing a Cash Drawer*

1. Determine the amount in your cash drawer before the start of business. Write this amount down and place your tally in a reliable location.

2. Count each form of currency. Write down the total number of bills and the total cash amount.

3. Calculate the total amount of coins.

4. Record all credit card and debit card transactions. Add to the total cash balance.

5. Record any checks received as payment. Add to the total cash balance.

6. Record any refunds. Subtract from the total cash balance.

7. Subtract your beginning balance from the total amount of payments received (sum of currency, credit and debit transactions, and checks with the refunds subtracted). This difference is your **net profit** (or **net loss** if the difference is negative). It is important to have a net profit in order to remain **solvent,** or capable of meeting financial obligations.

8. Document your final daily total.

*Example:*

At the start of business, your cash drawer has a total of $375.00. At 3:30 p.m., your shift is ending and you must balance the cash drawer. Based on the following information, complete the form below and determine the total net profit for your shift.

At the end of your shift, the following is in your cash drawer:

| *Denomination* | *Number of bills and coins* |
| --- | --- |
| $50.00 bills | 2 |
| $20.00 bills | 17 |
| $10.00 bills | 4 |
| $5.00 bills | 25 |
| $1.00 bills | 40 |
| $1.00 coins | 0 |
| Half dollars | 0 |
| Quarters | 13 |
| Dimes | 17 |
| Nickels | 5 |
| Pennies | 13 |

In addition, you have:

| | |
| --- | --- |
| Credit cards: | $135.00 |
| Checks: | $1030.62 |

Finally, the office manager authorized the following refunds to be paid from your drawer:

| | |
|---|---|
| Mrs. Erma Sick | $45.00 |
| Mr. U.R. Right | $25.00 |
| Ms. Tula Cross | $25.00 |
| Mr. Ox O'Gen | $85.00 |

Now, use this information to complete the form.

| Payment Methods | Total Amount |
|---|---|
| Beginning Cash Balance | |
| Total Amount of Cash | |
| Total Amount of Coins | |
| Total Amount of Checks | |
| Total Amount of Credit Card | |
| Total Amount of Refunds | |
| Total Revenue (Cash, Coins, Checks, Credit Cards) | |
| Total Expenses (Beginning Cash Balance, Refunds) | |
| Net Difference (Total Revenue – Total Expenses) | |
| Do you have a Net Profit OR Net Loss? | |

Calculate the total amount for the cash drawer *adding* the cash, coins, checks, and credit cards (revenue). From the total *subtract* the beginning cash balance and refunds (expenses).

| Payment Methods | Total Amount |
|---|---|
| Beginning Cash Balance | $375.00 |
| Total Amount of Cash | $645.00 |
| Total Amount of Coins | $5.33 |
| Total Amount of Checks | $1030.62 |
| Total Amount of Credit Card | $135.00 |
| Total Amount of Refunds | $180.00 |
| Total Revenue (Cash, Coins, Checks, Credit Cards) | Cash + Coins + Checks + Credit – Refunds = $1635.95 |
| Total Expenses (Beginning Cash Balance, Refunds) | Subtract beginning balance: |
| Net Difference (Total Revenue – Total Expenses) | $1635.95 – $375 = $1260.95 |
| Do you have a Net Profit or a Net Loss? | Net Profit |

Revenue:
$645.00 + $5.33 + $1030.62 + $135.00 = 1765.95

Expenses:
$375.00 + $180.00 = $555.00

Revenues – Expenses = Total amount

$1765.95 – $555.00 = $1210.95

 ## MATH IN THE REAL WORLD 6-5

Net Profit: Positive balance for the day.

Net Loss: Negative balance for the day.

Does this activity remind you of anything? Balancing your checkbook, or making the monthly family budget? If so, you are right. The business end of health care is very similar to activities we perform in our daily lives.

## PRACTICE THE SKILL 6-5

Use the following worksheet to assist with answering questions.

1. Beginning balance: $135.00

| Denomination | Number of bills and coins |
|---|---|
| $50.00 bills | 2 |
| $20.00 bills | 7 |
| $10.00 bills | 14 |
| $5.00 bills | 15 |
| $1.00 bills | 24 |
| $1.00 coins | 0 |
| Half dollars | 3 |
| Quarters | 10 |
| Dimes | 7 |
| Nickels | 15 |
| Pennies | 23 |

In addition, you have:

| | |
|---|---|
| Credit cards: | $135.00 |
| Checks: | $130.62 |

Finally, the office manager authorized the following refunds to be paid from your drawer:

| | |
|---|---|
| Gerry Edwin | $145.00 |
| Becca Gene | $125.00 |
| Ryan Mike | $25.00 |
| Shawn McGee | $185.00 |

Now, use this information to complete the form.

| Payment Methods | Total Amount |
|---|---|
| Beginning Cash Balance | |
| Total Amount of Cash | |
| Total Amount of Coins | |
| Total Amount of Checks | |
| Total Amount of Credit Card | |
| Total Amount of Refunds | |
| Total Amount from Calculations | |
| Do you have a Net Profit OR Net Loss? | |

*(Continued)*

## PRACTICE THE SKILL 6-5
*Continued from p. 144*

2. Beginning balance: $300.00

| Denomination | Number of bills/coins |
|---|---|
| $50.00 bills | 1 |
| $20.00 bills | 9 |
| $10.00 bills | 7 |
| $5.00 bills | 5 |
| $1.00 bills | 3 |
| $1.00 coins | 1 |
| Half dollars | 2 |
| Quarters | 4 |
| Dimes | 6 |
| Nickels | 8 |
| Pennies | 10 |

In addition, you have:

| | |
|---|---|
| Credit cards: | $235.00 |
| Checks: | $330.62 |

Finally, the office manager authorized the following refunds to be paid from your drawer:

| | |
|---|---|
| Kevin Hicks | $5.00 |
| Ben J. Men | $225.00 |
| S.P. Wall | $35.00 |
| Tara Georgia | $55.00 |

Now, use this information to complete the form.

| Payment Methods | Total Amount |
|---|---|
| Beginning Cash Balance | |
| Total Amount of Cash | |
| Total Amount of Coins | |
| Total Amount of Checks | |
| Total Amount of Credit Card | |
| Total Amount of Refunds | |
| Total Amount from Calculations | |
| Do you have a Net Profit OR Net Loss? | |

3. Beginning balance: $525.00

| Denomination | Number of bills/coins |
|---|---|
| $50.00 bills | 1 |
| $20.00 bills | 13 |
| $10.00 bills | 6 |
| $5.00 bills | 7 |
| $1.00 bills | 9 |
| $1.00 coins | 2 |
| Half dollars | 5 |

*(Continued)*

**PRACTICE THE SKILL 6-5**
*Continued from p. 145*

| Denomination | Number of bills/coins |
|---|---|
| Quarters | 8 |
| Dimes | 10 |
| Nickels | 13 |
| Pennies | 6 |

In addition, you have:

| | |
|---|---|
| Credit cards: | $535.00 |
| Checks: | $30.62 |

Finally, the office manager authorized the following refunds to be paid from your drawer:

| | |
|---|---|
| Pat S. | $65.00 |
| Mr. James | $225.00 |
| K.A. Matte | $25.00 |
| E.M. Gregg | $25.00 |

Now, use the information to complete the form.

| Payment Methods | Total Amount |
|---|---|
| Beginning Cash Balance | |
| Total Amount of Cash | |
| Total Amount of Coins | |
| Total Amount of Checks | |
| Total Amount of Credit Card | |
| Total Amount of Refunds | |
| Total Amount from Calculations | |
| Do you have a Net Profit OR Net Loss? | |

4. Beginning balance: $250.00

| Denomination | Number of bills/coins |
|---|---|
| $50.00 bills | 0 |
| $20.00 bills | 12 |
| $10.00 bills | 7 |
| $5.00 bills | 4 |
| $1.00 bills | 20 |
| $1.00 coins | 4 |
| Half dollars | 0 |
| Quarters | 17 |
| Dimes | 13 |
| Nickels | 13 |
| Pennies | 5 |

In addition, you have:

| | |
|---|---|
| Credit cards: | $715.00 |
| Checks: | $985.34 |

*(Continued)*

## PRACTICE THE SKILL 6-5
### Continued from p. 146

Finally, the office manager authorized the following refunds be paid from your drawer:

| | |
|---|---|
| Mrs. Snow | $15.00 |
| Mr. Mass | $5.00 |
| Ms. Bird | $35.00 |
| Ada Crutch | $45.00 |

Now, use the information to complete the form.

| Payment Methods | Total Amount |
|---|---|
| Beginning Cash Balance | |
| Total Amount of Cash | |
| Total Amount of Coins | |
| Total Amount of Checks | |
| Total Amount of Credit Card | |
| Total Amount of Refunds | |
| Total Amount from Calculations | |
| Do you have a Net Profit OR Net Loss? | |

5. Beginning balance: $600.00

| Denomination | Number of bills/coins |
|---|---|
| $50.00 bills | 1 |
| $20.00 bills | 7 |
| $10.00 bills | 2 |
| $5.00 bills | 5 |
| $1.00 bills | 4 |
| $1.00 coins | 0 |
| Half dollars | 0 |
| Quarters | 3 |
| Dimes | 7 |
| Nickels | 5 |
| Pennies | 3 |

In addition, you have:

| | |
|---|---|
| Credit cards: | $685.00 |
| Checks: | $454.43 |

Now, use the information to complete the form.

| Payment Methods | Total Amount |
|---|---|
| Beginning Cash Balance | |
| Total Amount of Cash | |
| Total Amount of Coins | |
| Total Amount of Checks | |
| Total Amount of Credit Card | |
| Total Amount of Refunds | |
| Total Amount from Calculations | |
| Do you have a Net Profit OR Net Loss? | |

## Day Sheets and Ledger Cards

Are you aware of all the different departments that require medical billing services? In many cases, billing for services is outsourced to different corporations and not done at the place of service. How is all of this information communicated from one department to another? **Encounter forms** (either paper or electronic) allow the health care professional to communicate with the billing professional on the type and price of services that occur during each visit. Once this information is documented, a day sheet can be generated. A day sheet will have similar information or could appear the same as a checkbook registry or an accounting spreadsheet (Figure 6-2). It is a recording of the daily business transactions. It delineates all charges, payments, and adjustments and shows that they are properly posted. The day sheet can assist when there is a discrepancy in balancing a cash drawer or bank statement.

Ledger cards can be generated for individual or family accounts. **Ledger cards** document all charges, payments, and adjustments made by the insurance company and the patient. Ledger cards should reflect a chronological snapshot of all services performed and who has made payment toward those services. Facilities use ledger cards (paper or electronic versions) when mailing monthly bills to patients (Figure 6-3).

## STRATEGY 6-7
### Ledger Cards

1. Record each procedure on a separate line.

2. Record dates of service in chronological order.

3. Record the date when a claim was submitted to the insurance company and for how much.

4. Record copayment, deductible, or coinsurance on the ledger card. This shows that the patient has met his or her financial responsibility.

5. When posting payment, always refer to the date of service to which the payment is being applied.

6. When posting payments from insurance companies, record payment for each procedure on a separate line (instead of a lump sum). This will reduce confusion if there are any discrepancies.

Once the receptionist or billing specialist receives the encounter forms, they are entered into an electronic database. There are many different billing programs, so if this becomes one of your responsibilities, you should receive computer training on the specific program you will be using. The electronic database is made up of large spreadsheets that can be manipulated so that the inputted information is displayed in different formats. Day sheets can be generated, as well as individual and family ledger cards. Accuracy is essential when inputting charges. An incorrect name or a decimal point in the wrong place will change the outcome of a claim. Errors equal loss of income to the practice.

## JOURNAL OF DAILY CHARGES & PAYMENTS

| | DATE | PROFESSIONAL SERVICE | FEE | | PAYMENT | | ADJUST-MENT | | NEW BALANCE | | OLD BALANCE | | PATIENT'S NAME | | |
|---|---|---|---|---|---|---|---|---|---|---|---|---|---|---|---|
| 1 | 04/11/08 | office visit, Est (Mary) | 65 | 00 | 25 | 00 | | | 246 | 73 | 206 | 73 | Bogert, Mary | | 1 |
| 2 | | | | | | | | | | | | | | | 2 |
| 3 | | | | | | | | | | | | | | | 3 |
| 4 | | | | | | | | | | | | | | | 4 |
| 5 | | | | | | | | | | | | | | | 5 |
| 6 | | | | | | | | | | | | | | | 6 |
| 7 | | | | | | | | | | | | | | | 7 |
| 8 | | | | | | | | | | | | | | | 8 |
| 9 | | | | | | | | | | | | | | | 9 |
| 10 | | | | | | | | | | | | | | | 10 |
| 11 | | | | | | | | | | | | | | | 11 |
| 12 | | | | | | | | | | | | | | | 12 |
| 13 | | | | | | | | | | | | | | | 13 |
| 14 | | | | | | | | | | | | | | | 14 |
| 15 | | | | | | | | | | | | | | | 15 |
| 16 | | | | | | | | | | | | | | | 16 |
| 17 | | | | | | | | | | | | | | | 17 |
| 18 | | | | | | | | | | | | | | | 18 |
| 19 | | | | | | | | | | | | | | | 19 |
| 20 | | | | | | | | | | | | | | | 20 |
| 21 | | | | | | | | | | | | | | | 21 |
| 22 | | | | | | | | | | | | | | | 22 |
| 23 | | | | | | | | | | | | | | | 23 |
| 24 | | | | | | | | | | | | | | | 24 |
| 25 | | | | | | | | | | | | | | | 25 |
| 26 | | | | | | | | | | | | | | | 26 |
| 27 | | | | | | | | | | | | | | | 27 |
| 28 | | | | | | | | | | | | | | | 28 |
| 29 | | | | | | | | | | | | | | | 29 |
| 30 | | | | | | | | | | | | | | | 30 |
| 31 | | | | | | | | | | | | | TOTALS THIS PAGE | | 31 |
| 32 | | | | | | | | | | | | | TOTAL PREVIOUS PAGE | | 32 |
| 33 | | | | | | | | | | | | | TOTALS MONTH TO DATE | | 33 |

COLUMN A    COLUMN B    COLUMN C    COLUMN D    COLUMN E

MEMO _____

| DAILY - FROM LINE 31 | | MONTH - FROM LINE 31 | | YEAR TO DATE - FROM LINE 33 | |
|---|---|---|---|---|---|
| **ARITHMETIC POSTING PROOF** | | **ACCOUNTS RECEIVABLE PROOF** | | **ACCOUNTS RECEIVABLE PROOF** | |
| Column E | $ | Accts. Receivable Previous Day | $ | Accts. Receivable beginning of Month | $ |
| Plus Column A | | Plus Column A | | Plus Column A MONTH TO DATE | |
| Sub-Total | | Sub-Total | | Sub-Total In C | |
| Minus Column B | | Minus Column B | | Minus Column B MONTH TO DATE | |
| Sub-Total | | Sub-Total | | Sub-Total | |
| Minus Column C | | Minus Column C | | Minus Column C MONTH TO DATE | |
| Equals Column D | | Accts. receivable End of Day | | Accts. receivable End of Day MONTH TO DATE | |

**Figure 6-2**    Day sheet. (From Buck C: *Practice kit for medical front office skills*, St. Louis, 2007, Saunders.)

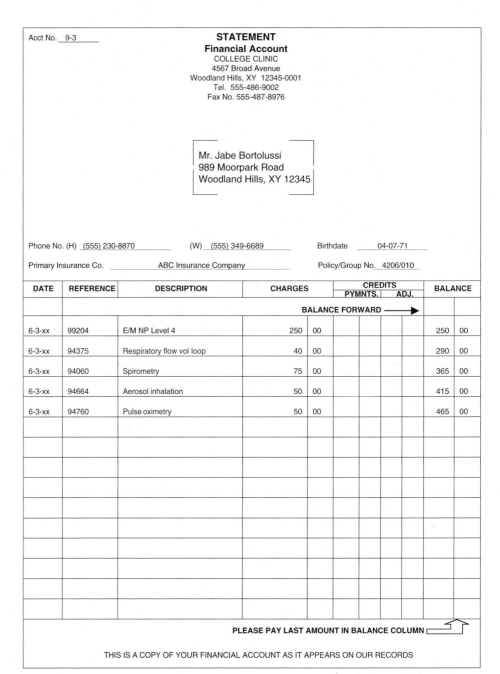

Acct No. __9-3__

**STATEMENT**
**Financial Account**
COLLEGE CLINIC
4567 Broad Avenue
Woodland Hills, XY  12345-0001
Tel.  555-486-9002
Fax No. 555-487-8976

Mr. Jabe Bortolussi
989 Moorpark Road
Woodland Hills, XY 12345

Phone No. (H) __(555) 230-8870__        (W) __(555) 349-6689__        Birthdate __04-07-71__

Primary Insurance Co. _____ABC Insurance Company_____        Policy/Group No. __4206/010__

| DATE | REFERENCE | DESCRIPTION | CHARGES | | CREDITS PYMNTS. | | ADJ. | | BALANCE | |
|------|-----------|-------------|---------|--|------------------|--|------|--|---------|--|
| | | | | | BALANCE FORWARD ➝ | | | | | |
| 6-3-xx | 99204 | E/M NP Level 4 | 250 | 00 | | | | | 250 | 00 |
| 6-3-xx | 94375 | Respiratory flow vol loop | 40 | 00 | | | | | 290 | 00 |
| 6-3-xx | 94060 | Spirometry | 75 | 00 | | | | | 365 | 00 |
| 6-3-xx | 94664 | Aerosol inhalation | 50 | 00 | | | | | 415 | 00 |
| 6-3-xx | 94760 | Pulse oximetry | 50 | 00 | | | | | 465 | 00 |
| | | | | | | | | | | |
| | | | | | | | | | | |
| | | | | | | | | | | |
| | | | | | | | | | | |
| | | | | | | | | | | |
| | | | | | | | | | | |
| | | | | | | | | | | |
| | | | | | | | | | | |
| | | | | | | | | | | |

PLEASE PAY LAST AMOUNT IN BALANCE COLUMN ⬑

THIS IS A COPY OF YOUR FINANCIAL ACCOUNT AS IT APPEARS ON OUR RECORDS

**Figure 6-3**   Ledger card. (From Fordney MT: *Workbook for insurance handbook for the medical office,* ed 10, St. Louis, 2008, Saunders.)

## PRACTICE THE SKILL 6-6

Document the following information on a ledger card. Maintain a running balance.

**1.** Denise L. Watson was seen on June 15, 20XX. The following charges are on the encounter form:

| Reference code | Description | Cost |
|----------------|-------------|------|
| 99202 | Office visit | $65.00 |
| 10060 | Incision and drainage (I&D) | $82.00 |
| 90703 | Tetanus shot | $25.50 |

*(Continued)*

## PRACTICE THE SKILL 6-6
*Continued from p. 150*

Record the information on the ledger card.

Acct No. ________

**STATEMENT**
**Financial Account**
COLLEGE CLINIC
4567 Broad Avenue
Woodland Hills, XY 12345-0001
Tel. 555-486-9002
Fax No. 555-487-8976

Phone No. (H) ____________ (W) ____________ Birthdate ____________

Primary Insurance Co. ____________ Policy/Group No. ____________

| DATE | REFERENCE | DESCRIPTION | CHARGES | CREDITS PYMNTS. | CREDITS ADJ. | BALANCE |
|---|---|---|---|---|---|---|
| | | | BALANCE FORWARD → | | | |
| | | | | | | |
| | | | | | | |
| | | | | | | |
| | | | | | | |
| | | | | | | |
| | | | | | | |
| | | | | | | |
| | | | | | | |
| | | | | | | |
| | | | | | | |
| | | | | | | |
| | | | | | | |
| | | | | | | |
| | | | | | | |
| | | | | | | |

PLEASE PAY LAST AMOUNT IN BALANCE COLUMN

THIS IS A COPY OF YOUR FINANCIAL ACCOUNT AS IT APPEARS ON OUR RECORDS

a. What is the total balance for this office visit? ____________

b. Continue using information from problem 1. Denise makes a $25.00 payment toward this office visit. Record this on the ledger card. What is the remaining balance? ____________

c. Continue using information from problem 1. On 6/23/XX, the insurance company pays $147.50 toward the above claim. Record this on the ledger card. What is the remaining balance? ____________

*(Continued)*

## PRACTICE THE SKILL 6-6
*Continued from p. 151*

**2.** Mr. Tad Mori is being seen on 5/18/XX for the following.

| Reference code | Description | Cost |
|---|---|---|
| 99202 | New patient | $65.00 |
| 28470 | Fracture care | $150.00 |
| 73620 | X-ray 2 view | $80.00 |
| 99070 | Supplies | $95.00 |

Complete a ledger card with a running balance.

Acct No. _____

**STATEMENT**
**Financial Account**
COLLEGE CLINIC
4567 Broad Avenue
Woodland Hills, XY 12345-0001
Tel. 555-486-9002
Fax No. 555-487-8976

Phone No. (H) _____ (W) _____ Birthdate _____

Primary Insurance Co. _____ Policy/Group No. _____

| DATE | REFERENCE | DESCRIPTION | CHARGES | CREDITS PYMNTS. | ADJ. | BALANCE |
|---|---|---|---|---|---|---|
| | | | BALANCE FORWARD ⟶ | | | |
| | | | | | | |
| | | | | | | |
| | | | | | | |
| | | | | | | |
| | | | | | | |
| | | | | | | |
| | | | | | | |
| | | | | | | |
| | | | | | | |
| | | | | | | |
| | | | | | | |
| | | | | | | |
| | | | | | | |
| | | | | | | |
| | | | | | | |
| | | | | | | |
| | | | | | | |

PLEASE PAY LAST AMOUNT IN BALANCE COLUMN

THIS IS A COPY OF YOUR FINANCIAL ACCOUNT AS IT APPEARS ON OUR RECORDS

Continue using information from problem 2. On 6/23/XX, the insurance company sends you a payment that covers 80% of the total charges from the 5/18/XX visit. Record this payment on the ledger card.

a. How much did the insurance company pay? _____

b. What amount is Mr. Mori's responsibility? _____

*(Continued)*

# PRACTICE THE SKILL 6-6
*Continued from p. 152*

c. On the day sheet below, record the following daily transactions:

Payment by Nathan Smith $25.00 cash

Payment by Lori Hertz $45.00 check 3354

Payment by M.R. Jones form $145.00

Payment for Nathan Smith by MediHealth Insurance for $32.67

Payment by Community Health Insurance for $436.58 for M.R. Jones

Refund to Lori Hertz for $20.00 overcharge

## JOURNAL OF DAILY CHARGES & PAYMENTS

| | DATE | PROFESSIONAL SERVICE | FEE | PAYMENT | ADJUST-MENT | NEW BALANCE | OLD BALANCE | PATIENT'S NAME | | |
|---|---|---|---|---|---|---|---|---|---|---|
| 1 | | | | | | | | | | 1 |
| 2 | | | | | | | | | | 2 |
| 3 | | | | | | | | | | 3 |
| 4 | | | | | | | | | | 4 |
| 5 | | | | | | | | | | 5 |
| 6 | | | | | | | | | | 6 |
| 7 | | | | | | | | | | 7 |
| 8 | | | | | | | | | | 8 |
| 9 | | | | | | | | | | 9 |
| 10 | | | | | | | | | | 10 |
| 11 | | | | | | | | | | 11 |
| 12 | | | | | | | | | | 12 |
| 13 | | | | | | | | | | 13 |
| 14 | | | | | | | | | | 14 |
| 15 | | | | | | | | | | 15 |
| 16 | | | | | | | | | | 16 |
| 17 | | | | | | | | | | 17 |
| 18 | | | | | | | | | | 18 |
| 19 | | | | | | | | | | 19 |
| 20 | | | | | | | | | | 20 |
| 21 | | | | | | | | | | 21 |
| 22 | | | | | | | | | | 22 |
| 23 | | | | | | | | | | 23 |
| 24 | | | | | | | | | | 24 |
| 25 | | | | | | | | | | 25 |
| 26 | | | | | | | | | | 26 |
| 27 | | | | | | | | | | 27 |
| 28 | | | | | | | | | | 28 |
| 29 | | | | | | | | | | 29 |
| 30 | | | | | | | | | | 30 |
| 31 | | | | | | | | TOTALS THIS PAGE | | 31 |
| 32 | | | | | | | | TOTAL PREVIOUS PAGE | | 32 |
| 33 | | | | | | | | TOTALS MONTH TO DATE | | 33 |

COLUMN A    COLUMN B    COLUMN C    COLUMN D    COLUMN E

MEMO _____

| DAILY - FROM LINE 31 | |
|---|---|
| ARITHMETIC POSTING PROOF | |
| Column E | $ |
| Plus Column A | |
| Sub-Total | |
| Minus Column B | |
| Sub-Total | |
| Minus Column C | |
| Equals Column D | |

| MONTH - FROM LINE 31 | |
|---|---|
| ACCOUNTS RECEIVABLE PROOF | |
| Accts. Receivable Previous Day | $ |
| Plus Column A | |
| Sub-Total | |
| Minus Column B | |
| Sub-Total | |
| Minus Column C | |
| Accts. receivable End of Day | |

| YEAR TO DATE - FROM LINE 33 | |
|---|---|
| ACCOUNTS RECEIVABLE PROOF | |
| Accts. Receivable beginning of Month | $ |
| Plus Column A MONTH TO DATE | |
| Sub-Total n | |
| Minus Column B MONTH TO DATE | |
| Sub-Total | |
| Minus Column C MONTH TO DATE | |
| Accts. receivable End of Day MONTH TO DATE | |

What was the ending balance on your day sheet? _____

## Petty Cash

Petty cash is a fund that can be used to buy small items or emergency items necessary for running the office. Examples of petty cash purchases include Post-It notes, postage, pens, Band-Aids, and photocopy paper. Many facilities have a petty cash form that must be partially filled out before the purchase is made and completed after the purchase. The form identifies for what the cash is used, what department is using the funds, and where the purchase is being made. Upon completion of the purchase, the total price of the purchase, a receipt, and change must be recorded. Petty cash *should not* be used to make change for customers without consent of the office manager. The petty cash drawer should be balanced at the end of each business day.

## PRACTICE THE SKILL 6-7

**Solve the following problems related to petty cash.**

1. The office manager completes a petty cash form to purchase birthday cards for the staff. She removes $20.00 from the petty cash drawer. A receipt and $1.98 in change has been returned to the petty cash drawer. How much did she spend? _____

2. The petty cash drawer has a beginning balance of $150.00. The following petty cash forms are in the drawer:

   The office manager used $67.45 to buy needed office supplies. The physician used $15.75 for lunch.

   The medical assistant (MA) used $42.68 for the purchase of gloves that have been delayed in shipping.

   How much money is currently in the petty cash drawer?

   _____

3. The petty cash drawer has a beginning balance of $200.00. The following petty cash forms are in the drawer:

   Removal of $25.00 for the purchase of kitchen supplies, Removal of $60.00 for the purchase of photocopy paper, Removal of $20.00 for the purchase of postage

   The following receipts and change have been accounted for:
   Kitchen supplies total cost: $23.44
   Photocopy paper purchase: $55.32
   Postage: $11.82

   In addition, the physician has written an IOU on a scrap piece of paper for $35.00 for gas.

   a. When balancing the cash drawer, are all withdrawals accounted for? If not, how much is outstanding? _____

   b. What is the balance of your petty cash drawer? _____

# COMPUTING WAGES

## Gross Pay

Even if you do not work in the human resources department, you should know how to calculate your wages. A common budgeting error occurs when a person bases their budget on gross salary instead of net salary. A realistic example could be that you have been hired as a phlebotomist at the local hospital. You have accepted an offer of $15.00 per hour. The first week, you work 30 hours. If you are expecting a check for $450.00, you will be disappointed. The $450.00 that you earned is referred to as your **gross income**, the total income before taxes and deductions are withheld. Common deductions could be payment for health, dental, eye insurance, or payment of outstanding charges (lunch, coffee, gift shop) that occur at your place of business, or garnishment of wages due to outstanding bills or child support.

Depending on the position and type of facility, staff may be hired to work 8-hour shifts, 10-hour shifts, 12-hour shifts, and occasionally 24-hour shifts (e.g., paramedics, emergency room physicians). Job descriptions should explain in detail when shift differential, overtime, and holiday pay will apply. In many jobs in the health care profession, employees receive additional compensation for working second or third shifts, weekend shifts, holidays, and overtime (anything over 40 hours in a week). Compensation varies from facility to facility and even department to department. A few common compensation benefits are described in the following paragraphs.

### Meal Breaks

Most employees *do not* receive a paid mealtime. The length of your meal break will be reflected in the hours you are scheduled to work. For example, a nurse is scheduled to work 8 hours with a ½-hour unpaid lunch. Her shift hours are 7:00 a.m. to 3:30 p.m. By subtracting the ½-hour lunch, her shift hours reflect that she will work 8 full hours.

### Shift Differential

Shift differential is compensation for working the difficult or nontypical work hours in a facility. These shifts, which typically include second shift (3:00 p.m. to 11:30 p.m.) and third shift (11:00 p.m. to 7:30 a.m.), can be hard to staff. Even with 12-hour shifts, differential compensation may apply after 3:00 p.m., depending on the facility.

*Example:*
A surgical tech's hiring wage is $16.35 per hour. How much will the surgical tech earn after working a 40-hour work schedule?

$16.35 × 40 = $654.00 *per week*

How much would the surgical tech earn if he worked second shift and received an additional $0.75 per hour? How much would he earn in a 40-hour week?

| | |
|---|---|
| $16.35 | Base pay |
| + 0.75 | Shift differential |
| $17.10 | *New hourly wage* |

$17.10 × 40 = $684.00 *per week*

How much would the surgical tech earn if he worked third shift and received an extra $1.50 per hour? How much would he earn in a 40-hour week?

| | |
|---|---|
| $16.35 | Base pay |
| + 1.50 | Shift differential |
| $17.85 | *New base pay* |

$17.85 × 40 = $714.00 *per week*

*Double Shift Compensation*

A double shift occurs when a staff member works back-to-back shifts (typically 8-hour shifts). It appears that the staff member is working 16 hours; however, as you will see in the following example, the staff member will be compensated for approximately $15\frac{1}{2}$ hours of work.

*Example:*

Joan has been asked to work a double shift from 7:00 a.m. to 3:30 p.m. and from 3:00 p.m. to 11:30 p.m.

1. What is the first thing you notice regarding the example? The shifts overlap by $\frac{1}{2}$ hour (3:00 to 3:30 p.m.), which means Joan has lost $\frac{1}{2}$ hour of pay.

2. The next thing to remember is that Joan will receive one meal break for each shift worked (lunch and dinner). Now Joan has lost $\frac{1}{2}$ hour for unpaid meals.

3. Now we can determine the total hours for which Joan will be paid:

   7:00 a.m. to 3:00 p.m. = 8 hours – $\frac{1}{2}$ hour for lunch = $7\frac{1}{2}$ hours

   3:00 p.m. to 11:30 p.m. = $8\frac{1}{2}$ hours – $\frac{1}{2}$ hour for lunch = 8 hours

   *Total hours paid for the double shift are $15\frac{1}{2}$ hours.*

An additional compensation for a double shift is that it may include shift differential compensation, depending on how the shifts fall.

## Weekend Differential

Weekend differential is monetary compensation for working the weekend, whether it be first, second, or third shift.

## Holiday Pay

Working a holiday can earn an employee either time and one-half or double time in pay. Each facility determines which shifts will be compensated at holiday pay.

*Example:*

Using the following information and the base pay of $18.56 per hour, we will figure out the answer to the questions below regarding differential and weekend pay.

| *Day of the week* | *Second shift* | *Third shift* | *Holiday* |
| --- | --- | --- | --- |
| M-F | $0.75/hour | $1.50/hour | Time and one-half |
| Weekend | $1.50/hour | $2.00/hour | Double time |

The License Practical Nurse (LPN) works second shift for 8 hours on Tuesday. Calculate the LPN's new hourly wage. Compute how much the LPN will earn after this 8-hour shift.

| *New hourly wage* | *Wage for 8-hour shift* |
| --- | --- |
| $18.56 | $19.31 |
| + 0.75 | ×    8 |
| $19.31 | $154.48 |

The LPN is working third shift on her mandatory Saturday coverage. This particular shift has designated as a holiday and the staff is eligible for additional compensation. Calculate how much the LPN will earn for this 8-hour shift.

$18.56          $20.56                    $41.12
+ 2.00          ×     2                    ×     8
$20.56/hour     $41.12/hour with holiday pay    $328.96

*Overtime*
Overtime is compensation for time worked over 40 hours in a 1-week period.
Overtime is usually at time and one-half pay.

## PRACTICE THE SKILL 6-8

Determine the start or end time for each of the following problems.
Calculate the amount earned for each shift.

1. The phlebotomist is scheduled to work an 8-hour shift with a 1/2 hour
   unpaid lunch. The phlebotomist will earn $14.50/hour. The shift starts at
   5:00 a.m. The worker does not receive any type of shift differential.

   a. What time will the shift end?
   b. Write the above answer in military time.
   c. How much will the phlebotomist earn for the 8-hour shift?

2. The urgent care facility opens at 10:00 a.m. The facility stays open for 10.5
   hours. What time will the facility close? _____ Write the answer
   using military time. _____

   The Medical Assistant (MA) works the whole 10 hour shift with one 1/2
   hour unpaid lunch. The MA receives $12.35/hour. This shift is not eligible
   for shift differential.

   a. What time will the facility close?
   b. Write the above answer using military time.
   c. How much will the MA earn for the shift?

3. An RN working in a long term care facility is scheduled to work a 12-hour
   shift. The shift starts at 7:00 a.m. and the staff received a 1/2 hour unpaid
   meal break at 1:00 p.m. The RN earns $23.00/hour. After 4:00 p.m. the
   RN earns an additional $0.45/hour.

   a. What times will the shift end?
   b. Write the above answer in military time.
   c. How much will the RN earn for the 12-hour shift?

4. A dialysis technician works a 10-hour shift with a 1/2 hour unpaid meal
   break. The shift ends at 2:00 pm. The dialysis technician earns $24.50/
   hour. This shift does not qualify for shift differential.

   a. What time must the dialysis technician report to work?
   b. Write the above answer in military time.
   c. How much will the dialysis technician earn for the 10-hour shift?

*(Continued)*

## PRACTICE THE SKILL 6-8
*Continued from p. 157*

5. The patient care assistant (PCA) reported to work at 2:00 pm for her scheduled 8-hour shift. Due to staffing shortage, the PCA has agreed to work a double shift. She will receive 1/2 hour unpaid meal break for each shift. With shift differential, the PCA will earn $13.25/hour.

   a. What time will the PCA's double shift be over?
   b. Write the above answer in military time.
   c. How much will the PCA earn for this double shift?

**Use the information below to answer the following questions.**

| Day of the week | Second shift | Third shift | Holiday |
|---|---|---|---|
| M-F | $0.75/hour | $1.50/hour | Time and one-half |
| Weekend | $1.50/hour | $2.00/hour | Double time |

6. The dietician earns $14.25 per hour. This week's work schedule is second shift on Monday, Tuesday, Wednesday, Friday, and Saturday for a total of 40 hours with a 1/2 hour unpaid lunch. Each shift works the same number of hours each day.

   a. Calculate the hourly wage.

   Weekday: _____

   Weekend: _____

   b. Calculate the daily wage.

   Weekday: _____

   Weekend: _____

   c. Compute the week's gross pay. _____

7. The third shift radiographic tech earns $19.47 per hour working third shift. She is scheduled to work on Saturday, Sunday, Monday, Thursday, and Friday for a total of 40 hours. She works equal number of hours a day and receives a 30-minute non-paid meal break.

   a. Calculate the hourly wage.

   Weekday: _____

   Weekend: _____

   b. Calculate the daily wage.

   Weekday: _____

   Weekend: _____

   c. Compute the week's gross pay. _____

*(Continued)*

## PRACTICE THE SKILL 6-8
*Continued from p. 158*

8. The healthcare professional earns $31.45 per hour. The healthcare professional is scheduled to work a 12-hour shift on Monday (a holiday), Tuesday, and Friday for a total of 36 hours. The shift runs from 7:00 a.m.-7:30 p.m. with a 1/2 hour non-paid meal time. Shift differential rate starts at 3:00 p.m.

    a. Compute the new wage with shift differential.

       Weekday: _____

       Weekend: _____

    b. Compute the typical daily wage.

       Weekday: _____

       Weekend: _____

    c. Calculate the daily holiday wage. _____

    d. Determine the week's gross pay. _____

9. The housekeeper is scheduled to work 11:00 p.m.-7:30 a.m. on Tuesday, Wednesday, and Thursday. On Friday the schedule changes to 3:00 p.m.-11:30 p.m. and on Sunday the schedule changes to 7:00 a.m.-3:30 p.m. The housekeeper receives a 30-minute non-paid meal break each shift. Friday's shift was one of the facilities designated holidays. The hourly wage for the housekeeper is $14.85/hr.

    a. Determine the new wage with third shift differential.

       Weekday: _____

       Weekend: _____

    b. Determine the new wage with second shift differential.

       Weekday: _____

       Weekend: _____

    c. Calculate the daily wage.

       Weekday: _____

       Weekend: _____

    d. Calculate how much was earned on the holiday. _____

    e. Compute the week's gross pay. _____

*(Continued)*

## PRACTICE THE SKILL 6-8
*Continued from p. 159*

10. The healthcare worker wants to make extra money during the holiday season. In order to accomplish this, they signed up for double shifts (2nd and 3rd) with starts at 3:00 p.m. The hourly wage is $35.00/hour with a 30 minute unpaid meal with each shift. Christmas Eve and New Year's Eve both fall on Sunday and Christmas Day and New Year's Day both fall on Monday.

    a. Calculate earnings with third shift differential.

       Weekday: _____

       Weekend: _____

    b. Calculate earnings with second shift differential.

       Weekday: _____

       Weekend: _____

    c. Compute holiday wages.

       Weekday: _____

       Weekend: _____

    d. Determine the gross pay for the 2-week pay period. _____

OBJECTIVE 5

## Net Wages

Unfortunately, payroll checks do not include the entire gross wage paid to you. Instead, payroll checks reflect the net wage. This is obtained by subtracting from your gross wage the total number of deductions mandated by the government and the cost of your benefits. Depending on the number of deductions and the cost of your benefits, the net pay could be significantly less than your gross pay.

*Example:*
You make $15.00 per hour and you worked 30 hours your first week. Your gross pay is **$450.00**. Based on the information you supplied on your payroll paperwork, the following taxes and deductions will be withheld:

| | |
|---|---|
| Federal tax: 6% | Withholding: $450.00 × 0.06 = $27.00 |
| State tax: 3% | Withholding: $450.00 × 0.03 = $13.50 |
| Medicare tax: 1% | Withholding: $450.00 × 0.01 = $4.50 |
| Worker's comp: 0.6235% | Withholding: $450.00 × 0.006235 = $2.81 |
| Health insurance | $45.00 |
| Total withholding | **$92.81** |

Gross pay – Deductions = Net pay   $450.00 – $92.81 = $357.19

Thus, your **net income** (the amount of your check) is **$357.19**.

# MATH IN THE REAL WORLD 6-6

State and federal taxes are always rounded to up and recorded in whole numbers.

Pay dates can vary from facility to facility. Commonly, organizations pay their employees every other week, or 26 pay periods per year. Recently, many facilities have begun paying employees twice a month (15th day of the month and the last day of the month), or 24 pay periods per year. Every other week versus twice a month doesn't sound like a big difference in pay until you map out the number of days you are being paid to work and when the 15th or the last day of the month falls.

# PRACTICE THE SKILL 6-9

Determine the amount of deductions for the problems below based on the following information.

| Deductions | Amount per gross earnings |
|---|---|
| Federal tax single | 9% |
| Federal tax married | 11% |
| State tax single | 6% |
| State tax married | 8% |
| Medicare tax | 2% |
| Worker's Compensation | 0.6325% |
| Insurance benefits single | $45.50 |
| Insurance benefits married | $95.78 |

1. Calculate the total amount of deductions based on a wage of $14.96/hour, a 40-hour work week, and the employee being single.

   a. What is the gross pay for the week? _____

   b. What is the total amount withheld for deductions? _____

   c. What is the net pay? _____

2. Calculate the total amount of deductions based on a wage of $23.44/hour, a 20-hour work week, and the employee being single.

   a. What is the gross pay for the week? _____

   b. What is the total amount withheld for deductions? _____

   c. What is the net pay? _____

*(Continued)*

## PRACTICE THE SKILL 6-9
*Continued from p. 161*

3. Calculate the total amount of deductions based on a wage of $38.77/hour, a 36-hour work week, and the employee being married.

   a. What is the gross pay for the week? _____

   b. What is the total amount withheld for deductions? _____

   c. What is the net pay? _____

4. Calculate the total amount of deductions based on a wage of $13.22/hour, a 40-hour work week, and the employee being married.

   a. What is the gross pay for the week? _____

   b. What is the total amount withheld for deductions? _____

   c. What is the net pay? _____

5. Your wage is $19.95/hour, and you work 80 hours per pay period. How much will you earn if you are single?

   a. What is the gross pay for the pay period? _____

   b. What is the total amount withheld for deductions? _____

   c. What is the net pay? _____

6. Your wage is $19.95/hour, and you work 80 hours per pay period. How much will you earn if you are married?

   a. What is the gross pay for the pay period? _____

   b. What is the total amount withheld for deductions? _____

   c. What is the net pay? _____

## BUILDING CONFIDENCE WITH THE SKILL 6-2

**Calculate the amount of coinsurance each party will pay.**

1. Medicare pays 80/20 coinsurance. The total bill is $178.55.

   a. How much will Medicare pay? _____

   b. How much will you collect from the patient? _____

*(Continued)*

## BUILDING CONFIDENCE WITH THE SKILL 6-2
### Continued from p. 162

2. The patient's insurance pays 90/10 coinsurance after a $200.00 deductible has been met. So far this year, the patient has paid $145.00 toward the deductible. Today's bill is $437.80.

   a. How much does the patient still owe towards the deductible? _____

   b. How much will the patient's insurance pay toward the bill? _____

   c. How much will the patient pay toward the bill (not including the deductible)? _____

   d. What is the total amount you will collect from the patient at the time of the visit? _____

3. The consumer has a $35.00 copayment for office visits. Today's charge is $45.00 for allergy shots. How much will you collect from the consumer?

   _____

4. A Medicare patient arrives at the office. Medicare has a $134.00 yearly deductible that must be met before the 80/20 coinsurance. The patient has paid $130.00 toward the deductible. Today's bill is $58.70.

   a. What is the remaining balance toward the deductible? _____

   b. How much will Medicare pay toward the bill? _____

   c. How much will the patient pay toward the bill (not including the deductible)? _____

   d. What is the total amount you will collect from the patient at the time of the visit? _____

5. The patient's managed care policy has a $25.00 copayment for all office visits. In addition, the patient is responsible for 20% of all radiology, laboratory test, and DME equipment costs. The patient is diagnosed with a dislocated clavical. The office visit is $85.00, the x-ray fee is $410.00, and the shoulder splint fee is $56.00.

   a. Calculate the billable amount for the insurance company. _____

   b. Compute the patient's financial responsibility for today's visit (not including the copay). _____

   c. Determine the total amount that the office will collect from the patient at the time of the visit. _____

## Using the following information, answer the questions.

| Day of the week | Second shift | Third shift | Holiday |
|---|---|---|---|
| M-F | $0.75/hour | $1.50/hour | Time and one-half |
| Weekend | $1.50/hour | $2.00/hour | Double time |

All shifts receive a 30-minute unpaid meal break.

*(Continued)*

## BUILDING CONFIDENCE WITH THE SKILL 6-2
*Continued from p. 163*

6. Wage: $21.40
   Shift worked: 8 hours, first shift
   Days worked: Tuesday, Thursday, Friday, Saturday, and Sunday

   a. What is the gross pay? _____

7. Wage: $16.75
   Shift worked: 8 hours, third shift
   Days worked: Tuesday, Thursday, Friday, Saturday, and Sunday

   a. What is the gross pay? _____

   b. How much was earned during the week? _____

   c. How much was earned on the weekend? _____

8. Wage: $8.75
   Shift worked: 8 hours, second shift
   Days worked: Monday (holiday), Thursday, Friday, Saturday, and Sunday

   a. What is the adjusted hourly pay for the holiday? _____

   b. How much was earned on the holiday? _____

   c. What is the adjusted hourly pay for the weekdays? _____

   d. What is the adjusted hourly pay for the weekends? _____

   e. What is the gross pay for the week? _____

9. Wage: $11.25
   Shift worked: 12 hours, first shift; received differential from 3:00 p.m. to
      7:00 p.m.
   Days worked: Tuesday, Thursday, Friday, Saturday (holiday), and Sunday
      (holiday)

   a. What is the adjusted weekday pay? _____

   b. What is the adjusted holiday pay? _____

   c. What is the gross pay? _____

10. Wage: $33.19
    Shift worked: 8 hours, third shift
    Days worked: Saturday and Sunday
    Shift worked: 8 hours, second shift
    Days worked: Wednesday, Thursday, and Friday

    a. What is the adjusted weekend pay? _____

    b. What is the adjusted weekday pay? _____

    c. What is the gross pay? _____

*(Continued)*

# BUILDING CONFIDENCE WITH THE SKILL 6-2
*Continued from p. 164*

Use the following information to answer the questions.

| Deductions | Amount per gross earnings |
| --- | --- |
| Federal tax single | 9% |
| Federal tax married | 11% |
| State tax single | 6% |
| State tax married | 8% |
| Medicare tax | 2% |
| Worker's Compensation | 0.6325% |
| Insurance benefits single | $45.50 |
| Insurance benefits married | $95.78 |

11. The employee works 80 hours/pay period. Deductions are determined at the married status and the hourly wage is $24.33/hour.

    a. Calculate the gross pay. _____

    b. Determine the deduction withholdings. _____

    c. Compute the net pay. _____

12. A new employee has been hired to work three 12-hour shifts per week. According to her payroll paperwork, the hiring wage is $28.00/hour and the employee is single.

    a. Calculate the gross pay for a 2-week pay period. _____

    b. Determine the deduction withholdings. _____

    c. Compute the net pay this 2-week pay period. _____

13. A paramedic has been hired at $18.00/hour and is scheduled to work two 24-hour shifts per week. According to the hiring agreement, the paramedic does not receive any shift differential but does receive 3 paid meal breaks a day. The payroll paperwork indicates that the paramedic is single.

    a. Calculate the gross pay for the 2-week pay period. _____

    b. Determine the total amount of deductions for this 2-week pay period.

    _____

    c. Compute the net pay for the 2-week pay period. _____

14. The healthcare worker has been hired as a part time employee (20 hour/week) at the rate of $33.00/hour. The payroll paperwork indicates that the employee is married.

    a. Calculate the gross pay for the 2-week pay period. _____

    b. Determine the total amount of deductions. _____

    c. Compute the net pay for this 2-week pay cycle. _____

*(Continued)*

## BUILDING CONFIDENCE WITH THE SKILL 6-2
*Continued from p. 165*

15. The healthcare worker just received a raise to $28.40/hour. According to the hiring contract this worker works three 12-hour shifts/week and has a married status. The worker submitted a payroll sheet that indicated that during the first week of the pay period, an additional 8 hours of overtime was approved at time and one half per hour.

   a. Calculate the amount the worker earned on the overtime shift.

   _____

   b. Compute the gross pay for the 2-week period. _____

   c. Compute the total amount of deductions. _____

   d. Calculate the net pay for the 2-week pay cycle. _____

 OBJECTIVE 6    PURCHASE ORDER

When counting inventory, whether it be for office supplies, medical supplies, or food for the kitchen, everyone is responsible for reporting what items need to be restocked. Depending on the facility, one or two employees may be in charge of ordering supplies. Accurately completing the **purchase order** (PO) involves writing legible numbers and description, the cost per item, and the total cost of the entire purchase. Preparation of POs can involve addition, subtraction, and multiplication to determine the total cost of the order.

## MATH IN THE REAL WORLD 6-7

Every time we order an item from a catalog, fundraising event, boy/girl scouts, or over the Internet, you are completing a purchase order.

*Example:*
You need to order the following supplies:

| Band-Aids | $0.99/box | 3 boxes |
| Alcohol | $2.39/bottle | 2 bottles |
| Slings | $5.67 each | 4 slings |

Shipping for orders under $50.00 is $12.35. Tax is 5.5%.

| Item | Description | Unit Price | Total Price |
|---|---|---|---|
| 3 boxes | Band-Aids | $0.99/box | $2.97 |
| 2 bottles | Alcohol | $2.39/bottle | $4.78 |
| 4 each | Sling | $5.67/each | $22.68 |
| | | **Subtotal Price** | $30.43 |
| | | **Tax 5.5%** | $1.68 |
| | | **Shipping** | $12.35 |
| | | **Total Price** | $44.46 |

## MATH IN THE REAL WORLD 6-8

Sales tax are always rounded up.

Sales tax varies from county to county and state to state.

*Example:*
Use the same information as in the above example. You have a $14.37 credit with this company from a previous order. Recalculate to determine the new cost of your order. Shipping for orders under $25.00 is $5.00.

| Item | Description | Unit Price | Total Price |
|------|-------------|------------|-------------|
| 3 boxes | Band-Aids | $0.99/box | $2.97 |
| 2 bottles | Alcohol | $2.39/bottle | $4.78 |
| 4 each | Sling | $5.67/each | $22.68 |
| | | **Subtotal Price** | $30.43 |
| | | **Credits or Refunds** | $14.37 |
| | | **New Subtotal** | $16.06 |
| | | **Tax 5.5%** | $0.89 |
| | | **Shipping** | $5.00 |
| | | **Total Price** | $21.95 |

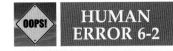

## HUMAN ERROR 6-2

*Credit is just another name for refund. Credits are subtracted from the subtotal prior to calculating the tax and shipping.*

## PRACTICE THE SKILL 6-10

Use the following chart to complete questions 1-3 regarding purchase orders.

| Item Description | Cost Per Item |
|------------------|---------------|
| Post-It Notes | $1.99 |
| Staples | $3.99 |
| Copy Paper | $56.79/box of 12 |
| Coffee Cups | $5.09 a dozen |
| Black Pens | $3.75/3 pack |
| Cotton Balls 100/package | $1.00 |
| Alcohol pads 150/box | $1.99 |
| Gloves (S, M, Lg) unsterile | $5.10 |
| Gloves XLG unsterile | $5.60 |
| Band-Aids assorted sizes | $4.12 |
| Face Shields 25/box | $11.54 |
| Tax | 5.5% |
| Shipping/Handling | |
| $0.00-$50.00 | $5.00 |
| $50.01-$100.00 | $12.00 |
| $100.01-$150.00 | $17.00 |
| $150.01-$200.00 | $21.00 |
| Over $200.01 | $30.00 |

*(Continued)*

# PRACTICE THE SKILL 6-10
*Continued from p. 167*

*Continued from p. 167*

1. Using the form below complete the PO for the following items.

    | | |
    |---|---|
    | 5 | boxes of medium unsterile gloves |
    | 3 | boxes of XL unsterile gloves |
    | 5 | boxes of alcohol swabs |
    | 2 | packages of cotton balls |
    | 100 | face shields |

2. Using the form below complete the PO for the following items.

    | | |
    |---|---|
    | 15 | Post-It notes |
    | 144 | coffee cups |
    | 4 | staples |
    | 18 | black pens |
    | 36 | packages of copy paper |

3. Using the form below complete the PO for the following items. According to the last shipping statement from this company, you have a $213.45 credit.

    | | |
    |---|---|
    | 10 | Post-It Notes |
    | 5 | Staples |
    | 60 | Copy Paper |
    | 96 | Coffee Cups |
    | 27 | Black Pens |
    | 300 | Cotton Balls |
    | 300 | Alcohol pads |
    | 12 | Band-Aids assorted sizes |
    | 75 | Face Shields |

**Purchase Order Form**

| Item | Description | Unit Price | Total Price |
|---|---|---|---|
| | | | |
| | | | |
| | | | |
| | | | |
| | | | |
| | | | |
| | | | |
| | | | |
| | | | |
| | | | |
| | | Subtotal Price | |
| | | Credits or Refunds | |
| | | New Subtotal | |
| | | Tax 5.5% | |
| | | Shipping | |
| | | Total Price | |

## CONCLUSION

Throughout this chapter, you have used information addressed in previous chapters. If you had difficulty following the processes, take some time to review the information on which you are weak. Remember: most errors occur because you are rushing through the calculations. Financial errors in dealings with patients and employees can be the cause of tension within the office. No one likes to open a paycheck and find an error. Health care facilities lose patients because of miscalculation of charges. As stated at the beginning of the chapter, health care is a business, so it must make a profit.

## MASTER THE SKILL

OBJECTIVES 3 4 5 6

Use the following chart to complete questions 1 to 3 regarding purchase orders.

| Item Description | Cost Per Item |
| --- | --- |
| Cotton balls 100/package | $0.99 |
| Alcohol pads 100/box | $1.99 |
| Glove (S,M,L) | $3.75/box |
| Gloves XL | $4.00/box |
| Syringe with $\frac{5}{8}$ needle | $18.75/box |
| Syringe with 1 inch needle | $18.75/box |
| Syringe with $1\frac{1}{2}$ inch needle | $19.00/box |
| Vacutainers red top | $23.50/box |
| Vacutainers blue top | $23.50/box |
| Vacutainers purple top | $23.50/box |
| Vacutainers SST top | $24.00/box |
| Multipurpose needles (18 g, 20 g, 21 g) | $18.00 |
| Butterfly needles | $37.95 |
| Sterile 4 × 4 gauze 100/box | $4.88 |
| Sterile 2 × 2 gauze 100/box | $4.00 |
| Ace wraps (2, 3, 4, 6 inch wraps) each | $3.22 |
| Crutches (all sizes) | $27.00/set |
| Sling | $6.50 |
| Ankle splint | $10.50 |
| Wrist splint | $8.76 |
| Thermometer probe covers 25/box | $2.32 |
| *Tax* | *5.5%* |
| *Shipping/Handling* | |
| *$0.00-$50.00* | *$7.50* |
| *$51.00-$100.00* | *$15.00* |
| *$101.00-$150.00* | *$22.50* |
| *$151.00-$200.00* | *$30.00* |
| *Over $200.00* | *$37.50* |

*(Continued)*

## MASTER THE SKILL
*Continued from p. 169*

1. The following items are needed for the office:
   2 sets of children's crutches
   2 sets of adults' crutches
   3 boxes of 4 × 4 gauze
   2 boxes of 2 × 2 gauze
   10 boxes of thermometer probe covers

**Purchase Order Form**

| Item | Description | Unit Price | Total Price |
|------|-------------|------------|-------------|
|  |  |  |  |
|  |  |  |  |
|  |  |  |  |
|  |  |  |  |
|  |  |  |  |
|  |  |  |  |
|  |  |  |  |
|  |  |  |  |
|  |  |  |  |
|  |  | Subtotal Price |  |
|  |  | Credits or Refunds |  |
|  |  | New Subtotal |  |
|  |  | Tax 5.5% |  |
|  |  | Shipping |  |
|  |  | Total Price |  |

2. The office manager has asked you to order the following supplies for the laboratory; there is a $125.00 credit with this vendor:
   2 boxes of butterfly needles
   4 boxes of red Vacutainers
   2 boxes of blue Vacutainers
   6 boxes of SST Vacutainers
   3 boxes of purple Vacutainers
   8 boxes of alcohol pads
   3 boxes of 2 × 2 gauze
   2 boxes of each size of multipurpose needles

**Purchase Order Form**

| Item | Description | Unit Price | Total Price |
|------|-------------|------------|-------------|
|  |  |  |  |
|  |  |  |  |
|  |  |  |  |
|  |  |  |  |
|  |  |  |  |
|  |  |  |  |
|  |  |  |  |
|  |  |  |  |
|  |  |  |  |
|  |  |  |  |

*(Continued)*

## MASTER THE SKILL
*Continued from p. 170*

| Item | Description | Unit Price | Total Price |
|------|-------------|------------|-------------|
|      |             | Subtotal Price |  |
|      |             | Credits or Refunds |  |
|      |             | New Subtotal |  |
|      |             | Tax 5.5% |  |
|      |             | Shipping |  |
|      |             | Total Price |  |

3. The medical assistant is in charge of restocking the supplies in the orthopedic room. After inventory of the room, the following order needs to be placed.
   6 wrist splints
   8 ankle splints
   4 slings
   2 children's crutches
   6 adults' crutches
   12 Ace wraps of each size
   Use the following shift differential and deductions information to answer questions 4 to 10.
   *Pay week*: Saturday-Friday
   *Overtime*: Anything over 40 hours per week

Use the following shift differential and deductions information to answer questions 4 to 10.

*Pay week:* Saturday-Friday

*Overtime:* Anything over 40 hours per week

|  | Second shift | Third shift | Holiday |
|--|--------------|-------------|---------|
| *Mon-Fri* 12-hour shift | $0.75/hour After 4:00 p.m. | $1.50/hour After 12:00 mid | Time and one-half |
| *Weekend* 12-hour shift | $1.50/hour After 4:00 p.m. | $2.00/hour After 12:00 mid | Double time |
| *Lunch* 8-hour shift 12-hour shift | Deduct: 30 min/shift 30 min/shift | | |

| | Amount/gross earnings dependents | | | |
|---|---|---|---|---|
| *Deductions* | *0* | *1* | *2* | *3+* |
| Federal tax single | 9% | 8.5% | 8% | 7.5% |
| Federal tax married | 11% | 10.5% | 9.5% | 9% |
| State tax single | 6% | 5.5% | 5% | 4.5% |
| State tax married | 8% | 7.5% | 7% | 6.5% |
| Medicare tax | 2% | | | |
| Worker's Compensation | 0.6325% | | | |
| Insurance benefits single | $45.50 | | | |
| Insurance benefits married | $95.78 | | | |

*(Continued)*

## MASTER THE SKILL
*Continued from p. 171*

4. Wage: $22.50/hour
   Shift worked: 7:00 a.m. to 7:30 p.m.
   Days worked: Monday, Tuesday, Wednesday, Sunday, Monday, and Tuesday
   Lunch break is taken from 1200-1230 hours.
   Deductions: single, insurance

   a. Calculate the daily pay per shift.

      Weekday: _____

      Weekend: _____

   b. Compute the gross pay. _____

   c. Compute the deductions. _____

   d. Compute the net pay for this pay period. _____

5. Wage: $28.75/hour
   Shift worked: 7:00 p.m. to 7:30 a.m. Meal is from 0300-0330.
   Days worked: Sunday, Monday, Tuesday, Thursday, Friday, and Saturday
   Deductions: married, two dependents, family insurance

   a. Determine the daily pay per shift.

      Weekday: _____

      Weekend: _____

   b. Calculate the gross pay. _____

   c. Determine the amount of deductions. _____

   d. Compute the net pay for this pay period. _____

6. Wage: $17.95/hour
   Shift worked: 7:00 p.m. to 7:30 a.m. Meal is taken from 0330-0400
   Days worked: Sunday, Monday, and Tuesday
   Shift worked: 3:00 p.m. to 11:30 p.m. Meal is taken from 1700-1730.
   Days worked: Thursday, Friday, and Saturday
   Deductions: married, three dependents, family insurance

   a. Determine the daily pay/shift.

      Weekday Shift A: _____

      Weekday Shift B: _____

      Weekend Shift A: _____

      Weekend Shift B: _____

*(Continued)*

## MASTER THE SKILL
*Continued from p. 172*

b. Calculate the gross pay? _____

c. Determine the deductible amount? _____

d. Compute the net pay. _____

7. Wage: $38.75/hour
Shift worked: 7:00 a.m. to 3:30 p.m.
Days worked: Saturday (holiday), Sunday (holiday), Wednesday, Thursday, Friday, Monday, Tuesday, Wednesday, Thursday, and Friday Deductions: single, two dependents, family insurance

   a. Calculate the daily wage per shift.

   Weekday: _____

   Weekend: _____

   b. Compute the gross pay. _____

   c. Determine the total amount of deductions. _____

   d. Compute the net pay for this pay period. _____

8. Wage: $37.82/hour
Shift worked: 3:00 p.m. to 11:30 p.m. Meal taken from 1730-1800.
Days worked: Sunday, Monday, and Tuesday
Shift worked: 11:00 p.m. to 7:30 a.m. Meal is taken from 0230-0300.
Days worked: Thursday, Friday, and Saturday
Deductions: married, two dependents, family insurance

   a. Determine the daily pay per shift.

   3:00 p.m. to 11:30 p.m. weekday: _____

   3:00 p.m. to 11:30 p.m. weekend: _____

   11:00 p.m. to 7:30 a.m. weekday: _____

   11:00 p.m. to 7:30 a.m. weekend: _____

   b. Calculate the gross pay. _____

   c. Determine the deductible amount. _____

   d. Compute the net pay for this pay period. _____

9. The administrative assistant works from 8:00 a.m.-5:00 p.m. Monday through Friday, with a 1 hour unpaid lunch each day. The gross salary is $38,560.00 per year. According to the payroll this is a single person with one deduction and has insurance.

*(Continued)*

## MASTER THE SKILL
*Continued from p. 173*

a. Determine the weekly salary. _____

b. Calculate the daily wage. _____

c. The administrative assistant is paid every other week. Calculate the net pay for the month. _____

10. The Director of Nursing (DON) in a long-term care facility and receives a gross yearly salary of $67,000. The DON is married with three dependents and has enrolled for the company's insurance family plan. The long-term care facility employees receive paychecks every other week.

   a. Calculate the gross salary per pay period. _____

   b. Compute the net salary per pay period. _____

11. Complete the following day sheet based on the provided information. Beginning balance of the cash drawer: $200.00

| Denomination | Number of bills/coins |
|---|---|
| $50.00 bills | 0 |
| $20.00 bills | 7 |
| $10.00 bills | 2 |
| $5.00 bills | 5 |
| $1.00 bills | 4 |
| $1.00 coins | 0 |
| Half dollars | 0 |
| Quarters | 3 |
| Dimes | 7 |
| Nickels | 5 |
| Pennies | 3 |

In addition, you have:

| | |
|---|---|
| Credit cards: | $485.00 |
| Checks: | $54.43 |

| Payment Methods | Total Amount |
|---|---|
| Beginning Cash Balance | |
| Total Amount of Cash | |
| Total Amount of Coins | |
| Total Amount of Checks | |
| Total Amount of Credit Card | |
| Total Amount of Refunds | |
| Total Amount from Calculations | |
| Do you have a Net Profit OR Net Loss? | |

*(Continued)*

## MASTER THE SKILL
*Continued from p. 174*

**12.** Beginning balance of the cash drawer: $300.00

| Denomination | Number of bills/coins |
|---|---|
| $50.00 bills | 1 |
| $20.00 bills | 2 |
| $10.00 bills | 7 |
| $5.00 bills | 4 |
| $1.00 bills | 14 |
| $1.00 coins | 0 |
| Half dollars | 0 |
| Quarters | 13 |
| Dimes | 9 |
| Nickels | 15 |
| Pennies | 13 |

In addition, you have:

| | |
|---|---|
| Credit cards: | $785.00 |
| Checks: | $154.43 |

The office manager has issued the following refunds from your drawer:

| | |
|---|---|
| Mr. Nichols | $55.00 |
| Mrs. Otis | $24.00 |
| Mr. Plant | $5.00 |

| Payment Methods | Total Amount |
|---|---|
| Beginning Cash Balance | |
| Total Amount of Cash | |
| Total Amount of Coins | |
| Total Amount of Checks | |
| Total Amount of Credit Card | |
| Total Amount of Refunds | |
| Total Amount from Calculations | |
| Do you have a Net Profit OR Net Loss? | |

**13.** A Medicare patient is being seen today. It has been determined that Medicare has a $124.00 yearly deductible which the patient has paid $110.00 towards the deductible. In addition, the patient has Blue Cross/ Blue Shield (BCBS) as a secondary insurance. Today's medical bill is $65.00.

a. Calculate the billable fee for Medicare. _____

b. Calculate the billable fee for BCBS. _____

c. Determine how much you will collect from the patient at this visit.

_____

*(Continued)*

## MASTER THE SKILL
*Continued from p. 175*

*Continued from p. 175*

14. The consumer's insurance will pay 70% of all medical expenses. Today's physical expenses total $435.67.

    a. Calculate the billable amount to the insurance company. _____

    b. Determine how much you will collect from the consumer. _____

15. The patient is being seen for their annual check up with the cardiologist. It has been determined that the patient has Medicare Part B which has a $134.00 yearly deductible. This is the first visit of a new insurance year. After the deductible has been satisfied, Medicare coinsurance will cover 80/20 of all outpatient medical bills. Today's bill is $108.00

    a. Calculate how much the office will collect from this patient. _____

    b. Compute the billable amount to Medicare. Explain your answer _____

# The Metric System

## CHAPTER OUTLINE

## LEARNING OBJECTIVES

*Upon completion of this chapter, the learner will be able to:*

1. Define the key terms that relate to the chapter.

2. Identify the key prefixes and word roots related to the metric system.

3. Convert between base unit metric measurements.

4. Convert between basic metric length, mass, and volume measurements.

5. Solve proportional problems using dimensional analysis theory.

6. Calculate mass and volume medication problems.

## KEY TERMS

OBJECTIVE 1

| | |
|---|---|
| Base Unit | Multidose Vial |
| Dimensional Analysis | PO |
| Equivalent | Prefix |
| IM | Prescription |
| IV | Units |
| Metric System | Word Root |

OBJECTIVE 1

Many of us have been exposed to the metric system since grade school. Through the years, knowledge of the metric system has become necessary in the fields of engineering, steel production, automotive manufacturing, and health care. The health care industry in the United States uses a combination of the metric system, household measurements, and the apothecary system in dispensing medications and educating patients about their medications. In this chapter, we focus on the metric system and common metric conversions.

## MATH TRIVIA 7-1

The metric system was established in France in the early 1800s.

OBJECTIVE **2**

# PREFIXES AND BASE UNITS (WORD ROOTS)

The metric system uses three **base units** (or **word roots**) to describe length, volume, and weight or mass. The three base units are as follows:

*Meter* (M, m) is used to describe length.
*Liter* (L) is used to describe volume. (The abbreviation for liter is always capitalized to avoid misinterpretation as the number 1.)
*Gram* (G, g) is used to describe mass.

The base word can be manipulated by changing the **prefix** to describe larger and smaller measurements. Prefixes are found before the base word, as described in the following examples:

| | | |
|---|---|---|
| *Kilo*meter | Kilo- is the prefix | Meter is the base word |
| *Milli*liter | Milli- is the prefix | Liter is the base word |
| *Micro*gram | Micro- is the prefix | Gram is the base word |

The following is a list of the prefixes used in the metric system and their meanings:

| Prefix | Symbol | Meaning | Multiplier (numerical) | Multiplier (exponential) |
|---|---|---|---|---|
| Kilo- | k | thousand | 1000 | $10^3$ |
| Hecto- | h | hundred | 100 | $10^2$ |
| Deka- | da, dk | ten | 10 | 10 |
| Base | M, L, or G | Base measurement | None | None |
| Deci- | d | tenth | 0.1 | $10^{-1}$ |
| Centi- | c | hundredth | 0.01 | $10^{-2}$ |
| Milli- | m | thousandth | 0.001 | $10^{-3}$ |
| Micro- | mc | millionth | 0.000001 | $10^{-6}$ |

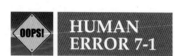

## HUMAN ERROR 7-1

*Until recently, the symbol µg was used as the abbreviation for micrograms. The symbol was based on the Greek letter mu (µ). This symbol has been discontinued in the pharmacy fields because of the confusion between µg and mg in handwritten documents.*

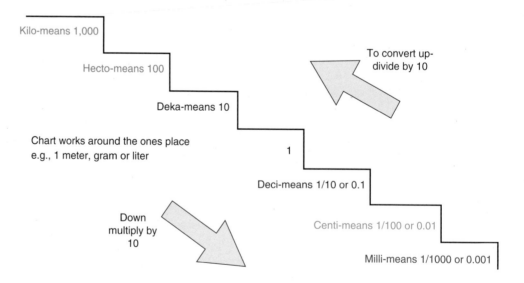

It is important to memorize these terms and the amounts they represent. A common mnemonic used to remember the prefix order from largest measurement to smallest is **K**angaroo **H**op **D**own **M**ountains **D**rinking **C**hocolate **M**ilk (Figure 7-1).

Miscommunication is a problem in the everyday world. Whether through written or spoken word, miscommunication results in errors. People's lives are in jeopardy when miscommunication occurs in the health care field. For this reason, measurements are documented in a manner that reduces the chance of miscommunication. If you have not been in the practice of labeling your answers, it is time to start. In health care, a number by itself means nothing; it must always be followed by an abbreviated label to avoid confusion.

## MATH TRIVIA 7-2

Other mnemonics to remember the metric system include:

Kings Have Dragons Because Dragons Melt Marshmallows

Kittens Hate Dogs But Do Chase Most Mice

King Henry Died Monday Drinking Chocolate Milk

Kilo, Hecto, Deka, Base (Measurement standard), Deci, Centi, Milli, Micro

*Example:*
A patient drank 250 mL at breakfast, 500 mL at lunch, and 525 mL at dinner. How much did the patient drink during his meals on this day? The correct answer is 1275 mL.

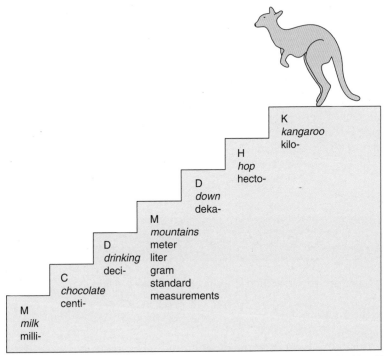

**Figure 7-1**    Mnemonic for remembering prefix order: **K**angaroo **H**op **D**own **M**ountains **D**rinking **C**hocolate **M**ilk.

## MATH QUICK TIP 7-1

If you are hopping down (descending) the stairs multiply by 10.

If you are hopping up (ascending) the stairs divide by 10.

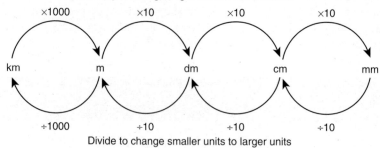

Multiply to change larger units to smaller units

Divide to change smaller units to larger units

## MATH QUICK TIP 7-2

1. A number is always accompanied by an abbreviation.
   Incorrect: 10
   Correct: 10 L

2. Metric abbreviations are always singular. Adding the "s" will change the meaning of the abbreviation.
   Incorrect: mLs
   Correct: mL

3. Periods are not used after metric abbreviations unless the abbreviation falls at the end of a sentence.
   Incorrect: 50 mL. of fluid
   Correct: 50 mL of fluid

4. If the amount is less than a whole number and is written as a decimal, a 0 is always placed before the decimal point.
   Incorrect: .03
   Correct: 0.03

## MATH QUICK TIP 7-3

The correct order to write metric **units** is as follows: **4 mg**.

1. Write the amount: **4**

2. Allow for a space between the amount and measurement.

3. Write the abbreviation for the prefix: **m**

4. Write the abbreviation for the word root: **g**

## PRACTICE THE SKILL 7-1

Write the correct prefix or word root described by each question.

1. What is the metric measurement for volume? _____

2. What is the prefix that means $\frac{1}{1000}$? _____

3. What is the metric measurement for length? _____

4. What is the prefix that means 10? _____

5. What is the metric measurement for weight or mass? _____

6. What is the prefix that means $\frac{1}{10}$? _____

7. What is the prefix that means 1,000? _____

8. What is the prefix that means $\frac{1}{1,000,000}$? _____

9. What is the prefix that means $\frac{1}{100}$? _____

10. What is the prefix that means 100? _____

## CONVERSION OF MEASUREMENTS IN THE METRIC SYSTEM    OBJECTIVES

There are many ways to convert measurements in the metric system in order to determine **equivalent** measurements. In this chapter, we will be using the strategies from Chapter 5 regarding proportions, cross multiplication, and dimensional analysis. Let's take a quick moment to review the steps for writing a proportion.

1. Read the problem.
2. Identify the known information.
3. Write your proportion so that the same units appear in the same location for each proportion.
4. Solve the problem using cross multiplication if your proportion is written as a fraction. If the problem is written in linear fashion, multiply the means ("inside" numbers) together and the extremes ("outside" numbers) together.

When you are working with equivalents, it is important to use the proper equivalent for the problem to be solved. If the improper equivalent is used, your answer will be off. Depending on the equipment and substance being measured, rounding may or may not be used in determining the final answer.

## STRATEGY 7-1
*Solving Equivalency Problems*

1. Establish what information is known.

2. Determine what is the known equivalent or conversion for which the problem is asking.

*(Continued)*

## STRATEGY 7-1
*Continued from p. 181*

3. Write down what is known on the left side of the equation.

4. Write down the remaining known information on the right side of the equation.

5. Identify the unknown information with an "X" in the equation.

6. If possible, reduce fractions before cross multiplication.

7. Cross multiply and solve for the unknown as discussed in Chapter 5.

*Example:*

How many meters are in 3,000 mm?

1. Establish what information is known.
   *The question is asking us to change millimeters to meters.*

2. Determine what is the known equivalent or conversion for which the problem is asking.
   *1,000 mm is equivalent to 1 meter.*

3. Write down what is known on the left side of the equation.
$$\frac{1000 \text{ mm}}{1 \text{ M}} =$$

4. Write down the remaining known information on the right side of the equation.
$$\frac{1000 \text{ mm}}{1 \text{ M}} = \frac{3000 \text{ mm}}{}$$

5. Identify the unknown information with an "X" in the equation.
$$\frac{1000 \text{ mm}}{1 \text{ M}} = \frac{3000 \text{ mm}}{X}$$

6. If possible, reduce fractions before cross multiplication.
$$\frac{1000 \text{ mm}}{1 \text{ M}} = \frac{3000 \text{ mm}}{X}$$

7. Cross multiply and solve for the unknown as learned in Chapter 5.
$$\frac{1000 \text{ mm}}{1 \text{ M}} = \frac{3000 \text{ mm}}{X}$$
$$1000X = 3000$$
$$\frac{1000X}{1000} = \frac{3000}{1000}$$
$$X = 3$$

*Answer:* 3 meters

Check your answer by substituting 3 for "X" and solving the problem.

*Further examples:*

1. How many cm are in 2.5 meters?
$$\frac{100 \text{ cm}}{1 \text{ M}} = \frac{X \text{ cm}}{2.5 \text{ M}} \quad \text{or} \quad 100 \text{ cm} : 1 \text{ M} :: X \text{ cm} : 2.5 \text{ M}$$

2. How many km are in 4000 meters?
$$\frac{1000 \text{ m}}{1 \text{ km}} = \frac{4000 \text{ m}}{X \text{ km}} \quad \text{or} \quad 1000 \text{ m} : 1 \text{ km} :: 4000 \text{ m} : X \text{ km}$$

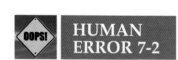

## HUMAN ERROR 7-2

*A common mistake when setting up equivalent or conversions problems is that the measurements are not in the same location. As in this example, it does not matter if mm is in the numerator or the denominator, but it does matter that mm is in the numerator or denominator on BOTH sides of the equation.*

**3.** How many meters are in 3.2 km?

$$\frac{1 \text{ km}}{1000 \text{ m}} = \frac{3.2 \text{ km}}{X \text{ m}} \quad \text{or} \quad 1 \text{ km} : 1000 \text{ m} :: 3.2 \text{ km} : X \text{ m}$$

## Dimensional Analysis

OBJECTIVE ⑤

The concept of **dimensional analysis** involves manipulating the base unit to obtain the desired answer by canceling out the unwanted units. This is an advanced form of ratios and proportions and is commonly used when comparing measurements having different base units.

To use the dimensional analysis concept, you must find the answers to three questions:

1. What are the original factors to convert?
2. What is the conversion formula or formulas?
3. What is the base unit of the answer?

## STRATEGY 7-2
### *Dimensional Analysis*

1. Read the question.

2. Identify which factors are to be converted.

3. Select the proper conversion formula or formulas.

4. Cancel unwanted units in a diagonal fashion.

5. Multiply across the problem.

6. Divide if necessary.

7. Label your answer with the desired base unit.

8. Check your answer.

*Example:*
3 feet = _____ inches

1. Read the question.
   *3 feet is equal to _____ inches.*
2. Identify what factors are to be converted.
   *3 feet*
3. Select the proper conversion formula or formulas.
   12 inches = 1 foot
4. Cancel unwanted units in a diagonal fashion.
   $$\frac{12 \text{ inches}}{1 \text{ \sout{foot}}} \times 3 \text{ \sout{feet}}$$
5. Multiply across the problem.
   $$\frac{12 \times 3}{1} = 36$$
6. Divide if necessary.
   *In this problem, division is not necessary because any fraction with 1 in the denominator represents a whole number.*
7. Label your answer with the desired base unit.
   *36 inches*

*Example:*

60 mL = _____ L

1. Read the question.
   *Find out how many liters are in 60 mL.*

2. Identify which factors are to be converted.
   *60 mL*

3. Select the proper conversion formula or formulas.
   *1000 mL equals 1 L*

4. Cancel unwanted units in a diagonal fashion.

$$\frac{1\ L}{1000\ \cancel{mL}} \times 60\ \cancel{mL}$$

5. Multiply across the problem.

$$\frac{1 \times 60}{1000} = 60$$

6. Divide if necessary.

$$\frac{60}{1000} = 0.06$$

7. Label your answer with the desired base unit.
   *0.06 liter or 0.06 L*

There are times when you need to use more than one conversion. This is the case in the following example.

*Example:*

5 kg = _____ mg

1. Read the question.
   *How many mg are in 5 kg?*

2. Identify what factors are to be converted.
   *5 kg*

3. Select the proper conversion formula or formulas.
   1 kg = 1000 G
   1 G = 1000 mg

4. Cancel unwanted units in a diagonal fashion.

$$\frac{1000\ mg}{1} \times \frac{1000\ \cancel{G}}{1\ \cancel{kg}} \times 5\ \cancel{kg}$$

5. Multiply across the problem.
   $1000 \times 1000 \times 5 = 5{,}000{,}000$

6. Divide if necessary.
   *Since the number 1 is in the denominator, division is not needed.*

7. Label your answer with the desired base unit.
   *5,000,000 mg*

## Meter

Table 7-1 provides abbreviations, measurements, and equivalent conversions regarding meters.

# MATH IN THE REAL WORLD 7-1

The most common measurements for length used in health care are the following:

- Millimeter (mm)—used in measuring incisions, lacerations, and tumors and in microscopic work

- Centimeter (cm)—used in measuring height of newborns and children, incisions, lacerations, and tumors

- Kilometer (km)—used in measuring the distance a person walks for exercise, in therapy, and in testing

| TABLE 7-1 | *Common Equivalencies for Length* |
|-----------|-----------------------------------|

| Metric Length | Length in Meters | Equal in Meters |
|---------------|------------------|-----------------|
| 1 millimeter (mm) | 0.001 of a meter | 1,000 mm = 1 M |
| 1 centimeter (cm) | 0.01 of a meter | 100 cm = 1 M |
| 1 decimeter (dm) | 0.1 of a meter | 10 dm = 1 M |
| 1 METER (M, m) | 1 METER | 1 M = 1 M |
| 1 dekameter (dam) | 10 meters | 1 dam = 10 M |
| 1 hectometer (hm) | 100 meters | 1 hm = 100 M |
| 1 kilometer (km) | 1,000 meters | 1 km = 1,000 M |

# PRACTICE THE SKILL 7-2

Complete the following table with the proper equivalent measurements.

| | Millimeters | Centimeters | Meters | Kilometers |
|-----|-------------|-------------|--------|------------|
| 1. | | 2,000 | | |
| 2. | | | 150 | |
| 3. | | | | 6 |
| 4. | | | 39 | |
| 5. | | 75 | | |
| 6. | 30 | | | |
| 7. | | | 4 | |
| 8. | | 2.5 | | |
| 9. | | | 12.5 | |
| 10. | 45,000 | | | |
| 11. | | | | 37 |
| 12. | 3,000 | | | |

As you continue through this chapter, you will see that the problems are set up in a consistent format. Get into the practice of labeling your answers. Start memorizing common measurement equivalents; this will make solving problems easier. The word base may change, but the prefixes will always remain the same.

## BUILDING CONFIDENCE WITH THE SKILL 7-1

1. There are _____ in a meter.
   a. 100 centimeters
   b. 1,000 kilometers
   c. 0.01 dekameter
   d. 10,000 millimeters

2. There are _____ in a kilometer.
   a. 10 hectometers
   b. 0.001 meter
   c. 1,000 meters
   d. 10 dekameters

3. There is _____ in a centimeter.
   a. 0.00001 meter
   b. 0.001 meter
   c. 0.0001 meter
   d. 0.01 meter

4. There is _____ in a millimeter.
   a. 0.00001 meter
   b. 0.001 meter
   c. 0.0001 meter
   d. 0.01 meter

5. There is (are) _____ in a decimeter.
   a. 0.1 meter
   b. 10 meters
   c. 100 meters
   d. 1,000 meters

**Write the metric prefixes from largest to smallest.**

deci, kilo, micro, deka, centi, hecto, milli

6. _____

7. _____

8. _____

9. _____

10. _____

*(Continued)*

## BUILDING CONFIDENCE WITH THE SKILL 7-1
*Continued from p. 186*

11. _____

12. _____

**Answer the following word problems.**

13. The incision is 25 mm. What is the equivalent measurement in cm?
_____

14. During his cardiac workout, the patient walked 9 meters. How many kilometers did he walk? _____

15. The surgeon stated that he made a 7.5 cm incision. How many mm was the incision? _____

16. You participated in a 5 K run. How many meters did you cover during the run? _____

17. The scar is 0.002 meter long. How many cm is the scar? _____

18. How many meters is 40 dekameters? _____

19. How many meters is 4,000 hectometers? _____

20. How many mm are in 12.5 meters? _____

## MATH TRIVIA 7-3

Can you identify the most common reference for a liter?

### Liter

The liter is the metric measurement for volume. In health care, liquid measurements include the following:

- Fluid intake—the amount that is drunk in a specified period; this will include IV fluids and any fluids given through a tube
- IV fluids—fluids given through or removed through a vein
- Irrigation fluids—fluids used during surgeries and postoperative treatments
- Urine output—the measurement of how the kidneys are working to keep the body healthy
- Dialysis—mechanical removal of waste products from the blood, which may result from kidney failure

Table 7-2 provides abbreviations, measurements, and equivalent conversions regarding liters.

| TABLE 7-2 | *Common Equivalencies for Volume* |
|-----------|-----------------------------------|

| Metric Volume | Volume in Liters | Equivalent in Liters |
|---------------|------------------|----------------------|
| 1 milliliter (ml) | 0.001 of a liter | 1,000 mL = 1 L |
| 1 centiliter (cL) | 0.01 of a liter | 100 cL = 1 L |
| 1 deciliter (dL) | 0.1 of a liter | 10 dL = 1 L |
| 1 LITER (L) | 1 LITER | 1 L = 1 L |
| 1 dekaliter (daL) | 10 liters | 1 daL = 10 L |
| 1 hectoliter (hL) | 100 liters | 1 hL = 100 L |
| 1 kiloliter (kL) | 1,000 liters | 1 kL = 1,000 L |

## MATH IN THE REAL WORLD 7-2

The most common liquid measurements in health care are the following:

- Milliliter (mL)—used in measuring IV fluids, liquid medication, intake of oral fluids, urine output, and the amount of fluid withdrawn from the body

- Deciliter (dL)—used in laboratory reports

- Liter (L)—used in measuring IV fluids, oral preparations for tests, and the amount of fluid withdrawn from the body

Using the same strategies as earlier in the chapter, work the following example problems.

*Example:*

How many L are in 5000 mL?

$$\frac{1000 \text{ mL}}{1 \text{ L}} = \frac{5000 \text{ mL}}{\text{X L}} \qquad 1000 \text{ mL} : 1 \text{ L} :: 5000 \text{ mL} : \text{X L}$$

How many mL are in 1.5 L?

$$\frac{1000 \text{ mL}}{1 \text{ L}} = \frac{\text{X mL}}{1.5 \text{ L}} \qquad 1000 \text{ mL} : 1 \text{ L} :: \text{X mL} : 1.5 \text{ L}$$

How many dL are in 4 L?

$$\frac{10 \text{ dL}}{1 \text{ L}} = \frac{\text{X dL}}{4 \text{ L}} \qquad 10 \text{ dL} : 1 \text{ L} :: \text{X dL} : 4 \text{ L}$$

## PRACTICE THE SKILL 7-3

Complete the following table with the proper equivalent measurements.

|     | Milliliters | Deciliters | Liters |
| --- | --- | --- | --- |
| 1. | 500 | | |
| 2. | | 15 | |
| 3. | | | 4 |
| 4. | | 45 | |
| 5. | 750 | | |
| 6. | | 7 | |
| 7. | | | 2 |
| 8. | 1500 | | |
| 9. | | 0.5 | |
| 10. | | | 12 |
| 11. | 0.008 | | |
| 12. | | 0.75 | |

## BUILDING CONFIDENCE WITH THE SKILL 7-2

Answer the following questions.

1. Write the abbreviation for liter. _____

2. Write the abbreviation for milliliter. _____

3. Write the abbreviation for kiloliter. _____

4. Write the abbreviation for deciliter. _____

5. At lunch, the patient drank 240 mL of milk, 240 mL of iced tea, and 500 mL of diet soda. What is the total amount the patient drank in mL?

   _____

6. Based on the answer from question 5, how many liters did the patient drink? _____

7. The nurse used 3,600 liters of irrigation fluid in a 24-hour period. How many kiloliters did the nurse use? _____

8. The nurse used 2,400 liters of irrigation fluid every 4 hours. At this rate, how many liters will the nurse use in a 24-hour period?

   _____

*(Continued)*

## BUILDING CONFIDENCE WITH THE SKILL 7-2
*Continued from p. 189*

9. At the end of dialysis treatment, 2.75 liters of fluid was removed from the patient. How many mL of fluid was removed from the patient?

   _____

10. The patient is scheduled for a colonoscopy in the morning. The patient must drink 2 Liters of preparation fluid. How many milliliters will the patient drink? _____

11. How many deciliters are in 3 liters? _____

12. How many mL are in 4.5 liters? _____

13. How many liters are in 300 deciliters? _____

14. How many liters are in 2575 mL? _____

15. How many mL are in 0.475 L? _____

16. A patient receives 6 units of blood during surgery. According to the bag, there was 325 mL of fluid in each bag. How many kL did the patient receive? _____

17. The chemist needs 4 daL to perform an experiment. In the storage room, the chemist finds a single 1 daL of the needed solution and 70 1 L bottles of the needed solution. What combination, using the least number of bottles, does the chemist need to complete the experiment?

   _____

18. The patient drank 75% of a 2 L bottle. How many hL did the patient drink? _____

19. The doctor wrote the following antibiotic order: 5 mL 4 times a day for 10 days. What is the total amount of medication that the pharmacy needs to dispense? _____

20. An infant drinks 120 mL of formula 6 times a day. Approximately how many liters does the infant drink in 1 week's time?

   _____

## Gram

Gram is the metric base unit for measuring weight or mass. Measurements that use grams include the following:

- Measurement of a person's weight
- Measurement of dry medication (pills, capsules, powders)
- Measurement of the weight of a tumor or body part

| TABLE 7-3 | Common Equivalencies for Weight | | |
|---|---|---|---|
| **Metric Weight** | **Weight/Mass** | **Equivalent in Grams** | |
| 1 microgram (mcG) | 0.000001 G | 1,000,000 mcg = 1 G | |
| 1 milligram (mG) | 0.001 of a G | 1,000 mg = 1 G | |
| 1 centigram (cG) | 0.01 of a G | 100 cg = 1 G | |
| 1 decigram (dG) | 0.1 of a G | 10 dg = 1 G | |
| 1 GRAM | 1 GRAM | 1 G = 1 G | |
| 1 dekagram (daG) | 10 G | 1 dag = 10 G | |
| 1 hectogram (hG) | 100 G | 1 hg = 100 G | |
| 1 kilogram (kG) | 1,000 G | 1 kg = 1,000 G | |

Table 7-3 provides abbreviations, measurements, and equivalent conversions regarding grams.

# MATH IN THE REAL WORLD 7-3

The most common measurements for weight or mass used in health care are the following:

- Microgram (mcg)—used in select (few) measurements of medication dosages
- Milligram (mg)—used to measure medication dosages and weight of organs from the body
- Gram (G or g)—used in medication dosages, weight of newborns and preemie infants, and weight of organs removed from the body
- Kilogram (kg)—used in determining correct medication dosage based on weight of patient

Using the gram as your base unit, try to solve the following example problems.

*Example:*
How many grams are in 500 mg?
$$\frac{1000 \text{ mg}}{1 \text{ g}} = \frac{300 \text{ mg}}{X \text{ g}} \quad \text{or} \quad 1000 \text{ mg} : 1 \text{ g} :: 500 \text{ mg} : X \text{ g}$$

*Example:*
How many kg are in 3500 g?
$$\frac{1 \text{ kg}}{1000 \text{ g}} = \frac{X \text{ kg}}{3500 \text{ g}} \quad \text{or} \quad 1 \text{ kg} : 1000 \text{ g} :: X \text{ kg} : 3500 \text{ g}$$

*Example:*

How many mg are in 6.7 g?

$$\frac{1000 \text{ mg}}{1 \text{ g}} = \frac{X \text{ mg}}{6.7 \text{ g}} \quad \text{or} \quad 1000 \text{ mg} : 1 \text{ g} :: X \text{ mg} : 6.7 \text{ g}$$

## MATH IN THE REAL WORLD 7-4
*Common Abbreviations*

The following are a few common abbreviations and terms used when physicians write medication orders and prescriptions.

**IM:** The abbreviation for intramuscular

**IV:** The abbreviation for intravenous

**PO:** The abbreviation for medication given by mouth

**mEq:** The abbreviation stands for milliequivalent and is used to measure potassium as a medication.

## PRACTICE THE SKILL 7-4

Solve the following mathematical conversions.

1. 0.2 G is equivalent to _____ mg.

2. 400 mg is equivalent to ___ grams.

3. 1.6 G is equivalent to _____ mg.

4. 5 mg is equivalent to _____ G.

5. 0.04 G is equivalent to _____ mg.

6. 5000 milligrams is equivalent to _____ mcg.

7. 2 mg is equivalent to _____ mcg.

8. 300 mcg is equivalent to ___ mg.

9. 1.8 mg is equivalent to ____ mcg.

10. 0.0002 G is equivalent to __ mcg.

11. 500,000 mcg is equivalent to _____ G.

12. 0.6 mg is equivalent to ____ mcg.

Complete the following table with the proper equivalent measurements.

|     | Micrograms | Milligrams | Grams |
| --- | --- | --- | --- |
| 13. | 20,000 | | |
| 14. | | 0.15 | |
| 15. | | | 3.5 |
| 16. | | 375 | |
| 17. | 2,500 | | |
| 18. | | | 0.006 |
| 19. | | 0.125 | |
| 20. | 3,000 | | |

# BUILDING CONFIDENCE WITH THE SKILL 7-3

**Answer the following questions.**

1. The physician orders 275 mg of medication. How many grams of medication are being given to the patient? _____

2. How many mg are in 60 mcg? _____

3. How many grams are in 3,500 mg? _____

4. The medicine is supplied in the amount 3,000,000 mcg. How many grams are in the medicine? _____

5. The patient's weight is 3,400 g. How many kilograms does the patient weigh? _____

**Convert the following metric equivalents.**

6. 0.08 mg is equal to _____ G

7. 0.007 kg is equal to _____ G

8. 4 mcg is equal to _____ mg

9. 7 kg is equal to _____ G

10. 3 G is equal to _____ mcg

11. 40 G is equal to _____ dag

12. 650 hg is equal to _____ G

13. 3,675 mg is equal to _____ kg

14. 1.5 g is equal to _____ mg

15. 14 G is equal to _____ mcg

16. 750 mg is equal to _____ G

17. 400 dag is equal to _____ G

18. 375 hg is equal to _____ G

19. 90 dg is equal to _____ G

20. 63 G is equal to _____ dkg

## Grams and Liters: Metric Concentrations

OBJECTIVE ⑥

When a dry medication is mixed in some type of liquid, the label will read mg/mL or G/L. This is commonly seen in the following:

• Premixed injections
• Multidose vials
• Liquid medications
• IV fluids

A slash mark divides the two measurements. The slash mark is read as *per*.

*Example:*
20 mg/5 mL is read as 20 mg per 5 mL.
Solving equivalent problems is done in the same manner as before, but the known proportion will be stated on the medication label or in the math problem.

## STRATEGY 7-3
*Solving Equivalent Problems*

1. Establish what information is known.

2. Determine what is the known equivalent or conversion for which the problem is asking.

3. Write down what is known on the left side of the equation.

4. Write down the remaining known information on the right side of the equation.

5. Represent the unknown information with an "X" in the equation.

6. If possible, reduce fractions before cross multiplication.

7. Cross multiply and solve for the unknown as learned in Chapter 5.

*Example:*
The physician has ordered 750 mg of liquid medication. The medication label reads 250 mg/5 mL. How many mL will you need to give?

1. Establish what information is known.
   *The medication comes 250 mg per 5 mL.*
   *The physician ordered 750 mg.*

2. Determine what is the known equivalent or conversion for which the problem is asking.
   $$\frac{250 \text{ mg}}{5 \text{ mL}} \qquad \text{or} \quad 250 \text{ mg} : 5 \text{ mL}$$

3. Write down what is known on the left side of the equation.
   $$\frac{250 \text{ mg}}{5 \text{ mL}} = \qquad \text{or} \quad 250 \text{ mg} : 5 \text{ mL} ::$$

4. Write down the remaining known information on the right side of the equation.
   $$\frac{250 \text{ mg}}{5 \text{ mL}} = 750 \text{ mg} \quad \text{or} \quad 250 \text{ mg} : 5 \text{ mL} :: 750 \text{ mg} :$$

5. Represent the unknown information with an "X" in the equation.
   $$\frac{250 \text{ mg}}{5 \text{ mL}} = \frac{750 \text{ mg}}{X \text{ mL}} \quad \text{or} \quad 250 \text{ mg} : 5 \text{ mL} :: 750 \text{ mg} : X \text{ mL}$$

6. If possible, reduce fractions before cross multiplication.
   $$\text{Divide by 5} \quad \frac{250 \text{ mg}}{5 \text{ mL}} = \frac{750 \text{ mg}}{X \text{ mL}}$$

   $$\frac{50 \text{ mg}}{1 \text{ mL}} = \frac{750 \text{ mg}}{X \text{ mL}}$$

7. Cross multiply and solve for the unknown as learned in Chapter 5.
   $$\frac{250 \text{ mg}}{5 \text{ mL}} = \frac{750 \text{ mg}}{X \text{ mL}} \quad \text{or} \quad \frac{50 \text{ mg}}{1 \text{ mL}} = \frac{750 \text{ mg}}{X}$$

   $$250x = 3750$$

   $$\frac{250X}{250} = \frac{3750}{250} \qquad \qquad \frac{750}{50} = \frac{50X}{50}$$

   $$X = 15 \qquad \qquad \qquad X = 15$$

*Answer:* 15 mL

## MATH QUICK TIP 7-4

When no number follows the slash mark, it is assumed that the number is 1.

*Example: 2 mg/mL is read as 2 mg per 1 mL.*

## PRACTICE THE SKILL 7-5

Solve the following calculations.

1. The medication comes in a multidose vial whose label reads 5 mg/mL. How many mg are in 10 mL? _____

2. The medication comes in a multidose vial whose label reads 30 mg/mL. How many mL would you need to give 45 mg of medication? _____

3. Mary is giving a pain shot of Torodol. The label reads 15 mg/0.5 mL. The physician orders 60 mg of Torodol. How many mL will they need to draw up? _____

4. The tetanus vaccine comes in a multidose vial with a total of 15 mL. Each dose is 0.5 mL. How many injections are in each vial? _____

5. The label on the medication vial reads 250 mg/5 mL. How many mg are being administered in 15 mL of medication? _____

6. The IV bag has 20 mEq of potassium in every liter of fluid. How much potassium will the patient receive after 3 L of IV fluid has been infused?

   _____

7. The antibiotic is supplied as 500 mg/mL. The physician orders 3 G of antibiotic. How many mL would you give? _____

8. The IV has 5,000,000 mcg/250 mL. How many G are in 250 mL? _____

9. The liquid medication label reads 35 mg/7.5 mL. How many mg are in 22.5 mL? _____

10. The medication order is 3 mcg/mL. How many mcg are in 500 mL? _____

# BUILDING CONFIDENCE WITH THE SKILL 7-4

Solve the following conversion problems.

1. How many mcg are in 25 mg? _____

2. How many mcg are in 0.5 mg? _____

3. How many g are in 250 mg? _____

4. A physician wrote an order for 0.1 G of penicillin. How many milligrams of penicillin are in 0.1 G? _____

5. How many mg are in 1500 mcg? _____

6. If a patient voids 2,400 mL of urine, how many L of urine has the patient voided? _____

7. How many meters are in 1 dekameter? _____

8. How many centimeters are in 4 meters? _____

Convert the following metric equivalents.

9. 25 mg/dL is equal to _____ mg/L

10. 4 mg/L is equal to _____ mg/dL

11. 12 G/L is equal to _____ mg/L

12. 250 mg/L is equal to _____ G/L

13. 2 cm is equal to _____ mm

14. 25.5 mcg is equal to _____ G

15. 30 mL is equal to _____ L

16. 75 mm is equal to _____ cm

17. 10 km is equal to _____ m

18. 10 L is equal to _____ dL

19. 35 m is equal to _____ km

20. 5 km is equal to _____ m

## CONCLUSION

This chapter discusses conversions between the three metric measurements used in health care. As we move on to Chapters 8 and 9, you will be asked to convert between the metric, household, and apothecary systems of measurement. Although we have primarily used the concept of ratio and proportion, there are other ways to solve this type of problem, and these are discussed in later chapters. As you are exposed to different methods, you will need to decide which conversion system works best for you, the student. When it comes to conversions, practice and memorization of equivalencies will build your confidence with the problem-solving process.

 **MASTER THE SKILL**

OBJECTIVES ① ② ③ ④ ⑤ ⑥

Write out the meaning for each abbreviation.

1. mg _____

2. dL _____

3. L _____

4. mcg _____

5. cm _____

6. mm _____

7. G _____

8. kg _____

9. mL _____

10. M _____

Write the correct abbreviation for each word.

11. hectometer _____

12. dekaliter _____

13. kilometer _____

14. decigram _____

15. microliter _____

16. centigram _____

17. hectoliter _____

18. millimeter _____

19. dekameter _____

Solve the following conversion problems.

20. How many kilometers are in 6,000 meters? _____

21. How many centimeters are in 4 meters? _____

22. How many centimeters are in 40 millimeters? _____

23. How many millimeters are in 3.5 centimeters? _____

24. How many millimeters are in 2 meters? _____

25. How many grams are in 2,500 milligrams? _____

26. How many milligrams are in 3.0 grams? _____

(Continued)

## MASTER THE SKILL
*Continued from p. 197*

27. How many kilograms are in 4,500 grams? _____

28. How many milligrams are in 5,000 micrograms? _____

29. How many micrograms are in 0.5 milligram? _____

30. How many deciliters are in 2 L? _____

31. How many mL are in 3.5 L? _____

32. How many L are in 6.5 kL? _____

33. How many L are in 4,500 mL? _____

34. How many kiloliters are in 1,500 mL? _____

35. How many L are in 7.6 kL? _____

36. How many liters are in 35 deciliters? _____

Solve the following word problems.

37. Tylenol is manufactured in 325 mg/tablets. The physician ordered 975 mg of Tylenol to the patient. How many tablets should you give? _____

38. The physician gave a verbal order to give Amoxil 450 mg PO. Amoxil is available in 100 mg/2 mL vials. How much should you give? _____

39. The physician orders 5 mEq of potassium/250 mL of normal saline. How many mEq of potassium are found in 1 L of normal saline? _____

40. The physician orders 12.5 mg/1 kg. The patient's weight is 100 kg. How much medication should you give? _____

41. The school has asked you to bring in 4 kL of soda for a party. Soda comes in 2 L containers. How many containers do you need? _____

42. The patient's weight is 100 kg. You are to give 5 mg/kg of cough medicine. How many mg of cough medicine should you give? _____

43. The physician orders Torodol 60 mg injection. The label reads 20 mg/mL. How many mL should you give? _____

44. The multidose vial label reads 5 mcg/0.1 mL. The vial holds 1 mL. How many doses can be given from a full vial? _____

45. The physician orders a steroid injection for the treatment of poison ivy. The vial reads 4 mg/mL. How many mg has the physician ordered if you are to give 2 mL? _____

*(Continued)*

## MASTER THE SKILL
*Continued from p. 198*

46. The IV has 500 mg of antibiotic in a 250 mL bag. The patient receives this antibiotic three times a day.

   a. How many mg of medication has the patient received in a 24-hour period? _____

   b. How many mL have been infused into the patient in a 24-hour period?
   _____

47. The physician orders 10 mg/3 mL of medication to be given four times a day.

   a. How many mg of medication will be given? _____

   b. How many mL will be given in a 24-hour period?
   _____

48. The physician orders 150 mg/7.5 mL twice a day for 10 days.

   a. How many mg of medication does the patient receive each day? _____

   b. How many mL does the patient receive each day? _____

   c. How many mg will the patient have received at the end of the treatment? _____

   d. How big a bottle (mL) should the pharmacy give the patient when the prescription is filled? _____

49. The tumor weight was 25 kg.

   a. How many dg does the tumor weigh? _____

   b. How many G does the tumor weigh? _____

   c. How many mg does the tumor weigh? _____

50. The surgical rod was 56 mm long.

   a. How long will it be in centimeters? _____

   b. How long would it be in meters? _____

# US Customary Units and the Apothecary System

## CHAPTER OUTLINE

Apothecary System

US Customary System (Household Measurements) and Avoirdupois System
  Fractions and Cross Multiplication

Conclusion

## LEARNING OBJECTIVES

*Upon completion of this chapter, the learner will be able to:*

1. Define the key terms that relate to the chapter.

2. Identify base measurement units used in the apothecary system.

3. Calculate equivalent measurements between the apothecary and metric systems.

4. Identify base measurement units used in household measurements (US Customary System, avoirdupois system).

5. Compute equivalent measurement utilizing the avoirdupois system with 100% accuracy.

6. Compute equivalent measurements between household and apothecary measurements.

OBJECTIVE **1**

## KEY TERMS

Apothecary System
Avoirdupois System
Units

US Customary System (Household
  Measurements)

OBJECTIVE **1**

Working with medications has always been a challenge in the United States. Physicians, based on their educational background, may use the metric system, the apothecary system, or the **US Customary System (household measurements)** and the **avoirdupois** system when prescribing medications.

As metric measurements become the predominant format for medication packaging, the use of the apothecary system will become minimal. The apothecary system is an approximate system and is less accurate than the metric system. Furthermore, the use of abbreviations and symbols in the apothecary system has a greater potential for error.

In this chapter, we continue to use ratio, proportion, and solving for *X* (see Chapter 5) to set up our conversion problems. In addition, we refer to the metric conversions from Chapter 7. Conversion between the metric system and the US Customary System (household measurements), or the avoirdupois system, is needed by caregivers who are dispensing liquid medication in a home setting. Figure 8-1 demonstrates measuring tools commonly used in health care and home settings for dispensing liquid medication.

OBJECTIVE **2**

## APOTHECARY SYSTEM

The **apothecary system** is an old English system of measurement that became popular in the United States in the 18th century. The base units in the apothecary system are the grain (weight), minim (volume), and inch (length) (Box 8-1). A grain

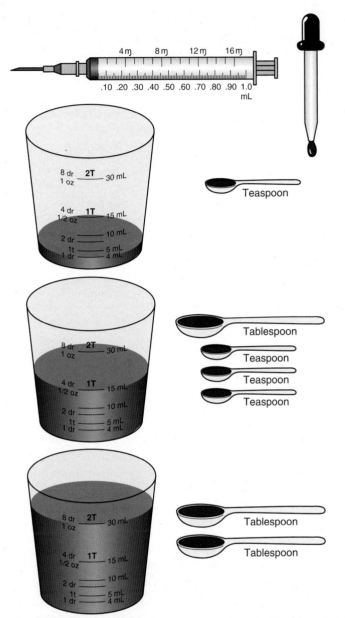

**Figure 8-1    Common measuring tools for dispensing liquid medication.** (From Fulcher RM, Fulcher EM: *Math calculations for pharmacy technicians: A worktext*, St. Louis, 2007, Saunders.)

| BOX 8-1 | *Apothecary Measurements* | |
|---|---|---|
| **Weight*** | **Volume*** | **Length*** |
| Grain | Minim | Inch |
| *Scruple*† | Fluid dram | Yard |
| Dram | Fluid ounce | Mile |
| Ounce | Pint | |
| Pound | Quart | |
| | Gallon | |

*From smallest measurement to greatest measurement.
†Scruples were never used as a pharmacology measurement.

| TABLE 8-1 | Equivalents in the Apothecary System | | |
|---|---|---|---|
| Type of Substance | Abbreviation | Unit of Measure | Common Equivalents |
| Volume/liquid | ɱ | minim | — |
| | flʒ | fluid dram | ɱ lx (60) |
| | flʒ | fluid ounce | ʒ viii (8) |
| Mass | gr | grain | — |
| | ʒ | dram | gr lx (60) |
| | ʒ | ounce | ʒ viii (8) |
| | # | pound | ʒ xii (12)* |

From Fulcher RM, Fulcher EM: Math calculations for pharmacy technicians: A worktext, St. Louis, 2007, Saunders.
*Note that in the apothecary system a pound is only 12 ounces.

## HUMAN ERROR 8-1

*The apothecary system is quickly being replaced by the metric system. Common errors that occur between the apothecary and metric systems include:*

- *Confusing G (gram) for gr (grain)*
- *Confusing minims for milliliters*
- *Confusing micrograms (mcg) for grains (gr)*
- *Confusing the dram symbols for Roman numerals*

is the dry weight measurement equal to a large grain of wheat. Minims are based on the amount of liquid that equals the weight of a grain, and the inch is the approximate length of two wheat grains.

The apothecary system is a familiar measurement system in the United States because household equivalents were developed for conversion from apothecary measures (Table 8-1). Because of the lack of consistent accuracy, however, the apothecary system is being phased out in favor of the metric system in the field of pharmacology.

## MATH TRIVIA 8-1

Minims must be measured in a minim glass or syringe that is calibrated for minims.

In the apothecary system, *12* ounces is equal to 1 pound, whereas the US Customary System (household measurements), or the avoirdupois system, recognizes *16* ounces as equal to 1 pound. To avoid confusion, always follow the established equivalent utilized by your place of employment. Table 8-2 provides further apothecary-to-metric conversions.

## MATH QUICK TIP 8-1

kg to lbs: multiply by 2.2

lbs to kg: divide by 2.2

| TABLE 8-2 | Apothecary-to-Metric Conversion | | |
|---|---|---|---|
| Apothecary | Metric | | Metric |
| ½ grain | 30 mg | | |
| 1 grain | 60 mg | | |
| 15 grains | 1,000 mg | | 1 G |
| 2.2 pounds | 1,000 G | | 1 kg |

*Because of rounding, the conversions are approximate and are not intended to provide exact conversions between the metric system and the apothecary system.*

## MATH QUICK TIP 8-2

Grains are written with the abbreviation gr followed by a Roman numeral to represent the amount.

**Example:** gr v is read as grains 5.

## MATH TRIVIA 8-2

The Roman numeral used for ½ is s̄s.

Once again, let's work with conversion problems. The box Strategy 8-1 is a reminder of how to set up the problems.

## STRATEGY 8-1
*Writing Proportions*

1. Read the problem.

2. Identify the known information.

3. Write your proportion so that the same units appear in the same location for each proportion.

4. Solve the problem using cross multiplication if your proportion is written as a fraction. If your problem is written in linear fashion, multiply the means ("inside numbers") together and the extremes ("outside numbers") together.

OBJECTIVE 3

## PRACTICE THE SKILL 8-1

Solve the following equivalents.

1. 2 G is equal to _____ mg.

2. gr x is equal to _____ G.

3. gr v is equal to _____ G.

4. 3 L is equal to _____ mL.

5. gr xv is equal to _____ mg.

6. 6 G is equal to _____ mg.

7. 240 mg is equal to _____ G.

8. 30 mL is equal to _____ L.

9. 4 dram is equal to _____ mL.

10. 45 mL is equal to _____ drams.

11. 200 pounds is equal to _____ kg.

12. 75 pounds is equal to _____ kg.

13. 150 pounds is equal to _____ kg.

14. 225 pounds is equal to _____ kg.

15. 42 pounds is equal to _____ kg.

16. 1,640 G is equal to ____ pounds.

17. 3,650 G is equal to ____ pounds.

18. 75 kg is equal to _____ pounds.

19. 100 kg is equal to _____ pounds.

20. 4 kg is equal to _____ pounds.

OBJECTIVE 4

## US CUSTOMARY SYSTEM (HOUSEHOLD MEASUREMENTS) AND AVOIRDUPOIS SYSTEM

The **avoirdupois system**, which is used to measure weight, and the US Customary System, commonly known as household measurements, are the way we measure quantities at home. The base units for these systems can be found in any kitchen— ounces, pounds, teaspoons, tablespoons, cups, pints, quarts, inches, feet, and yards. Most of you will find household measurements very user friendly. In the health care system, it is common to see prescriptions written with a mix of metric and household measurements.

*Example:*
Amoxicillin 250 mg/5 mL
1 teaspoon three times a day
Dispense 180 mL

Before the pharmacy provided calibrated dispensing droppers and measuring spoons, families had to use what was available to dispense medication. Can you think of complications that might result from using household measurements rather than a calibrated measuring utensil? Whether the person is using a cooking measuring spoon or one out of the silverware drawer will change the amount of medication the patient is receiving.

Tables 8-3 and 8-4 and Box 8-2 reflect common conversions used in household measurements.

| TABLE 8-3 | *Linear Measurements* | | |
| --- | --- | --- | --- |
| Inches | Feet | Yards | Miles |
| 12 inches | 1 foot | | |
| 36 inches | 3 feet | 1 yard | |
| | 5,280 feet | 1,760 yards | 1 mile |

| TABLE 8-4 | *Mass and Liquid Equivalency* | |
| --- | --- | --- |
| Household Measurement | Equivalents | Additional Equivalents |
| 60 drops (gtt) | 1 teaspoon (t or tsp) | 60 minims |
| 3 teaspoons | 1 tablespoon (T or Tbsp) | 180 gtt |
| 1 tablespoon | ½ ounce (oz) | 180 gtt |
| 2 tablespoons | 1 ounce | 6 teaspoons |
| 1 ounce | ⅛ cup (c) | 2 tablespoons |
| 4 ounces | ½ cup | 1 juice glass |
| 6 ounces (oz) | ¾ cup | 1 teacup |
| 8 ounces | 1 measuring cup | 16 tablespoons |
| 2 cups | 1 pint (pt) | 16 ounces |
| 2 pints | 1 quart (qt) | 32 ounces |
| 4 cups | 1 quart | 32 ounces |
| 4 quarts | 1 gallon | 128 ounces |

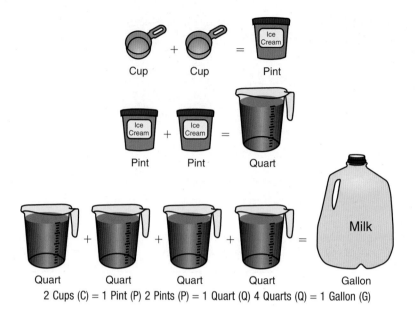

2 Cups (C) = 1 Pint (P)  2 Pints (P) = 1 Quart (Q)  4 Quarts (Q) = 1 Gallon (G)

## MATH TRIVIA 8-3

12 ounces = 1 pound Apothecaries measurement
2.2 pounds = 1 kg Apothecaries to Metric

## MATH IN THE REAL WORLD 8-1
### Real World Measurements in Health Care

| | |
|---|---|
| Height | Feet and inches |
| Weight | Pounds and ounces |
| Liquid intake | Ounces, cups, pints, quarts, and gallons: |
| | 2 Cups (C) = 1 Pint (P) |
| | 2 Pints (P) = 1 Quart (Q) |
| | 4 Quarts (Q) = 1 Gallon (G) |
| Dietary intake | Ounces and cups |

Using Tables 8-3 and 8-4 and Box 8-2, as well as your knowledge of solving for X (see Chapter 5), work through the following Practice the Skill exercises.

# PRACTICE THE SKILL 8-2

OBJECTIVE 4

Solve for the correct equivalency.

1. 6 Tbsp is equal to _____ tsp.

2. 4 oz is equal to _____ Tbsp.

3. 64 oz is equal to _____ pt.

4. 384 ounces is equal to _____ gallons.

5. 16 qt is equal to _____ gallons.

6. 6 gallons is equal to

   a. _____ quarts.

   b. _____ pints.

   c. _____ cups.

   d. _____ ounces.

7. 360 gtt is equal to _____ Tbsp.

8. 12 T is equal to _____ tsp.

9. 3 tsp is equal to _____ Tbsp.

10. 16 cups is equal to _____ qt.

11. 12 pt is equal to _____ cups.

12. 72 inches is equal _____ ft.

13. 7 yd is equal to _____ ft.

14. 180 inches is equal to _____ ft.

15. 180 inches is equal to _____ yd.

*(Continued)*

## PRACTICE THE SKILL 8-2
*Continued from p. 207*

**16.** 48 pints is equal to

a. _____ oz.

b. _____ cups.

c. _____ quarts.

d. _____ gallons.

**17.** 27 tsp is equal to _____T or _____ozs.

**18.** 66 inches is equal to _____ft and _____inches.

**19.** 77 inches is equal to _____ft and _____inches.

**20.** 4 ft and 3 inches is equal to _____inches.

## Fractions and Cross Multiplication

What happens when there is a fraction in the conversion equation? Do we just ignore the fraction or round the answer to a whole number? No, we need to add the fractional amount to the solution of our conversion problem.

## STRATEGY 8-2
*Working with Fractions*

**1.** Read the problem.

**2.** Identify the known information. ("What do we have?")

**3.** Identify the proper conversion ratio. ("What do we know?")

**4.** Identify the unknown information. ("What are we trying to find?")

**5.** Set up the proportion.

**6.** Solve for *X*.

**7.** Add the fractional amount to the solution of the conversion problem.

**8.** Label the answer with the correct measurement.

*Example:*
An infant measures 2 feet $2\frac{1}{2}$ inches. What is the infant's total length in inches?

**1.** Read the problem.
  *An infant is measured at 2 feet $2\frac{1}{2}$ inches. What is the infant's total length in inches?*

**2.** Identify the known information. ("What do we have?")
  *The infant's length is 2 feet $2\frac{1}{2}$ inches. The fractional part of the problem is $2\frac{1}{2}$ inches.*

**3.** Identify the proper conversion ratio. ("What do we know?")
  1 foot = 12 inches

**4.** Identify the unknown information. ("What are we trying to find?")
*The total length of the infant in inches*

**5.** Set up the proportion.

$$\frac{1 \text{ ft}}{12 \text{ in}} = \frac{2 \text{ ft}}{X \text{ in}} \quad 1 \text{ ft} : 12 \text{ in} :: 2 \text{ ft} : X \text{ in}$$

**6.** Solve for $X$

$$1 \times X = 12 \times 2 \qquad 12 \times 2 :: 1 \times X$$

$$\frac{1X}{1} = \frac{24}{1} \qquad\qquad \frac{24}{1} :: \frac{1X}{1}$$

$$X = 24 \text{ inches} \qquad X = 24 \text{ inches}$$

**7.** Add the fractional amount to the solution of the conversion problem.
24 inches + 2½ inches = 26½ inches

**8.** Label your answer with the correct measurement.
*inches*

*Answer:* The infant is 26½ inches long.

*Example:*
The child's height is 43½ inches. How tall is the child in feet and inches?

**1.** Read the problem.
*The child's height is 43½ inches. How tall is the child in feet and inches?*

**2.** Identify the known information. ("What do we have?")

**3.** Identify the proper conversion ratio. ("What do we know?")

**4.** Identify the unknown information. ("What are we trying to find?")

**5.** Set up the proportion.

$$\frac{1 \text{ ft}}{12 \text{ in}} = \frac{X \text{ ft}}{43 \text{ in}}$$

$$12 \times X = 1 \times 43$$

$$\frac{12X}{1} = \frac{43}{1}$$

Divide both sides by 12 in order to isolate the $X$.

$X = 43/$(division symbol)$12$

$X = 3$ remainder 7

**6.** Solve for "$X$"
$X = 3$ *feet with a remainder of* 7

**7.** Add the fractional amount to the solution of the conversion problem.
3 feet *with* 7 inches + 1/2 inches = 3 feet 7 1/2 inches.

**8.** Label your answer
*feet and inches*

*Answer:* The child's height is 3 feet and 7½ inches.

1 ft : 12 in :: $X$ ft : 43 inches

$12 \times X :: 1 \times 43$

$12X :: 43$

$$\frac{12X}{12} :: \frac{43}{12}$$

$X = 3$ with a remainder of 7

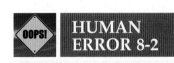

**HUMAN ERROR 8-2**

*Remember to check to make sure your result answers the questions. Does the answer make sense? This will decrease the chances of math errors.*

I realize that many of you used **mental math** to figure out this problem, and that's fantastic. There are many problems for which you will be able to use mental math or rationalize. Frequently, however, when converting between different measurement systems, you will need to write out the problem, at least for visualization.

OBJECTIVES

## BUILDING CONFIDENCE WITH THE SKILL 8-1

1. 15 gtt = _____ tsp

2. 6 Tbsp = _____ oz

3. 15 tsp = _____ Tbsp

4. 4 c = _____ oz

5. 6 pt = _____ qt

6. 3 Tbsp = _____ oz

7. 60 inches = _____ ft

8. 2 feet = _____ inches

9. 44 lbs = _____ oz

10. 6 T = _____ tsp

11. 60 gtt = _____ tsp

12. 6 c = _____ oz

13. 6 c = _____ pt

14. 9 tsp = _____ Tbsp

15. 39 inches = ___ ft and ____ inches

16. 2 qt = _____ gal

17. 6 Tbsp = _____ oz

18. 6 oz = _____ c

19. 5 c = _____ oz

20. 9 tsp = _____ Tbsp

21. 75 gtt = _____ tsp

22. 24 Tbsp = _____ c

23. 4 c = _____ pt

24. 20 oz = _____ lb

25. 3½ lbs = _____ oz

26. 52 inches = _____ft and _____inches

27. 84 inches + 3 feet 5 inches = _____feet and _____inches

28. 8 dr + 45 mL + 1 oz = _____pint(s)

29. 3 cups + 4 pints + 2 quarts = _____gallon(s)

30. 1 gallons – 1 quart – 3 pints – 4 cups = _____ounces

## CONCLUSION

In this chapter, we discuss equivalent measurements between the apothecary system and the US Customary System (household measurements) or the avoirdupois system. Until the apothecary system has been completely phased out, it is important to understand the basic relationship of grains to milligrams and drops to minims. Health care providers in a variety of jobs use conversions between metric and household measurements. Chapter 9 continues our discussion of conversions between all three systems of measurement: metric, apothecary, and household.

## MASTER THE SKILL

OBJECTIVES

Give the correct abbreviation for each term.

1. Cups _____

2. Pounds _____

3. Yards _____

4. Teaspoons _____

5. Quarts _____

Give the correct term for each abbreviation.

6. T or Tbsp _____

7. gtt _____

8. gr _____

9. oz _____

10. ft _____

Solve the following conversions.

11. 4′6″ = _____ inches

12. 6′1″ = _____ inches

13. 5′10″ = _____ inches

14. ½ Tbsp = _____ tsp

15. ½ T = _____ gtt

16. 3 pt = _____ qt

17. 6 qt = _____ gal

18. 3 tsp = _____ gtt

19. 45 gtt = _____ tsp

20. 30 oz = _____ lb

21. 24 oz = _____ c

22. 10 c = _____ oz

23. 200 kg = _____ lb

24. 75 kg = _____ lb

25. 300 lb = _____ kg

26. 45 lb = _____ kg

27. 90 mg = _____ gr

28. 45 gr = _____ mg

29. 60 gr = _____ G

30. 60 gtt = _____ minims

31. 3 tsp = _____ minims

32. 120 mg = _____ grains

Answer the following word problems.

33. The pediatric patient measures 39 inches. How tall is the patient in feet and inches? _____.

34. The physician orders 6 tsp of cough syrup. The patient's caregiver asks how many tablespoons that is. Your response is _____.

35. The preparation for a radiographic test includes drinking 64 oz of clear liquids. The healthcare provider instructs the patient to drink _____ cups of clear liquids in order to prepare for the test.

*(Continued)*

## MASTER THE SKILL
*Continued from p. 211*

36. The tumor's weight is 112 oz. What is the weight of the tumor in pounds?
_____ .

37. How much does a 12.4-lb organ weigh in kg? _____

38. How many ounces are in 8 Tbsp? _____

39. How many cups are in 4 gallons? _____

40. How many grains are in 60 grams? _____

41. How many pounds are in 80 kg? _____

42. How many pints are in 5 gallons? _____

43. How many grains are in 2 G? _____

44. How many gtt are in 4 Tbsp? _____

45. How many gtt are in 3 tsp? _____

46. How many pints are in 4 gallons? _____

47. If 2 gallons serves six people, how many gallons are needed to serve 90 people? _____

48. The juice container holds 160 ounces. How many 4-ounce juice glasses will the container fill? _____

49. The physical therapist has asked the patient to walk 15 feet with his walker. How many yards should the patient walk? _____

50. How many Tbsp are in a 12-oz bottle of cough medicine? _____

# Application of Measurement and Dose Conversion

## CHAPTER OUTLINE

## LEARNING OBJECTIVES

*Upon completion of this chapter, the learner will be able to:*

1. Define the key terms that relate to the chapter.

2. Identify common abbreviations used in the health care field.

3. Interpret basic physician's orders.

4. Use the appropriate equivalents to solve conversion problems using the metric, apothecary, and U.S. Customary (household measurements) systems.

5. Convert temperature measurements between Fahrenheit and Celsius.

## KEY TERMS

OBJECTIVE **1**

| | |
|---|---|
| Celsius (or Centigrade) | Quantity |
| Dosage Strength | Refills |
| Fahrenheit | Route |
| Inscription | Signa (Sig) |
| Medication Order | |

OBJECTIVE **1**

Have you ever read the label on a pill bottle after a prescription has been filled? Many times, you will see a mixture of metric and U.S. Customary (household) measurements (Figure 9-1). Then the pharmacist hands you a measuring device with both metric and U.S. Customary (household) measurements on it (Figure 9-2). You want to give or take the correct dose, but which do you use—milliliters or teaspoons?

In the previous chapters, all of the questions dealt with the same base measurements. In this chapter, however, we practice converting between metric, apothecary, and U.S. Customary (household) measurements. The chapter also discusses common abbreviations used in the health care field, interpretation of physician orders, and conversion of temperature measurements from Fahrenheit to Celsius.

## COMMON ABBREVIATIONS USED IN THE HEALTH CARE FIELD

OBJECTIVE **2**

Have you ever taken a foreign language class? Medical terms and abbreviations used in the health care field can be compared to a foreign language. Because the medical field has a Latin word base, translations may not be obvious.

Lawrence Merry, M.D.
4th Street and Jones Ave.
Holly, GA 00111
phone# - 001-555-2176

Patient Name_____ Date _____
Address_____ Age _____

℞  Amoxicillin 250 mg/5 ml
    1 teaspoon three times a day x 10 days
    Amount: 180 ml

_____    Refill _____
DEA#_____

**Figure 9-1** Script with medication order. (Modified from Fulcher RM, Fulcher E: *Math calculations for pharmacy technicians: A worktext*, St. Louis, 2007, Saunders.)

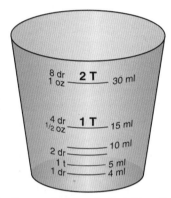

**Figure 9-2** Measuring cup used to dispense liquid medication. (From Kee J, Hayes E: *Pharmacology: A nursing process approach*, St. Louis, 2004, Saunders.)

Tables 9-1 and 9-2 identify common abbreviations that are used when giving orders in the health care field. It is important that all health care professionals understand and can interpret common abbreviations—these abbreviations are not exclusive to the study of pharmacology.

The frequency of an order can be confusing. The abbreviation *BID*, which means "twice a day," is *not* the same as *q2h*, which means "every 2 hours." When requesting that a procedure, therapy, or medication be given at a specific time interval, the physician writes the hour frequency as a number.

## MATH QUICK TIP 9-1

Only use facility-approved abbreviations when documenting in charts.

*Example:*
Unasyn 500 mg IV
Q8H × 3 days
The above example Q8H means to give the medication every 8 hours. This order is more specific than *tid* (three times a day), which is more flexible with the time intervals between dosages.

| TABLE 9-1 | *Abbreviations Commonly Used by Pharmacology and Nursing Health Care Workers* |
|---|---|
| **Abbreviation Number or Quantity** | **Meaning** |
| a.c. | Before meals |
| Ad lib | As desired; as tolerated |
| a.m. | Morning |
| bid | Twice a day |
| BP | Blood pressure |
| $\overline{c}$ | With |
| d | Day |
| d/c | Discontinue |
| H, hr | Hour |
| hs | Hour of sleep |
| IM | Intramuscular |
| IV | Intravenous |
| K | Potassium |
| Na | Sodium |
| npo | Nothing by mouth |
| p.c. | After meals |
| p.m. | Afternoon |
| PO | Per oral or by mouth |
| prn | As needed |
| Q, q | Every |
| qid | Four times a day |
| qs | Quantity sufficient |
| ℞ | Prescription |
| $\overline{s}$ | Without |
| # | number or quantity |
| SC, SQ, Subq | Subcutaneous |
| Sig | Directions |

*(Continued)*

| TABLE 9-1 | Abbreviations Commonly Used by Pharmacology and Nursing Health Care Workers—cont'd |
|---|---|
| Abbreviation Number or Quantity | Meaning |
| SL | Sublingual, under the tongue |
| STAT | Immediately |
| Tab | Tablet |
| tid | Three times a day |
| TPR | Temperature, pulse, respiration |
| VO | Verbal order |
| VS | Vital signs |

| TABLE 9-2 | Abbreviations Commonly Used by Laboratory and Nursing Health Care Workers |
|---|---|
| Abbreviation | Meaning |
| BM | Bowel movement |
| CBC | Complete blood count |
| CMP | Comprehensive metabolic panel |
| FBS | Fasting blood sugar |
| Hct | Hematocrit |
| Hgb | Hemoglobin |
| H/H | Hemoglobin and hematocrit |
| Plat. | Platelets |
| WBC | White blood count |

## PRACTICE THE SKILL 9-1

Match the following abbreviations with the correct meaning.

_____1. every                       **A.** bid

_____2. before meals                **B.** a.c.

_____3. intramuscular               **C.** CBC

(Continued)

## PRACTICE THE SKILL 9-1
### Continued from p. 216

| | |
|---|---|
| _____4. intravenous | D. q |
| _____5. twice a day | E. IV |
| _____6. complete blood count | F. IM |
| _____7. every 4 hours | G. STAT |
| _____8. after meals | H. tid |
| _____9. every 6 hours | I. p.c. |
| _____10. as desired | J. Hgb |
| _____11. Hematocrit | K. qid |
| _____12. white blood count | L. VO |
| _____13. three times a day | M. WBC |
| _____14. every day | N. CMP |
| _____15. immediately | O. ad lib |
| _____16. four times a day | P. prn |
| _____17. hemoglobin | Q. Hct |
| _____18. verbal order | R. q4h |
| _____19. as needed | S. qd |
| _____20. comprehensive metabolic panel | T. q6h |

## INTERPRETATION OF PHYSICIAN'S ORDERS

OBJECTIVE ③

Physician's orders are given by the physician either in writing or orally to communicate what medication, tests (e.g., laboratory, radiology and/or nuclear medicine), or therapy he or she would like to have implemented. Orders are written in the patient's chart by designated health care personnel. Medical abbreviations are commonly mixed in with longhand descriptions of the orders.

*Example:*
CBC q6h × 3 days then D/C.
Interpretation: Draw blood for a complete blood count every 6 hours for 3 days, then discontinue.

All physician's orders should have the same basic information—what is to be done and how often.

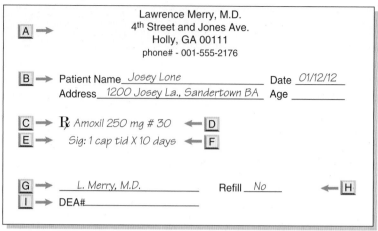

Figure 9-3    Examples of prescription blanks and their components. A, Single-line prescription. B, Multiple-line prescription. The five major components of a prescription are the superscription (C); the inscription (D); the signa (E); the subscription (F); and the signature (G). Use of multiple-line prescription blanks is dependent on state statutes in the state of practice. (From Fulcher EM, Soto CD, Fulcher RM: *Pharmacology: Principles & Applications,* ed 3, St. Louis, Saunders, 2012.)

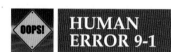

## HUMAN ERROR 9-1

*To prevent medication errors, more prescriptions are being written electronically and sent directly to the pharmacy.*

*In addition, with the increase of electronic health records (EHR) many facilities are prohibiting the use of abbreviations.*

**Medication orders** and prescriptions must include specific information (Figure 9-3):

| Elements of the prescription | Description |
|---|---|
| Inscription | Name of the medication |
| Inscription | Dosage strength of the medication |
| Route | How the medication should be taken |
| Frequency or Signa (Sig) | How often the medication should be taken |
| Quantity | How much medication should be dispensed |
| Refill | How many refills of the medication are allowed |

Let's look at the prescription in Figure 9-3 and identify the required information.

| | |
|---|---|
| 1. Name of the medication | Pen-V-K (correct name: Pen-Vee K) |
| 2. Dosage strength of the medication | 250 mg |
| 3. How the medication should be taken | Tablets (by mouth) route |
| 4. How often the medication should be taken | Every 6 hours |
| 5. How much medication should be dispensed | 40 tablets |
| 6. How many refills of the medication are allowed | Refills are not specified so there would be no refills |

If there is ever a question regarding the medication order, or the order does not make sense, the physician *must* be contacted. The physician writes the order in a specific manner that will affect the care of the patient. Clarification of any order should come from the physician or the physician's representative.

## MATH IN THE REAL WORLD

DEA number are assigned by the Drug Enforcement Administration (DEA) to qualified health care workers who prescribe controlled substances.

Depending on the medication orders written, math may be involved in determining the correct amount of medication to be dispensed, the way to reconstitute the medication, and the amount of medication to be given over a specified period of time.

## MATH QUICK TIP 9-2

In today's society, patients commonly fill their routine medication prescriptions through the mail. Mail order prescriptions are usually dispensed in a 90-day supply (3 months). In the calculation of how much medication to dispense, 1 month equals 30 days.

## PRACTICE THE SKILL 9-2

Interpret the following orders.

1. VS q1h times 6 h

2. FBS qam times 7 d

3. Epinephrine STAT

4. Zithromax 250 mg qd

5. CBC q12h

6. Premarin 1.25 mg tab qd times 21 d

7. Amoxil 500 mg tid times 10 d

8. H/H q6h times 4 then q12h times 2 d

9. Aspirin (ASA) 500 mg bid prn

10. 1000 mL IV q8h

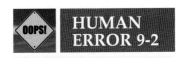

## HUMAN ERROR 9-2

*Once you have joined the workforce, have your calculations checked by a coworker. Many medication errors have been the result of incorrect math computations.*

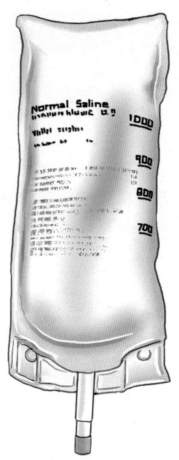

**Figure 9-4**    Intravenous fluids.

Once the physician has written an order, it is up to the health care personnel to determine the proper procedure for completing that order. *This* is where math is involved.

*Example:*
The physician writes: 1000 mL IV q8h (Figure 9-4).
Dilemma: How fast must the IV drip in order for 1000 mL to infuse in 8 hours?
Math: Divide 1000 mL by 8 hours.
*Solution:* The IV must drip at 125 mL/hr for 1000 mL to be given in 8 hours.

*Example:*
The physician writes: Pen-V-K 2.5 mg/kg tid (Figure 9-5). The patient's weight is 35 kg.
Dilemma: How much medication should the physician have prescribed?
Math: Multiply 2.5 mg × 35 kg.
*Solution:* 87.5 mg of medication three times a day.

As you progress through this chapter, you will encounter computations that require a multistep approach to solving the problem. Before you start your math computations, make sure you understand what the question is asking. Check that your answer makes sense. Take your time—accuracy is the key.

Lawrence Merry, M.D.
4th Street and Jones Ave.
Holly, GA 00111
phone# - 001-555-2176

Patient Name_____ Date _____
Address_____ Age _____

℞          Pen-V-K 2.5 mg/kg tid




_____ Refill _____
DEA#_____

**Figure 9-5**   Physician order. (Modified from Fulcher RM, Fulcher E: *Math calculations for pharmacy technicians: A worktext*, St. Louis, 2007, Saunders.)

# BUILDING CONFIDENCE WITH THE SKILL 9-1

## Interpret the following orders.

**1.** Pencillin 250 mg po qid × 10 days

_____

**2.** Nitroglycerin 0.4 mg sl q5minutes prn

_____

**3.** Diuril 0.25 mg 1 tab qam prn swelling

_____

**4.** Phenergan 25 mg po q4-6 prn nausea and vomiting

_____

## Identify the different parts of the following prescriptions.

**5.**

Lawrence Merry, M.D.
4th Street and Jones Ave.
Holly, GA 00111
phone# - 001-555-2176

Patient Name_____ Date _____
Address_____ Age _____

℞          atorvastatin 10 mg
            #30
            sig: i tab qhs

_____ Refill _____
DEA#_____

(From Fulcher RM, Fulcher E: *Math calculations for pharmacy technicians: A worktext*, St. Louis, 2007, Saunders.)

a. Inscription: _____

b. Dosage: _____

*(Continued)*

# BUILDING CONFIDENCE WITH THE SKILL 9-1
*Continued from p. 221*

c. Route: _____

d. Quantity: _____

e. Sig: _____

6.

> **Lawrence Merry, M.D.**
> 4th Street and Jones Ave.
> Holly, GA 00111
> phone# - 001-555-2176
>
> Patient Name_____ Date _____
> Address_____ Age _____
>
> ℞          hydrocodone w/APAP 5/500
>            #20
>            sig: i or ii tab q6-8h prn pain
>
> _____ Refill _____
> DEA# XX112233

(From Fulcher RM, Fulcher E: *Math calculations for pharmacy technicians: A worktext*, St. Louis, 2007, Saunders.)

a. Inscription: _____

b. Dosage: _____

c. Route: _____

d. Quantity: _____

e. Sig: _____

7.

> **Lawrence Merry, M.D.**
> 4th Street and Jones Ave.
> Holly, GA 00111
> phone# - 001-555-2176
>
> Patient Name_____ Date _____
> Address_____ Age _____
>
> ℞          Premarin 0.625 mg
>            #30
>            sig: i tab daily at approximately same hour
>
> _____ Refill _____
> DEA#_____

(From Fulcher RM, Fulcher E: *Math calculations for pharmacy technicians: A worktext*, St. Louis, 2007, Saunders.)

a. Inscription: _____

b. Dosage: _____

*(Continued)*

# BUILDING CONFIDENCE WITH THE SKILL 9-1
*Continued from p. 222*

c. Route: _____

d. Quantity: _____

e. Sig: _____

8.

> Lawrence Merry, M.D.
> 4th Street and Jones Ave.
> Holly, GA 00111
> phone# - 001-555-2176
>
> Patient Name_____ Date _____
> Address_____ Age _____
>
> ℞　Prednisone 10 mg
> 　　#40
> 　　sig: i tab qid x 4 d ; i tab tid x 4 d ; i tab bid x 4 d ;
> 　　i tab daily x 4
>
> _____ Refill _____
> DEA#_____

(From Fulcher RM, Fulcher E: *Math calculations for pharmacy technicians: A worktext*, St. Louis, 2007, Saunders.)

a. Inscription: _____

b. Dosage: _____

c. Route: _____

d. Quantity: _____

e. Sig: _____

## Based on the order, determine what quantity should be given.

9. The patient was admitted for dehydration. The physician has ordered 0.9NS 1000 mL q6h. How many mLs will the patient receive in 24 hours?

Solution: _____

10. The physician is writing a 4-month supply of Lasix 40 mg 1 tablet po bid with 0 refills. The patient will be spending the winter in Texas and will have all 4 months filled at one time. How many pills will the patient receive?

Solution: _____

11. The physician writes: Vancomycin 3 mg/kg q8h. The patient's weight is 75 kg.

a. How many mg of Vancomycin will the patient receive with each dose?

Solution: _____

OBJECTIVE **4**

## CONVERSION BETWEEN METRIC, APOTHECARY, AND US CUSTOMARY (HOUSEHOLD MEASUREMENTS) SYSTEMS

Many health care careers require you to convert between the metric system and the U.S. Customary (household measurements) system. In addition, on rare occasion it may be necessary to convert between all three systems of measurement. Unless you know the decimal conversion factor between the metric system and the U.S. Customary system, computations will produce an approximate answer. Many facilities provide employees with a table for conversion between metric and household measurements. Table 9-3 shows common equivalents among the three systems of measurements.

This text has discussed several methods to establish equivalency, including ratios and proportions, cross multiplication, and dimensional analysis. During the next exercises, you are encouraged to try the different methods to establish which method works best for you. Once you have found a methodology with which you are comfortable, stick with it. Accuracy is based on the way you set your problem up for computation.

OBJECTIVE **4**

# BUILDING CONFIDENCE WITH THE SKILL 9-2

---

**Solve the following conversion problems.**

1. How many millimeters are in 12 inches? _____

2. How many grams are in 5,000 micrograms? _____

3. How many pounds are in 80 Kg? _____

4. How many pints are in 5 gallons? _____

5. How many inches are in 35 mm? _____

6. How many hours are in 5,400 seconds? _____

7. How many mcg are in 5.5 G? _____

8. How many meters are in 50 inches? _____

9. How many liters are in 8 gallons? _____

10. How many mL are in 8 oz of tea? _____

11. How many pounds are in 60 kg? _____

12. How many mm are in 1 inch? _____

13. How many meters are in 30 yards? _____

---

*(Continued)*

| TABLE 9-3 | Metric Equivalents Frequently Used in Health Care |
|-----------|---------------------------------------------------|

| Metric | Apothecary | U.S. Customary (Household Measurements) |
|--------|------------|------------------------------------------|
| | 1 minim* | 1 gtt |
| 1 mL† | 15 minims | 15 gtt |
| 5 mL | | 1 tsp |
| 15 mL | | 3 tsp<br>1 Tbsp<br>½ ounce |
| 30 mL | | 6 tsp<br>2 Tbsp<br>1 ounce |
| 240 mL | 8 oz | 8 oz<br>1 cup |
| 500 mL | 16 oz | 16 oz<br>1 pt |
| 1,000 mL<br>1 liter | 32 oz | 32 oz<br>2 pt<br>1 qt |
| 4 liters | 128 oz | 1 gallon<br>4 qt |
| 2.5 cm | 1 inch | 1 inch |
| 1 decimeter | | 4 inches |
| 1 meter | | 39 inches |
| 1 km | | 0.6 mile |
| 1 mg | $\frac{1}{60}$ grain | |
| 30 mg | ½ grain | |
| 60 mg | 1 grain | |
| 1 gram | 15 grains | ¼ tsp |
| 4 grams | 60 grains | 1 tsp |
| 15 grams | | 1 Tbsp |
| 30 grams | | 2 Tbsp<br>1 oz |
| 1 kg | | 2.2 pounds |

*Because of rounding, the conversions are approximate and are not intended to provide exact conversions between the metric system and the apothecary system.*
*\*Minims and grains are not commonly used in pharmaceutical preparations.*
*†Cubic centimeter (cc) and milliliter (mL) are equal measurements; mL is the common measurement in health care practice.*

## BUILDING CONFIDENCE WITH THE SKILL 9-2
*Continued from p. 224*

14. Each DVD costs $13.50.

   a. How many DVDs could you purchase with a $125.00 gift certificate?
   _____

   b. What amount would remain on the gift certificate? _____

15. Mrs. Julie pays $30.00 per prescription. She buys six prescriptions a month. How much will Mrs. Julie pay for 6 months of prescriptions? _____

16. The nursing home staffs four nurses for every 15 beds and two nurse aides for every 20 beds. Currently, the nursing home has 98 residents.

   a. How many nurses are needed? _____

   b. How many nurse aides are needed? _____

17. The hospital staffs six phlebotomists for every 30 patients at the hospital. Currently, there are 420 patients. How many phlebotomists are needed?
   _____

18. How many tsp are in 3 oz of fluid? _____

19. How many mL are in 15 tsp of fluid? _____

20. How many mL are in 8 qt? _____

OBJECTIVE ⑤

## CONVERSION BETWEEN FAHRENHEIT AND CELSIUS TEMPERATURES

The **Fahrenheit** thermometer is based on a temperature scale proposed by Daniel Gabriel Fahrenheit in 1724. The Fahrenheit thermometer has an 180 degree separation between freezing and boiling points of water, where the freezing point of water is defined to be 32° and the boiling point of water is defined to be 212°.

The **Celsius (or Centigrade)** thermometer uses a temperature scale with a 100 degrees between boiling and freezing points of water, where water is defined to freeze at 0° and boil at 100°.

## MATH QUICK TIP 9-3
*Temperature Conversions*

A rise in temperature of 5° on the Celsius scale represents a rise in temperature of 9° on the Fahrenheit scale (Figure 9-6). Therefore, there is a 5 : 9 ratio between the Celsius and Fahrenheit scales.

$$\text{Celsius} = (F - 32) \times \frac{5}{9}$$

*(Continued)*

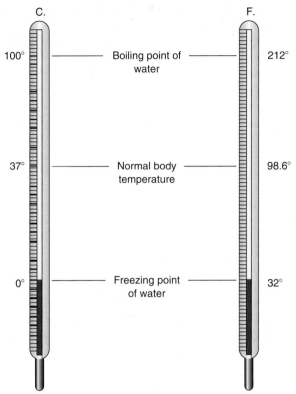

**Figure 9-6** Comparison of Celsius (left) and Fahrenheit (right) scales on a mercury thermometer. (From Asperheim MK: *Introduction to pharmacology*, ed 10, St. Louis, 2005, Saunders.)

## MATH QUICK TIP 9-3
*Continued from p. 226*

$$\text{Fahrenheit} = \left(\frac{9}{5} \times C\right) + 32$$

$$\text{Celsius} = (F - 32) \div 1.8$$

$$** \frac{5}{9} = 1.8$$

$$\text{Fahrenheit} - (C \times 1.8) + 32$$

## STRATEGY 9-1
*Converting between Celsius and Fahrenheit*

1. Use either the proportional formula,

   $$C : F - 32 :: 5 : 9$$

   or the ratio formula,

   $$C = (F - 32) \times \frac{5}{9}$$

   $$F = \frac{9 \times C}{5} + 32$$

*(Continued)*

## STRATEGY 9-1
*Continued from p. 227*

Or the decimal formula:

$C = (F - 32) \div 1.8$

$F = C \times 1.8 + 32$

2. Insert the known temperature into your formula.

3. Solve your equations for the unknown temperature.

4. Label your answer.

*Example:*

40°C is equal to _____ °F

1. Use either the proportional formula, ratio formula, or decimal formula.

$C : F - 32 :: 5 : 9$

2. Insert the known temperature into your formula.

$40 : F - 32 :: 5 : 9$

3. Solve your equations.

$40 : F - 32 :: 5 : 9$

$(F - 32) \times 5 :: 40 \times 9$

$5F - 160 :: 360$

$5F :: 520$      *By adding 160 to the left side of the equation, the −160 is canceled out, leaving only 5F. What is done to the left side must be done to the right side, so 160 was added to 360 for a total of 520.*

$\dfrac{5F}{5} :: \dfrac{520}{5}$      *Divide both sides by 5 to isolate F.*

$F = 104$

4. Label your answer.

*40°C is equal to 104°F.*

If you are still not confident with your skills with fractions use the *decimal* 1.8

$\frac{9}{5} = 1.8$

## MATH QUICK TIP 9-4

When rounding temperature values remember to round to the nearest tenth of a degree.

*Example:*

40°C is equal to _____°F.

_____ °F = (1.8 × 40°C) + 32

°F = (1.8 × 40) + 32

°F = 72 + 32

°F = 104

*Example:*

97°F is equal to _____ °C.

°C = (F − 32) × 9/5          Remember order of operations

°C = (97 − 32) × 9/5

°C = (65) × 9/5

°C = 325/9

°C = 36.1          Rounded to the nearest tenth

Here is the same problem using the decimal 1.8.

97°F is equal to _____ °C.

°C = (97 − 32) ÷ 1.8

°C = 65 ÷ 1.8

°C = 36.1

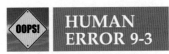

## HUMAN ERROR 9-3

*Make sure to remember to change the F to C conversion formula from multiplying by ⅖ to dividing by 1.8 if you switch from fraction to decimal.*

## PRACTICE THE SKILL 9-3

Convert the following temperatures from Celsius to Fahrenheit.

1. −20°C = _____ °F    6. −5°C = _____ °F

2. 20°C = _____ °F    7. 75°C = _____ °F

3. 32°C = _____ °F    8. 0°C = _____ °F

4. 28°C = _____ °F    9. 100°C = _____ °F

5. 45°C = _____ °F    10. 97°C = _____ °F

Convert the following temperatures from Fahrenheit to Celsius.

11. −7°F = _____ °C    16. 85°F = _____ °C

12. −2°F = _____ °C    17. 97°F = _____ °C

13. 32°F = _____ °C    18. 102°F = _____ °C

14. 55°F = _____ °C    19. 105°F = _____ °C

15. 70°F = _____ °C    20. 212°F = _____ °C

Solve the following word problems.

21. Normal body temperature is between 97°F and 99°F. What is the normal body temperature in Celsius? _____

22. The medical assistant obtains a reading of 37.8°C on the thermometer. The patient's mother would like to know what her daughter's temperature is in F. _____

23. The laboratory refrigerator is to be kept between −3 and 0 degrees C. What range would you need to keep the refrigerator with a Fahrenheit thermometer? _____

*(Continued)*

## PRACTICE THE SKILL 9-3
*Continued from p. 229*

24. The laboratory needs to incubate specimens at 99°F. What temperature would you need to incubate the specimens using a Celsius thermometer?

_____

25. The meteorologist is predicting a high temperature of 40°C. He is also projecting a heat index of 106°F.

a. What is the high temperature in F? _____

b. What is the heat index in C? _____

## CONCLUSION

Ratio and proportion computations are used on a daily basis in the clinical setting. Every division—from nursing to pharmacy to scheduling—encounters conversion problems in some form. To ensure accuracy with your computations, it is important that you establish which methodology works for you in solving equations. As this text progresses, additional methods for solving metric conversions will be introduced. Each strategy is designed to provide you with the necessary tools for accuracy in your mathematical computations.

OBJECTIVES ② ③ ④ ⑤

## MASTER THE SKILL

1. The incision is 6.5 inches long. How many centimeters is the incision?

_____

2. The drive is 7500 meters. How many kilometers is it? _____

3. The playing field is 6000 feet in length. How many yards is it?

_____

4. The incision is 45 cm. How many inches is the incision? _____

5. How many centimeters are in 6 meters? _____

6. How many drops are in 8 tsp? _____

7. How many drops are in 8 Tbsp? _____

8. How many tsp are in 3 ounces? _____

9. How many tsp are in 2 cups? _____

10. How many cups are in 4 gallons? _____

11. 750 mL is the same as _____ liters.

*(Continued)*

## MASTER THE SKILL
*Continued from p. 230*

**12.** 5.5 grams is the same as _____ milligrams.

**13.** 6 mL is the same as _____ cc.

**14.** How much will the baby weigh in lb if he weighs 10.5 kg?

_____

**15.** 10 mL is the same as _____ tsp.

**16.** 2 cups is the same as _____ ounces.

**17.** 10 lb is the same as _____ kg.

**18.** 60 mL is the same as _____ ounces.

**19.** 22 pounds is the same as _____ kg.

**20.** 3 ounces is the same as _____ G.

**21.** 60 mL is the same as _____ tsp.

**22.** 6 tsp is the same as _____ fluid ounces.

**23.** 9 ounces is the same as _____ tsp.

**24.** 70 kg is the same as _____ lb.

**25.** 3 pints is the same as _____ qt.

**26.** 6 decimeters is the same as _____ inches.

**27.** 6 yards is approximately _____ meters.

**28.** 6 tsp is the same as _____ mL.

**29.** 2 Tbsp is the same as _____ mL.

**30.** 14 quarts is the same as _____ gallons.

Convert the following temperatures.

**31.** 3°C = _____ °F    **36.** 98.6°F = _____ °C

**32.** −5°C = _____ °F    **37.** 101°F = _____ °C

**33.** 45°C = _____ °F    **38.** 103° F = _____ °C

**34.** 32°C = _____ °F    **39.** 97°F = _____ °C

**35.** 80°C = _____ °F    **40.** −10°F = _____ °C

*(Continued)*

## MASTER THE SKILL
*Continued from p. 231*

Solve the following word problems.

41. The physician orders Mylanta 1 oz.

    a. How many tsp should you give? _____

    b. How many mL should you give? _____

42. The physician orders 1 gallon of liquid preparation to be given over a 3-hour period.

    a. How many 8-ounce glasses does the patient need to drink in the 3-hour period? _____

    b. How many milliliters of liquid preparation does the patient drink in the 3-hour period? _____

    c. Approximately how many liters are in 1 gallon? _____

43. The physician is monitoring the fluid intake of the patient during mealtime. Based on the following information, how many milliliters did the patient drink at breakfast? _____

    | | |
    |---|---|
    | Juice | 4 ounces |
    | Milk | 4 ounces |
    | Coffee | 8 ounces |

44. Based on the following information, what is the total amount of milliliters did the patient consumed in a 24-hour period? _____

    | Breakfast | Lunch | Snack | Dinner | Snack |
    |---|---|---|---|---|
    | Juice 8 oz | Soda 4 oz | Water 8 oz | Soda 8 oz | Milk 4 oz |
    | Milk 4 oz | Tea 8 oz | | Tea 8 oz | |
    | Coffee 8 oz | Frozen ice 8 oz | | Broth 8 oz | |

45. The consumer receives 2 Tbsp of cough medicine three times a day (tid). How many mL will the consumer receive in a 24-hour period?

    _____

46. You have Tylenol, 325 mg/tablet. You need to give 650 mg of Tylenol. How many tablets do you give? _____

47. You are to give Amoxil 450 mg PO. You have a liquid suspension of Amoxil 100 mg/2 mL. How much should you give?

    _____

48. The school asked you to bring in 1 kL of soda for a party. The soda comes in 2 L containers. How many containers do you need?

    _____

*(Continued)*

## MASTER THE SKILL
*Continued from p. 232*

**49.** The patient's weight is 200 lb. You are to give 5 mg/kg of cough medicine. How many mg of cough medicine should you give?

_____

**50.** The patient is to receive 2½ tsp of medication four times a day. The medication label reads: 15 mg/5 mL.

    a. How many mg does the patient receive with each dose?

    _____

    b. How many tsp of medication are given in a 24-hour period?

    _____

    c. How many mg of medication does the patient receive in a 24-hour period? _____

Identify the common abbreviations for the following descriptions.

**51.** Hour of sleep _____

**52.** Once a day _____

**53.** Four times a day _____

**54.** Twice a day _____

**55.** Every 8 hours _____

Identify how often (the frequency) for each of the following orders.

**56.** Lasix 80 mg p.o. bid _____

**57.** Digoxin 0.125 mg p.o. qd _____

**58.** Slow-K 10 mEq p.o. bid _____

**59.** CBC qid × 4 days _____

**60.** Cephalexin 500 mg tid × 10 d _____

## CHAPTER OUTLINE

## LEARNING OBJECTIVES

*Upon completion of this chapter, the learner will be able to:*

1. Define the key terms that relate to the chapter.

2. Describe movement of the decimal when working with the metric system.

3. Multiplication and Division by the Power of 10.

4. Define significant figures.

5. Rewrite problems using standard scientific notation.

6. Use a calculator to solve problems written in standard scientific notation.

OBJECTIVE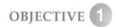

## KEY TERMS

| | |
|---|---|
| Exponent | Significant Figures |
| Mental Math | Standard Scientific Notation |

OBJECTIVE

In this chapter, we discuss strategies for reducing very large or very small numbers by using the principles of power of 10 or writing numbers in scientific notation. **Exponents** are used to represent large base 10 numbers and when writing numbers in scientific notation. If you are unsure of how to manipulate exponents or negative numbers, you might want to review the relevant sections in Chapter 1.

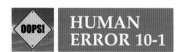

### HUMAN ERROR 10-1

*When dealing with very small numbers scientific notation is written in negative exponents.*

$0.000003 = 3 \times 10^{-6}$
OR
$0.0000000000234$
$= 2.34 \times 10^{-11}$

### MATH QUICK TIP 10-1

Scientific notation is shorthand for writing really large or small numbers.
    Which number would you like to deal with?
    3,400,000 or $3.4 \times 10^{6}$
    34,000,000,000,000 would be converted into $3.4 \times 10^{13}$

# POWER OF 10

In Chapter 7, you learned the prefixes that are used in the metric system. Because the metric system is based on the power of 10, it is common to solve the conversion problems using **mental math** or manipulation of the decimal point. Table 10-1 demonstrates the power of 10 written as an exponent and as the multiplier.

Because the metric system is based on the factor 10, conversion problems are often solved by simply moving the decimal point to either the right or the left.

## PRACTICE THE SKILL 10-1

Write the following numbers as exponents.

1. 100 _____

2. 10,000 _____

3. 1,000,000 _____

4. 1,000 _____

5. 100,000 _____

6. 0.001 _____

7. 0.000001 _____

8. 0.00001 _____

9. 0.01 _____

10. 0.000000001 _____

## TABLE 10-1    *Metric Prefixes as Power of 10*

| Prefix | Multiplier | Power of 10 |
|--------|------------|-------------|
| Micro- | 0.000001 | $10^{-6}$ |
| Milli- | 0.001 | $10^{-3}$ |
| Centi- | 0.01 | $10^{-2}$ |
| Deci- | 0.1 | $10^{-1}$ |
| Deka- | 10 | 10 |
| Hecto- | 100 | $10^{2}$ |
| Kilo- | 1,000 | $10^{3}$ |

OBJECTIVE **3**    ## MULTIPLICATION AND DIVISION BY THE POWER OF 10

Before we begin our discussion on multiplication and division of exponents, we should review the Laws of Exponents.

| Law of exponents | Example |
|---|---|
| When multiplying exponents, with the same bases, **ADD** the exponents. | $X^3$ times $X^4 = X^{3+4} = X^7$ |
| When dividing exponents, with the same bases, **SUBRTACT** the exponents. | $\dfrac{X^7}{X^5} = X^{7-5} = X^2$ |
| When you raise a power to a power, **MULTIPLY** the exponents. | $(X^3)^5 = X^{3 \cdot 5} = X^{15}$ |
| When a product or a quotient is raised to a power, **RAISE** each factor to the power. | $(XY)^4 = X^4 \cdot Y^4$ |
| | $\left(\dfrac{X}{Y}\right)^4 = \dfrac{X^4}{Y^4}$ |
| Any non-zero number with a **ZERO** power is 1. | $X^0 = 1$ |
| Any number with a **NEGATIVE** power is written as a fraction. 1 in the numerator and the number raised to a positive power in the denominator. | $X^{-6} = \dfrac{1}{X^6}$ |
| 1 divided by any number raised to a **NEGATIVE** power is that number raised to a **POSITIVE** power. | $\dfrac{1}{X^{-9}} = X^9$ |
| A fraction raised to the **NEGATIVE** power is the reciprocal of the fraction raised to the **POSITIVE** power. | $\left(\dfrac{X}{Y}\right)^{-4} = \left(\dfrac{Y}{X}\right)^4$ |

When working with two numbers expressed using exponents, if their *bases are the same* then you can easily compute multiplication and division of the numbers. To obtain the result of multiplying the two numbers, simply *add* their exponents. Similarly, to divide the two numbers, you would *subtract* the exponents to obtain the answer.

| Scientific notation | Expanded form |
|---|---|
| $1 \times 10^{-9}$ | 0.0000000001 |
| $1 \times 10^{-6}$ | 0.000001 |
| $1 \times 10^{-3}$ | 0.001 |
| $1 \times 10^{-2}$ | 0.01 |
| $1 \times 10^{0}$ | 1 |
| $1 \times 10^{3}$ | 1,000 |
| $1 \times 10^{6}$ | 1,000,000 |
| $1 \times 10^{9}$ | 1,000,000,000 |

## MATH QUICK TIP 10-2

When counting zeros, the student must remember to include the zero in front of the decimal in order to get the correct number of zeros.

$10^{-2} = 0.01$ (Hundredths place)

Incorrect answer would be .001 (Thousandths place)

*Example:*

$100 \times 1,000$

1. Write the equation as a power of 10.
   $10^2 \times 10^3$

2. The operation is multiplication; add the exponents to obtain the answer.
   $10^{2+3}$

3. The answer is $10^5$.

*Example:*

$10,000 \div 100$

1. Write the equation as a power of 10.
   $10^4 \div 10^2$

2. The operation is division; subtract the exponents to obtain the answer.
   $10^{4-2}$

3. The answer is $10^2$.

## PRACTICE THE SKILL 10-2

Rewrite the problems using the power of 10. Solve the problem, keeping your answer in the power of 10 format.

1. $10 \times 100$ _____

2. $1,000 \times 10,000$ _____

3. $100 \times 100,000$ _____

4. $10 \times 10 \times 100$ _____

5. $1,000 \times 1,000,000$ _____

6. $1,000 \times 100 \times 10$ _____

7. $0.1 \times 0.001$ _____

8. $0.00001 \times 10$ _____

9. $0.001 \times 0.000001$ _____

10. $0.001 \times 0.0001 \times 0.1$ _____

11. $1,000,000 \div 1,000$ _____

12. $100 \div 1,000,000$ _____

13. $10 \div 0.001$ _____

14. $0.01 \div 0.001$ _____

15. $100 \div 10,000$ _____

*(Continued)*

# PRACTICE THE SKILL 10-2
*Continued from p. 237*

**16.** 0.001 ÷ 100 _____

**17.** 0.00000001 ÷ 0.00001 _____

**18.** 100,000 ÷ 100,000,000 _____

**19.** 100,000,000 ÷ 1,000 _____

**20.** 0.001 ÷ 100 _____

Another way to calculate with positive powers is to count the number of 0s and move your decimal point the same amount to the right (multiply) or left (division). Like many people, you may be able to perform this operation in your head. However, explaining how you solved the problem can be difficult. Let's break down the steps that you may be doing in your head.

# STRATEGY 10-1
*Multiplication of Positive Powers*

1. Identify which operation is being performed—multiplication or division.

2. Count the number of 0s in the multiplier.

3. Move the decimal point that number of places to the right.

   *Example:*
   14.118 × 100
   1. Identify which operation is being performed—multiplication or division.
      *multiplication*
   2. Count the number of 0s in the multiplier.
      *100 is the multiplier, and it has two 0s.*
   3. Move the decimal point two places to the right.
      14.118 = 1411.8

The correct answer is 1411.8.

# STRATEGY 10-2
*Division of Positive Powers*

1. Identify which operation is being performed—multiplication or division.

2. Count the number of 0s in the divisor.

3. Move the decimal point that number of places to the left.

*(Continued)*

## STRATEGY 10-2
*Continued from p. 238*

*Example:*

$310199.1 \div 10,000$

1. Identify which operation is being performed—multiplication or division.
   *division*

2. Count the number of 0s in the divisor.
   *10,000 is the divisor, and there are four 0s.*

3. Move the decimal point four places to the left.
   310199.1

The correct answer is 31.01991.

## STRATEGY 10-3
*Multiplication and Division by Negative Exponents*

*Example:* $3 \times 10^{-3}$    $0.001 = 10^{-3}$

Multiplying by 0.001 would mean you move the decimal to the **left** 3 digits.
$3 \times 0.001 = 0.003$

Dividing by 0.001 would mean you move the digit to the **right** 3 digits.
$3 \div 0.001 = 3,000$

## PRACTICE THE SKILL 10-3

Complete the following table.

Do not use a calculator; this is a mental math skill.

| Problem | Which Direction is the Decimal Moving? | How Many Places Will the Decimal Move? | Answer |
|---|---|---|---|
| 1. 892.0491 × 100 | | | |
| 2. 45.00872 × 1,000 | | | |
| 3. 275632.1 ÷ 100,000 | | | |
| 4. 517199.5 ÷ 1,000 | | | |
| 5. 11.44 × 10 | | | |
| 6. 92519.64 ÷ 100 | | | |
| 7. 621.3589 × 100 | | | |
| 8. 6213.589 ÷ 100 | | | |
| 9. 321.557 × 10 | | | |
| 10. 873259.3 ÷ 100,000 | | | |

*(Continued)*

## PRACTICE THE SKILL 10-3
*Continued from p. 239*

Find the solution for the following problems:

**11.** $4.56 \div 10^{-5} =$ _____

**12.** $3.22 \div 10^{-3} =$ _____

**13.** $7.8931 \div 10^{-6} =$ _____

**14.** $985.4611 \div 10^{-2} =$ _____

**15.** $0.002 \div 10^{-7} =$ _____

**16.** $5.7316459 \times 10^{-8} =$ _____

**17.** $0.008971 \times 10^{-6} =$ _____

**18.** $2.0056 \times 10^{-2} =$ _____

**19.** $3.4521 \times 10^{-9} =$ _____

**20.** $6754.234169 \times 10^{-8} =$ _____

## Conversion between Metric Units

Chapter 5 discussed the way to set up proportions and ratios so that you could convert between metric measurements to find the equivalent value. Since the metric system is based on the power of 10, many students find it easier to convert similar measurements by manipulating the decimal point rather than setting up the problem as a proportion. When the conversion is from a larger to a smaller metric unit, the decimal point moves to the right. When a smaller metric unit is being converted to a larger one, the decimal point moves to the left (Table 10-2).

## MATH IN THE REAL WORLD 10-1
*Conversions Found in Health Care*

- Millimeters to centimeters
- Centimeters to meters
- Milliliters to liters
- Milligrams to grams
- Grams to kilograms

See Figure 7-1.

| TABLE 10-2 | *Movement of Decimal Points* |
|---|---|

| Direction of Movement in Problem | Movement of Decimal | Multiply by Multiplier? | Divide by Multiplier? |
|---|---|---|---|
| From a larger metric unit to a smaller metric unit | Right | Yes | No |
| From a smaller metric unit to a larger metric unit | Left | No | Yes |

*Example:*

How many micrograms are in 0.5 mg?

1. We know that micrograms are smaller than milligrams, so move the decimal to the right.

2. Micrograms are represented as $10^{-6}$.

3. Milligrams are represented as $10^{-3}$.

4. Move the decimal over three places to the right.
   0.500

5. Answer: There are 500 mcg in 0.5 mg.

Many times people have difficulty not with the actual calculation, but with the proper way to set up the problem. In the next exercise, the goal is to assist you in applying strategies that will build your confidence in setting up math problems.

## BUILDING CONFIDENCE WITH THE SKILL 10-1

Complete the following table.

| Problem | Movement of Decimal: Right or Left | Mathematical Operation: Multiplication or Division |
|---|---|---|
| 1. 0.15 g to mg | | |
| 2. 0.25 mL to dL | | |
| 3. 500 mg to G | | |
| 4. 1.75 cm to mm | | |
| 5. 5 mm to m | | |
| 6. 2 L to dL | | |
| 7. 3500 mL to L | | |
| 8. 0.04 mg to mcg | | |
| 9. 2.5 G to mg | | |
| 10. 1500 mL to L | | |
| 11. 300 hm to m | | |
| 12. 4.5 km to m | | |
| 13. 750 mg to G | | |
| 14. 800 mcg to G | | |
| 15. 2 L to mL | | |

OBJECTIVE  **SIGNIFICANT FIGURES**

To what place value should answers be rounded? Significant figures are utilized when reporting scientific data obtained during testing or research. However, using significant figures will depend on what the problem is asking. In other words, report the answer to the question in a value that not only makes sense but also answers the question.

*Example:*
While at the grocery store, Ashley purchases the following items:

| | | |
|---|---|---|
| Bananas | 3 pounds | Cost: $0.59/pound |
| Bread | 2 loaves | $1.89/loaf |
| Potatoes | 5 pound bag | $1.50/pound |
| Chicken soup | 3 cans | $0.79/can |

What is the total cost of the bill before sales tax? What is the price of the bill with a 6.5% sales tax?

The question discusses money (dollars and cents), which indicates that the answer should be reflected in the hundredths place value.

**Significant figures** represent the precision of the measurement with which you are working. Your answer should reflect the least precision that is necessary or have the same number of significant figures as your smallest value. Whether rounding is appropriate in calculating a dosage depends on the medication, the method of delivery, and the way in which the medication is manufactured.

 **MATH QUICK TIP 10-3**

1. All non-zero numbers are always significant.
   *Example:* 1, 2, 3, 4, 5, 6, 7, 8, 9

2. If a number contains a 0, the 0 is considered a significant figure.
   *Example:* 456,709,288   There are nine significant figures.

3. In a number without a decimal point, only zeros between non-zero digits are significant.
   *Example:* 39,800   There are three significant figures, and the zeros are placeholders.

4. In a number with a decimal point, all zeros to the right of the first non-zero digits are significant.
   *Example:* 0.009310   There are only four significant figures.

 **MATH IN THE REAL WORLD 10-2**
*Devices for Measurement*

- Distance: rulers, tape measures, height charts

- Weight: scales

- Volume: beakers, medicine cups, measuring cups, test tubes

- Temperature

# MATH IN THE REAL WORLD 10-3

Areas that use significant figures:

- Laboratory
- Pharmacology
- Engineering development and manufacturing of devices
- Research
- Biomedical areas

# PRACTICE THE SKILL 10-4

Identify how many significant figures are in the following numbers.

1. 4,506,132 _____
2. 132,567,901 _____
3. 1,254 _____
4. 600 _____
5. 12,768,000 _____
6. 12.4056 _____
7. 0.0398 _____
8. 1.320 _____

9. 0.00460 _____
10. 0.79801 _____
11. 12,009 _____
12. 5.0670 _____
13. 1,450 _____
14. 876,092,356,000 _____
15. 78.02330 _____

## Performing Mathematical Computations with Significant Figures

# MATH QUICK TIP 10-4

OBJECTIVE **4**

1. When significant figures are added or subtracted, the answer is expressed in the same place value as the least significant figure.
   *Example:* 2.34 + 1.5 + 6.789 = 10.629   The answer is 10.6.

2. Multiplication and division answers should contain the same number of significant figures as the smallest significant in the problem.
   *Example:* 0.53 × 0.0475 = 0.025175   The answer is 0.025.

3. Depending on the purpose of the calculation, the answer may be rounded off.

## PRACTICE THE SKILL 10-5

Solve the following problems. Identify the place value in which the answer is expressed.

**a.** Write your answers in significant figures *without* rounding.

**b.** Write your answers in significant figures *with* rounding.

**1.**    2.354
        6.34
      + 7.08

        a. _____

        b. _____

**2.**    4567.0980
            2.345
      +      1.65456

        a. _____

        b. _____

**3.**    0.25
        0.40
        0.333
      + 1.5

        a. _____

        b. _____

**4.**    5.76
        2.35
        0.15
      + 2.2

        a. _____

        b. _____

**5.**      56.78
         4670.12
            9.0089
      +      0.5478

        a. _____

        b. _____

**6.**    123.7866
      −   23.005

        a. _____

        b. _____

**7.**    0.892
      − 0.0012

        a. _____

        b. _____

**8.**    12.45
      −  6.3

        a. _____

        b. _____

**9.**    25.5
      −  3.569

        a. _____

        b. _____

**10.**    0.0795
      −  0.00254

        a. _____

        b. _____

**11.**    4.67
      × 0.025

        a. _____

        b. _____

*(Continued)*

## PRACTICE THE SKILL 10-5
*Continued from p. 244*

12.　15.67
　　× 9.87

a. _____

b. _____

13.　0.975
　　× 1.250

a. _____

b. _____

14.　0.5423
　　× 0.0027

a. _____

b. _____

15.　0.009013
　　× 2.5

a. _____

b. _____

16.　75.25
　　÷ 3.32

a. _____

b. _____

17.　450.009
　　÷ 0.33

a. _____

b. _____

18.　6798.002
　　÷ 12.44

a. _____

b. _____

19.　0.0045
　　÷ 0.015

a. _____

b. _____

20.　2.008
　　÷ 0.804

a. _____

b. _____

## STANDARD SCIENTIFIC NOTATION

OBJECTIVE 5

**Standard scientific** notation is commonly used to avoid errors when calculations have very small or large numbers. Scientific notation uses the power of 10 as an exponent and a number that is greater than 1 and less than 10. Numbers that are less than 1 can be written using a negative exponent.

　Standard scientific notation is written with the number (less than 10) multiplied by 10 to a specific power.

*Example:*

23,600,000 can be written as $2.36 \times 10^7$.

First, we need to determine a number less than 10. In this case, place a decimal between 2 and 36. Second, count how many place values the decimal moved to obtain 2.36. In this case, it was 7. Thus, 7 is now our exponent.

Let's try a few examples using positive and negative exponents.

*Example:*

25,000

Move the decimal four spaces and place it between the 2 and 5.

$2.5 \times 10^4$ is the answer.

*Examples:*

1. 210

   $2.1 \times 10^2$

   For negative exponents, the decimal is moved to the left.

2. 0.00004

   $4 \times 10^{-5}$

   Start with 4 and move 5 decimal places to the left. Results in 0.00004.

3. 0.0015

   $1.5 \times 10^{-3}$

## MATH QUICK TIP 10-5

Numbers that are less than 1 use a negative exponent.

*Example:* 0.005   $5 \times 10^{-3}$

10 to the 0 power is equal to 1.
10 to the first power is equal to 10.

## MATH QUICK TIP 10-6

1. When multiplying numbers with exponents, the numbers are multiplied and the exponents are added.

   *Example:* $(5 \times 10^2) \times (4 \times 10^3) =$

   Numbers:     $5 \times 4 = 20$
   Exponents:   $2 + 3 = 5$
   Answer:      $20 \times 10^5$

2. When dividing numbers with exponents, the exponents are subtracted.

   *Example:* $(9 \times 10^4) \div (3 \times 10^2)$

   Divide:      $9 \div 3 = 3$
   Exponents:   $4 - 2 = 2$
   Answer:      $3 \times 10^2$

## PRACTICE THE SKILL 10-6

Rewrite the following equations using scientific format.

1. 3,500 _____     6. 0.0002 _____

2. 6,230,000,000 _____     7. 0.056 _____

3. 5,670,000 _____     8. 0.000003 _____

4. 220 _____     9. 0.00037 _____

5. 6,700,000,000 _____     10. 0.000054 _____

If you need to refresh your skills with positive and negative numbers, refer to Chapter 1 of this text or speak to your instructor for assistance.

## BUILDING CONFIDENCE WITH THE SKILL 10-2

Solve the following problems. Write your answers in Arabic format.

1. $9.62 \times 10^3 =$ _____

2. $76.89 \times 10^{-5} =$ _____

3. $5.67 \times 10^2 =$ _____

4. $12.54 \times 10^{-6} =$ _____

5. $1345.2 \times 10 =$ _____

6. $0.0045 \times 10^4 =$ _____

7. $0.00000098 \times 10^7 =$ _____ $=$ _____

8. $1.32 \times 10^{-6} =$ _____

9. $8.9 \times 10^{-9} =$ _____

10. $6.55 \times 10^6 =$ _____

Solve the following problems.

11. $(4.45 \times 10^3) + (2.25 \times 10^2) =$ _____

12. $(3.15 \times 10^3) + (0.02 \times 10) =$ _____

*(Continued)*

# BUILDING CONFIDENCE WITH THE SKILL 10-2
*Continued from p. 247*

13. $(0.002 \times 10^{-3}) + (1.2 \times 10^{3}) =$ _____

14. $(0.0015 \times 10^{4}) - (0.00007 \times 10^{2}) =$ _____

15. $(2.7 \times 10^{5}) \div 0.66 =$ _____

16. $(0.33 \times 10^{-3}) \times (0.2 \times 10) =$ _____

17. $(4.5 \times 10^{3}) \div (2.2 \times 10^{-2}) =$ _____

18. $(3.4 \times 10^{7}) \div (2.2 \times 10^{5}) =$ _____

19. $(8.1 \times 10^{9}) \div (2.7 \times 10^{3}) =$ _____

20. $(3.5 \times 10^{-5}) - (5.7 \times 10^{-3}) =$ _____

OBJECTIVE **6**    ## COMPUTATIONS WITH CALCULATORS

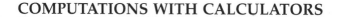

Scientific calculators are useful tools for performing calculations written in scientific notation. They can be confusing because of the multitude of functions and symbol keys. In addition, calculator buttons and functions are not universal. Before you complete the next practice session, find the directions for your calculator. Read over the sections regarding inputting exponents and scientific notation. Play around with your calculator to solve the questions. Make sure you are comfortable. Your calculator can be your best friend or the most infuriating piece of equipment in the office.

# MATH IN THE REAL WORLD 10-4

How to enter scientific notation in a scientific calculator:

1. Enter the digit number into your calculator.

2. Press the EE or EXP button. Do not use the multiplication button.

3. Enter the exponent number. If the exponent is negative, use the +/– button to make the exponent negative.

4. The answer should appear.

*Example:*
$6.0 \times 10^{5}$ times $4.0 \times 10^{3}$
If you entered the problem into the computer correctly, your answer should be $2.4 \times 10^{9}$.

## PRACTICE THE SKILL 10-7

Using a calculator, compute the following problems. Write your answers in Arabic format.

1. $3.56 \times 10^{-4} =$ _____

2. $5.78 \times 10^{6} =$ _____

3. $0.009 \times 10^{-2} =$ _____

4. $3.469 \times 10^{-5} =$ _____

5. $0.000304 \times 10^{3} =$ _____

6. $[(3.22 \times 10^{5})(0.891 \times 10^{-2})] =$ _____

7. $[(6.75 \times 10^{4})(2.33 \times 10^{2})] =$ _____

8. $[67.8 \times 10]^{3} =$ _____

9. $[5.556 \times 10]^{2} =$ _____

10. $[0.025 \times 10]^{2} =$ _____

11. $(3.45 \times 10^{-2}) \div (1.23 \times 10^{1}) =$ _____

12. $8 \times 10^{9} =$ _____

13. $0.005 \times 10^{4} =$ _____

14. $0.0009 \times 10^{-3} =$ _____

15. $(45.2 \times 10^{6}) + (2.35 \times 10^{-4}) + (0.008 \times 10^{2}) =$ _____

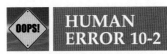

### HUMAN ERROR 10-2

*Make sure to use the parenthesis when entering the problems into your calculator. Order of operations matter to the calculator too, and if you forget them, your answers will be incorrect.*

## BUILDING CONFIDENCE WITH THE SKILL 10-3

Solve the following problems with the use of your calculator. Write your answers in Arabic format (a) and scientific notation (b).

1. $(9.4 \times 10^{4}) \times (8.2 \times 10^{2}) =$

   a. _____

   b. _____

2. $(6.73 \times 10^{2}) \times (8.2 \times 10^{3}) =$

   a. _____

   b. _____

*(Continued)*

## BUILDING CONFIDENCE WITH THE SKILL 10-3
*Continued from p. 249*

*Continued from p. 249*

**3.** $(3.1 \times 10^2)^2 =$

   a. _____

   b. _____

**4.** $(7.25 \times 10)^3 =$

   a. _____

   b. _____

**5.** $(6.1 \times 10^2) \div (3.4 \times 10) =$

   a. _____

   b. _____

**6.** $(4.7 \times 10^{-2}) \div (9.38 \times 10^{-3}) =$

   a. _____

   b. _____

**7.** $(9.3 \times 10^3) + (7.2 \times 10^2) =$

   a. _____

   b. _____

**8.** $(1.1 \times 10^{-2}) + (8.9 \times 10^{-4}) =$

   a. _____

   b. _____

**9.** $(8.0 \times 10^2) - (7.3 \times 10^3) =$

   a. _____

   b. _____

**10.** $(4.1 \times 10^{-1}) - (3.7 \times 10^{-1}) =$

   a. _____

   b. _____

**11.** $(8.6 \times 10^4) \div (3.1 \times 10^2) =$

   a. _____

   b. _____

**12.** $(2.31 \times 10^2) \div (8.9 \times 10) =$

   a. _____

   b. _____

**13.** $(9.235 \times 10^{-3}) \div (1.814 \times 10^{-3}) =$

   a. _____

   b. _____

**14.** $(2.6 \times 10^{-4}) \div (6.2 \times 10^{-3}) =$

   a. _____

   b. _____

**15.** $(6.66 \times 10) + (2.25 \times 10^2) =$

   a. _____

   b. _____

**16.** $(2.7 \times 10^{-2}) + (8.9 \times 10^{-3}) =$

   a. _____

   b. _____

**17.** $4.5 \times 10^3 =$

   a. _____

   b. _____

**18.** $6.3 \times 10^2 =$

   a. _____

   b. _____

**19.** $3.5 \times 10^{-2} =$

   a. _____

   b. _____

**20.** $5.7 \times 10^{-3} =$

   a. _____

   b. _____

## CONCLUSION

In this chapter, we have introduced you to the basic use of the concepts regarding the power of 10 and standard scientific notation and principles for rounding. With the evolution and expansion of the biomedical fields, research, biomedical engineering, and pharmacology, the use of scientific notation and significant figures are becoming more prevalent in the health care arena. It is important that all health care workers know of how and when to use this form of computation.

## MASTER THE SKILL

OBJECTIVES ③ ④ ⑤ ⑥

Determine the number of significant figures in the following numbers.

1. 2,580,593 _____

2. 9587.0083 _____

3. 9107.022 _____

4. 354,500 _____

5. 86,510.0 _____

6. 871.0 _____

7. 0.0913 _____

8. 0.04312 _____

9. 0.000128 _____

10. 926.9 _____

11. 707 _____

12. 132.005 _____

13. 0.86120 _____

14. 833.009 _____

15. 20 _____

Solve the following problems. The correct answer should reflect the correct significant figure.

16.    65.23
      2.345
      0.098
  + 23.11

17.    13.2456
     0.809766
     3.4456
  + 0.0023654

18.    567.009
      2.34432
  + 78.099

*(Continued)*

## MASTER THE SKILL
*Continued from p. 251*

19.    502.100
       43.5000
    + 206.43300

20.    892.0491
       520.8383
    + 504.5988

21.    439.008
    −    6.54

22.    0.10954
    − 0.00321

23.    67.80900
    −  0.453000

24.    90.34
    −  6.789

25.    1678.044
    −  348.220

26.    211.5
    ×   2.48

27.    1.395
    × 2.898

28.    13.25
    ×   2.2

29.    0.75
    × 0.020

30.    0.008
    × 0.0225

31.    3.68
    ÷ 0.94

32.    15.2
    ÷   3.7

33.    2.103
    ÷ 0.03

34.    5.609
    ÷ 9.03

35.    0.12159
    ÷ 0.009

Express the following numbers using standard scientific notation.

36. 0.00037 _____

37. 1,400,000 _____

38. 0.00766 _____

39. 3.57000 _____

40. 0.000009 _____

41. 20 _____

42. 600 _____

43. 75,000 _____

44. 0.00065 _____

Solve the following problems.

45. $(9.62 \times 10^3) (4.21 \times 10^2) =$ _____

46. $(3.95 \times 10^4) (4.44 \times 10) =$ _____

*(Continued)*

## MASTER THE SKILL
*Continued from p. 252*

47. $(6.91 \times 10^{-3})(9.58 \times 10) =$ _____

48. $(8.6 \times 10^4) \div (3.1 \times 10^2) =$ _____

49. $(2.31 \times 10^2) \div (8.9 \times 10) =$ _____

50. $(9.235 \times 10^{-3}) \div (1.814 \times 10^{-3}) =$ _____

Using your calculator, solve the following problems.

51. $(5.5 \times 10^3)^2 =$ _____

52. $(7.7 \times 10^{-2})^2 =$ _____

53. $(1.7 \times 10^{-3})^3 =$ _____

54. $(2.6 \times 10^{-4}) \div (6.2 \times 10^{-3}) =$ _____

55. $(6.66 \times 10) + (2.25 \times 10^2) =$ _____

56. $(3.5 \times 10^{-2}) - (5.7 \times 10^{-3}) =$ _____

Solve the following word problems, using the power of 10. Write your answers in Arabic (a) and scientific notation (b).

57. In a 24-hour period, the patient drank 4.5 L of fluid. How many mL did the patient drink?

    a. _____

    b. _____

58. The patient is receiving the following IV fluids:
    Antibiotics 0.1 L × 3 doses
    IV for hydration 1 L × 2 bags
    Blood pressure medication 0.5 L

    Calculate the total amount of IV fluids in mL that the patient has received.

    a. _____

    b. _____

59. The patient has received 150,000 mg of antibiotics in a 24-hour period. How many grams has the patient received?

    a. _____

    b. _____

*(Continued)*

## MASTER THE SKILL
*Continued from p. 253*

60. A premature infant's weight is 3,500 G. How many kg does the infant weigh?

    a. _____

    b. _____

61. The patient's incision is 4 cm in length. How many mm long is the incision site?

    a. _____

    b. _____

62. The physician wrote the following order for antibiotics: 3 mg/kg three times a day × 10 days. The patient's weight is 25 kg. How much medication will the patient receive in a 24-hour period?

    a. _____

    b. _____

63. What is the total amount of antibiotics the patient from question 62 will receive over the 10-day period?

    a. _____

    b. _____

64. The patient's wound drained 0.35 L of fluid in a 12-hour period. How many mL has the wound drained?

    a. _____

    b. _____

65. An infant is receiving 15 mg/kg of antibiotics twice a day. The infant's weight is 18 lbs. How many milligrams of antibiotic will the infant receive in one dose?

    a. _____

    b. _____

# Algebraic Equations and Introduction to Statistics

## CHAPTER OUTLINE

## LEARNING OBJECTIVES

*Upon completion of this chapter, the learner will be able to:*

1. Define the key terms that relate to the chapter.

2. Identify the difference between like and unlike terms.

3. Solve algebraic equations with like terms with 100% accuracy.

4. Solve algebraic equations with unlike terms with 100% accuracy.

5. Compute mean, median, and mode with 100% accuracy.

6. Identify how samples can be obtained.

7. Determine the probability of an occurrence.

8. Discuss how basic statistics are utilized in the health care fields.

9. Establish variances and standard deviation for a data set.

## KEY TERMS

Arithmetic Average
Bimodal
Census
Coefficients
Continuous Data
Discrete Data
Exponents
Mean
Median
Mode
Outlier
Polymodal

Probability
Qualitative Data
Quantitative Data
Random Sampling
Range
Sample
Standard Deviation
Statistics
Target Sampling
Terms
Variables
Variance

Throughout the majority of this textbook, you have been asked to solve problems with only one variable "X." We are now going to discuss how to solve Algebraic equations with one or more variables. **Terms in an algebraic equation** are numbers and variables, letters which represent unknown values, that are combined into numeric expressions using rational number operations such as +, −, ×, and ÷. Where the frustration occurs with students is trying to decide where to start with a problem.

## LIKE TERMS

When two terms have the same variables and/or the same variables with the same exponents they are considered **Like Terms**.

Examples of Like Terms: x and 6x          or          $7xy^2z^3$ and $-3xy^2z^3$
Examples of Non Like Terms: 3x and 3y          or          $12x^2y$ and $6xy^2$

When adding or subtracting like terms, first you should add or subtract the coefficients, and keep the variables and exponents the same.

*Examples:*
**a.** $x + 2x = 3x$                **b.** $7xy^2z^3 - 3xy^2z^3 = 4xy^2z^3$
**c.** $12x + 3y - 7x = 5x + 3y$                **d.** $3(2x - 5) - x = 6x - 15 - x = 5x - 15$

## SOLVING EQUATIONS

Equations are two (or more) expressions that are equivalent separated by an equal sign. To solve equations for a variable, use inverse operations to "undo" operations on the variable. To keep the equation "balanced," whatever operation is done to one side of the equal sign must also be done to the other side.

 **STRATEGY 11-1**

Strategy for solving equations.

*Example:* x − 6 = 18
1. What is the equation really saying?
   *What number minus 6 equals 18*
   Keep the equation "balanced" by adding 6 to both sides. Why are we adding 6 to each side? In order to solve for x we must get x by itself.
2. x − 6 = 18
   x = 24
3. Check Solution by placing answer into the equation.
   24 − 6 = 18
   Strategy for solving equations with more than one variable:

*Example:* 12x + 3y − 7x = 5x + 3y
1. Identify your variables.
   X and Y
2. Combine your variables if possible.
   12x − 7x + 3y = 5x + 3y
3. Simplify your equation.
   5x + 3y = 5x + 3y
4. Solution to problem is: 5x + 3y = 5x + 3y

## PRACTICE THE SKILL 11-1

Solving equations with one variable.

**1.** X – 3 = 4 _____

**2.** 10t = 50 _____

**3.** W/7 = 3 _____

**4.** (3/4)y = 12 _____

**5.** 2x + 3 = 5 _____

**6.** (4x + 1)/3 = 7 _____

**7.** 25t = 125 _____

**8.** 125y = 875 _____

**9.** 2x + 15 = 90 _____

**10.** 3t – 48 = –3 _____

**11.** x – 4 = 13 _____

**12.** f + 7 = 19 _____

**13.** 3 – x = 12 _____

**14.** –v + 6 = 13 _____

**15.** t ÷ 8 = 64 _____

**16.** w/4 = –13 _____

**17.** 5x = 420 _____

**18.** 26 = –3x _____

**19.** 7d – 8 = 41 _____

## STRATEGY 11-2

Variables on both sides of the equation.

*Example:* $3x + 1 = 5x + 9$

**1.** Get the variable you are solving for on one side of the equal sign; get all other terms on the other side using the inverse operations.
$3x + 1 = 5x + 9$
Using the distributive property     $3x + 1 - 3x - 9 = 5x + 9 - 3x - 9$

**2.** Combine all like terms.
$-8 = 2x$

**3.** Divide both sides by the coefficient in front of the variable so that the variable is alone.
$$\frac{-8}{2} = \frac{2x}{2}$$
$-4 = x$

**4.** Insert the answer into the equation as the variables to check results
$3x - 4 + 1 = 5x - 4 + 9$
$-12 + 1 = -20 + 9$
$11 = 11$

## MATH QUICK TIP 11-1

Reminder for Order of Operations: Please Excuse My Dear Aunt Sally
   Other mnemonic devices that will help you to remember the Order of Operations could be:
   **BODMAS:** Brackets, Order (powers and/or square roots), Division, Multiplication, Addition, Subtraction
   **BEDMAS:** Brackets, Exponents, Division, Multiplication, Addition, Subtraction
   **PEMDAS:** Parenthesis, Exponents, Multiplication, Division, Addition, Subtraction

## PRACTICE THE SKILL 11-2

1. $5 - 3c - 2 = c$ _____

2. $-(x + 3) = 2(-3 + 4x)$ _____

3. $\dfrac{x}{3} - 6 = \dfrac{2x}{12}$ _____

4. $2(x + 5) = 5(-2x - 5)$ _____

5. $4y + 10 - 2y = 4y + 12 - y$ _____

6. $7x - 28 + 4x = 9x - 36 - 4x$ _____

## SOLVE LITERAL EQUATIONS FOR ONE VARIABLE

Get the variable you are solving for on one side of the equal sign; get all other terms on the other side using the inverse operations. Because there are multiple variables, the answer will not look like x = 6, but as long as the variable you are solving for is isolated on one side of the equal sign, the problem is solved. Be sure to reduce fractions and move any negatives from the denominator to the numerator using the equivalent fraction −1/1 = 1/−1.

*Examples:* Solve the following equations for the specified variable.

a. $6x - 2 = 3 + y$ for x
   The goal is to have x on one side of the equation by itself. Start by adding 2 to each side of the equation.
   $6x - 2 = 3 + y$   $6x - 2 + 2 = 3 + 2 + y = 6x = 5 + y$
   Now divide by both sides of the equation. This will allow the x to be alone on one side of the equation.
   $$\dfrac{6x}{6} = \dfrac{5 + y}{6}$$
   *Answer:* $x = \dfrac{5 + y}{6}$

**b.** ab = 3cd Solve for c

The goal is to have c on one side of the equation by itself. This can be accomplished by dividing both sides of the equation by 3d

$$\frac{ab}{3d} = \frac{3cd}{3d}$$

*Answer:* $c = \dfrac{ab}{3d}$

Using the above principles, explain the steps to solve the following examples:

**c.** $x = 2z^2 + 3y$ Solve for y

$y = (x - 2z^2)/3$

**d.** 3/4 b − 2 = a Solve for b

$b = (4(a + 2))/3 = (4a + 8)/3$

**e.** xy = 3/z Solve for z

$z = 3/xy$

**f.** T=1/5 qpr Solve for r

$r = 5\ T/qp$

# PRACTICE THE SKILL 11-3

1. Solve y = mx + b for x. _____

2. Solve y = (1/3) x + 5 for x. _____

3. Solve Ax + By = C for y. _____

4. Solve Ax + By = C for x. _____

5. Solve C = (5/9)(F − 32) for F. _____

6. Solve F = (9/5) C + 32 for C. _____

7. Solve A = 1/2 bh for b. _____

8. Solve A = 1/2 bh for h. _____

9. Solve V = 4/3 πr² h for h. _____

10. Solve V = 1/3 πr² h for h. _____

# BUILDING CONFIDENCE WITH THE SKILL 11-1

**Solve the equation for the unknown variable.**

1. 2 = 4b + 8 _____

5. 3/8 d = 24 _____

2. 2y + 29 − 8y = 5 _____

6. −1/2 b = 21 _____

3. 7x + 2 = 5x + 2_____

7. −2 = 1/6 y _____

4. 2 1/5 h = 2 _____

8. 21 = (−2)/3 g _____

*(Continued)*

## BUILDING CONFIDENCE WITH THE SKILL 11-1
*Continued from p. 259*

9. y/6 = 6/9 _____    15. k/2 – 9 = –11 _____

10. (x – 15)/4 = –6 _____    16. Solve P = 2l + 2w for w. _____

11. (m – 1)/8 = 3 _____    17. Solve P = 2l + 2w for l. _____

12. 15 = (4x – 2)/5 _____    18. Solve V = l w h for w. _____

13. 10 = –6 – (3/4) d _____    19. Solve V = 1/3 l h w for w _____

14. 2/3 x + 2 = 4/5 _____    20. Solve 5x – 4 = 3z + 5y for x. ____

**OBJECTIVE 1**

How do we know what the average salary is for nurses in your region? How do we know who the best pitcher is in the major leagues? How do we know what the number one rated TV show is? All this information is based on statistics. In this chapter, we break down the common elements used in the health care field.

## MATH IN THE REAL WORLD 11-1
*How Statistical Information Is Used in Health Care*

- To establish quality control levels for equipment
- To establish range for normal blood test
- To determine insurance reimbursement based on treatment plans
- To determine payment for procedures
- To determine which vaccinations are beneficial and at what ages
- To conduct research on medications
- To conduct research on cures for diseases
- To determine mortality rate
- To determine morbidity rate

**OBJECTIVE 5**

## ARITHMETIC AVERAGE AND MEAN

When trying to analyze data, it is often useful to try to understand and describe what the "middle" or "center" of your data set looks like. There are three common measurements used in statistics to describe the center of your data: the arithmetic mean (or average), the median, and the mode. Determining which measurement to use will be based on how you are using the information you are studying.

The terms arithmetic mean and the average are used interchangeably in statistics. The process includes adding a series of numbers and dividing the sum by the count of the numbers in the series. Since the mean is a measure of the center of the data, the result of your mean should always be larger than the smallest value in your set of data and smaller than the largest value in your set of data. Also, it is possible that the mean may not be equal to a number from the original series.

Example: The average of the numbers 3, 5, and 10 is 6.
6 is greater than 3
6 is smaller than 10
6 is not one of the numbers in the original set (3, 5, 10)

## MATH IN THE REAL WORLD 11-2
### *Everyday Averages*

- The average gas price is $3.86.

- The pitcher's ERA is 2.37.

- Your grade point average is 3.75.

- The average person's age at retirement is 63.5 years.

- The average number of students in the third grade classes is 31.

## STRATEGY 11-3
### *Computing the Mean When All Values Are Equally Weighted*

*Example:* Find the mean of the following numbers: 8, 9, 10, 12, 15, 20, 25, 32

1. Determine the sum of all the values.
   $8 + 9 + 10 + 12 + 15 + 20 + 25 + 32 = 131$

2. Divide the sum by the total number of values.
   $131 \div 8 = 16.375$

If your professor uses a weighted grading scale (Figure 11-1), this strategy will not accurately compute your grade. The student must take into account each component's percentage in relationship to the whole. A quick explanation for computing weighted grades is to:

1. Determine your percentage by dividing the total number of points you received by the total number of points available for each weighted component separately.
2. Multiply the grade percentage for each of the components by their respective weighted value.
3. Add the weighted value scores together to determine your grade percentage.

Suppose a class's grading categories are assignments, test, and exams. The categories are weighted as follows:

| | |
|---|---|
| Assignments | 30% |
| Test | 30% |
| Exams | 40% |

Suppose your averages are as follows:

| | |
|---|---|
| Assignment | 89% |
| Test #1 | 79% |
| Exam | 87% |

*How is your grade calculated?*
Multiply percentages by respective weights (written as decimals)

$$0.3(89) + 0.3(79) + 0.4(87) = 26.7 + 23.7 + 34.8$$

$$= 85.2\% \text{ final grade}$$

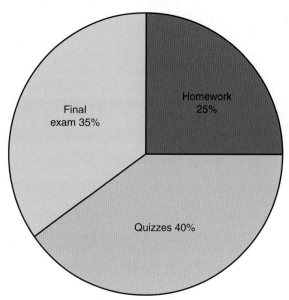

**Figure 11-1**   Example of weighted grades.

## PRACTICE THE SKILL 11-4

Determine the mean for each set of numbers. Write your answers using significant figures.

**1.** 22, 35, 67, 99, 108, 151, 223, 67, 59, 42 _____

**2.** 0.08, 1.09, 2.27, 4.3, 0.007, 0.55, 6.6 _____

**3.** 325, 130, 65, 95, 128, 42, 140, 35, 240 _____

**4.** 45, 90, 55, 120, 150, 38, 15 _____

**5.** 2.25, 4.75, 3.33, 8.92, 6.79, 10.89, 2.02 _____

**6.** $44.55, $23.55, $89.90, $145.67, $203.11, $571.22 _____

**7.** 0.003, 1.003, 0.006, 2.27, 0.8907, 1.5779, 2.267, 4.334 _____

**8.** 10, 12, 15, 9, 11, 8, 4, 14, 7, 6, 3, 8 _____

**9.** 98, 93, 88.5, 84.5, 76, 50, 99, 76.5 _____

**10.** 444, 333, 555, 666, 222, 111, 888, 999, 777 _____

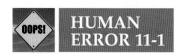

### HUMAN ERROR 11-1

*The most common error involves inaccurate computations in addition and division. Look at your answer. Does it make sense? If not, recompute.*

# MEDIAN

Unlike mean, median indicates what number is in the middle of a data set when the numbers are put in either ascending or descending order. This comes in handy when you have a large set of numbers—too large to use mental math in determining the middle value. The median will have an equal number of data values above and below the median. The median may or may not be the same as the mean.

## STRATEGY 11-4
*Determining the Median: Even Number in Data Set*

*Example:* 25, 24, 12, 15, 18, 28, 17, 21

1. Write your number set from least to greatest value.
   *12, 15, 17, 18, 21, 24, 25, 28*

2. Divide the total number of data entries by 2.
   $$\frac{8}{2} = 4$$

3. Add 1 to the value determined in step 2.
   $$4 + 1 = 5$$

4. The median will be determined by averaging the numbers in this data set found in the places determined by step 2 and step 3. In this case, we will average the fourth and fifth numbers in the series.
   $$18 + 21 = 39$$
   $$39 \div 2 = 19.5$$

5. The median for this data set is 19.5.

When the data set contains an odd number of values, the median can be determined by following the steps in the box Strategy 11-5.

## STRATEGY 11-5
*Determining the Median and Mean*

Determining the median: Odd number in a data set

*Example:* 33, 24, 18, 15, 36, 28, 30

1. Write the number set from lowest to highest value.
   *15, 18, 24, 28, 30, 33, 36*

2. Since this data set has an odd number, add 1 to the total number of data values.
   $$7 + 1 = 8$$

3. Divide the answer from step 2 by 2.
   $$\frac{8}{2} = 4$$

*(Continued)*

## STRATEGY 11-5
*Continued from p. 263*

4. Starting from the lowest values, count over (or down, if your list is vertical) to the value of the list corresponding to the answer you found in step 3. (In this case, we count to the fourth value.) This is your median.

*15, 18, 24, 28, 30, 33, 36*

Or vertically:

15

18

24

28

30

33

36

5. The median is 28.

### Determining the mean with negative values in a data set

*Example:* –7, –5, –2, 3, 7, 12, 13

1. First add all the number together.
   –7 + (–5) + (–2) + 3 + 7 + 12 + 13 =

2. Combine like values:
   –7 + (–5) + (–2) = –14
   3 + 7 + 12 + 13 = 35

3. Rewrite your problem:
   –14 + 35 = 21

4. Now divide the total by the number of values
   21/7 = 3

5. The mean is equal to 3

### Determining the median with negative values in a data set

*Example:* –5, –2, 3, 7, 12,

1. First place in ascending order
   –5, –2, 3, 7, 12,

2. Count the data points + 1 divide by 2
   5 + 1 = 6/2 = 3

3. Count over 3 to get median: Median is 3

## PRACTICE THE SKILL 11-5

Determine the median for the following set of numbers.

1. 4, 6, 2, 1, 3, 5, 9, 8, 7 _____

2. 31, 35, 37, 31, 30, 34, 36 _____

3. 21, 24, 19, 20, 22, 23, 21, 25 _____

4. 3, 5, 7, 2, 4, 6 _____

5. 2.22, 2.25, 2.23, 2.24, 2.26, 2.27, 2.29, 2.28 _____

6. 24, 26, 28, 30, 32, 34, 36, 38, 40, 42, 44, 46, 48, 50 _____

7. −10, −9, −5, −3, −2, −6, −12, −14, −4, −8 _____

8. 0.02, 0.1, 0.04, 0.09, 0.07, 0.05, 0.01, 0.03, 0.06, 0.001 _____

9. 456, 400, 419, 428, 437, 450, 440, 411, 413, 417, 448, 432

_____

10. 5, 3, 1, −5, −3, −1, 4, 2, −2, −4 _____

## MODE

OBJECTIVE 5

Mode can be described as the value that occurs most frequently in a data set. Let's look at an example of mode.

## STRATEGY 11-6
*Determining the Mode*

1. List the data set from least to greatest value.

2. Count the occurrence of each value.

3. The data value with the highest occurrence is the mode.

## MATH TRIVIA 11-1

**Bimodal** occurs when there are 2 sets of modes in a data set.
**Polymodal** occurs when there are more than 2 sets of modes in a data set.

*Example:*

The instructor has posted the grades for the last exam:

99, 97, 89, 89, 90, 92, 93, 89, 89, 87, 80, 84, 84, 84, 89, 95

1. List the data set from least to greatest value.

   80, 84, 84, 84, 87, 89, 89, 89, 89, 89, 90, 92, 93, 95, 97, 99

2. Count the occurrence of each value.

   *80 occurrence*
   *84 occurrences*
   *87 occurrence*
   *89 occurrences*
   *90 occurrence*
   *92 occurrence*
   *93 occurrence*
   *95 occurrence*
   *97 occurrence*
   *99 occurrence*

3. The data value with the highest occurrence is the mode.
   The mode is 89 because this value occurred five times within the data set.

## PRACTICE THE SKILL 11-6

Determine the mode for each of the following data sets.

1. 35, 34, 31, 40, 36, 33, 33332, 31 _____

2. 104, 110, 120, 110, 115, 118, 119, 106 _____

3. 99, 98, 95, 94, 95, 99, 97, 98, 95, 94, 95, 95, 99, 98, 97, 96, 99 _____

4. 0.09, 0.07, 0.01, 0.02, 0.09, 0.02, 0.01, 0.03, 0.01, 0.08, 0.07, 0.02, 0.02, 0.03, 0.04

   _____

5. 33, 22, 33, 45, 33, 55, 46, 33, 72, 78, 88, 90, 33, 11, 12, 33, 22, 22, 45, 33, 40

   _____

6. 12.99, 10.99, 12.99, 14.99, 39.99, 12.99, 9.99 _____

7. 19.99, 109.99, 9.99, 99.99, 19.99, 14.99, 9.99, 109.99, 109.99, 9.99, 9.99, 9.99, 109.99

   _____

8. 1, 2, 3, 4, 5, 4, 3, 2, 2, 3, 4, 5, 6, 5, 4, 3, 3, 2, 3, 6, 7, 8, 2, 2, 3, 2, 2, 2, 3

   _____

9. −2, −4, −4, −5, −6, −3, −3, −2, −2, −1, −1, −1, −2, −6, −6, −6 _____

10. 60, 65, 67, 69, 60, 65, 65, 67, 69, 60, 60, 60, 68, 60 _____

*(Continued)*

## PRACTICE THE SKILL 11-6
*Continued from p. 266*

3 Ways to Measure "Center" of Data Distribution

| Series of Numbers | Mean: The sum of the number set divided by the total number of data points in the set. | Median: Middle value in an ordered number set. Determine by listing numbers least to greatest. | Mode: Number(s) that occurs the most often in a number set. |
|---|---|---|---|
| 12, 14, 2, 6, 17, 12, 12, 2, 6, 1 | 12 + 14 + 2 + 6 + 17 + 12 + 12 + 2 + 6 + 1 = 84/10 = 8.4 or **8 is the mean** If using significant figures. | 17, 14, 12, 12, **12**, 6, 6, 2, 2, 1 = 12 + 6 = 18 18/2 = 9 **9 is the median** | 17, 14, **12, 12, 12**, 6, 6, 2, 2, 1 **12 is the mode** |
| 12, 3, 15, 15, 12, 12, 13, 3, 1, 15, 2, 15, 1, 15, 15 | 12 + 3 + 15 + 15 + 12 + 12 + 13 + 3 + 1 + 15 + 2 + 15 + 1 + 15 + 15 = 149/15 = 9.93 or **10 is the mean** If using significant figures. | 15, 15, 15, 15, 15, 15, 13, 12, 12, 12, 3, 3, 2, 1, 1 = The middle value is the 8th number. **12 is the median** | **15, 15, 15, 15, 15, 15,** 13, 12, 12, 12, 3, 3, 2, 1, 1 **15 is the mode** |
| 3, 3, 8, 10, 12, 12, 12, 15 | 3 + 3 + 8 + 10 + 12 + 12 + 12 + 15 = 75/8 = 9.375 or **9 is the mean** If using significant figures. | 15, 12, 12, 12, 10, 8, 3, 3 = 12 + 10 = 22 22/2 = 11 **11 is the median** | 15, **12, 12, 12**, 10, 8, 3, 3 = **12 is the mode** |

## BUILDING CONFIDENCE WITH THE SKILL 11-2

Determine the mean, median, and mode for each of the following number sets.

1. 35, 33, 31, 31, 32, 33, 34, 35, 33, 35, 33, 35, 31, 33

   Mean: _____

   Median: _____

   Mode: _____

2. 185, 182, 183, 190, 191, 183, 185, 188, 189, 187, 185, 185

   Mean: _____

   Median: _____

   Mode: _____

*(Continued)*

## BUILDING CONFIDENCE WITH THE SKILL 11-2
*Continued from p. 267*

**3.** 1.2, 0.9, 0.8, 1.4, 1.5, 0.8, 0.7, 0.8

Mean: _____

Median: _____

Mode: _____

**4.** 14, 18, 16, 13, 11, 19, 20, 10, 18, 13, 15, 13, 13, 18

Mean: _____

Median: _____

Mode: _____

**5.** 2.62, 2.62, 2.56, 2.58, 2.60, 2.61, 2.64, 2.61, 2.62, 2.63, 2.64, 2.64, 2.62, 2.62

Mean: _____

Median: _____

Mode: _____

## Solve the following word problems.

**6.** The following grades were posted for the medical math midterm exam:

99, 98.5, 97, 96, 99, 98, 98.5, 97, 97, 97, 96, 50, 77, 84, 77, 76, 85, 85, 85, 85, 85.

What is the class average for the midterm exam? _____

What is the median grade for the midterm exam? _____

What is the mode for the midterm exam? _____

**7.** You conducted a study regarding birth order. You asked students in four of your classes to participate. Students were allowed to participate only once in the survey. Following are your results:

| | | | |
|---|---|---|---|
| Oldest: | 25 | 5th Child: | 3 |
| Youngest: | 31 | 6th Child: | 0 |
| 2nd Child: | 14 | 7th Child: | 1 |
| 3rd Child: | 9 | 8th Child: | 2 |
| 4th Child: | 11 | Only Child: | 20 |

Mode: _____

*(Continued)*

## BUILDING CONFIDENCE WITH THE SKILL 11-2
*Continued from p. 268*

8. What is the average number of children born during a multiple birth?

    (sum up all answers to number of children born during multiple birth)/
    total number of multiple births

    $= ((2+2+2+\dots+2)+(3+3+\dots+3)+(4+4+4)+6+(7+7))/27$

    $= ((2\times12)+(3\times9)+(4\times3)+6+(7\times2)/27$

    $= 83/27$

    $= 3.074$ children on average during a multiple birth

    $= 4$ children (must round up since can't have partial child)

9. The following data set includes days of stay for a patient with an appendectomy:

    3, 4, 5, 4, 3, 3, 3, 3, 2, 3, 5, 4, 5, 3, 3, 2, 3, 2, 3, 2, 3, 3, 2, 3, 4, 4, 5, 3, 5, 4, 3, 3

    What is the mean number of days a patient stays with an appendectomy?

    _____

    What is the median number of days a patient stays with an appendectomy?

    _____

    What is the mode number of days a patient stays with an appendectomy?

    _____

10. The following counties reported an outbreak of meningitis:

    | | | | |
    |---|---|---|---|
    | Butler: | 12 | Montgomery: | 5 |
    | Warren: | 10 | Clinton: | 3 |
    | Hamilton: | 8 | Greene: | 6 |
    | Preble: | 6 | | |

    What is the mean number of outbreaks in a county? _____

    What is the median number of outbreaks in a county? _____

    What is the mode number of outbreaks in a county? _____

## DATA TYPES

Most people believe that the collection of data is the easiest part of research. In many cases, you ask people to complete a survey and, with the use of statistics, you compare the results. But did you know there are different types of data? In this section we are going to discuss 4 major types of data:

- Qualitative data: descriptive (Example: color of marbles)
- Quantitative data: specific numerical information (Example: number of marbles in a jar)
- Discrete data: can only use specific values (whole numbers) (Example: number of students in a classroom)

- Continuous data: can use any value within a range (Example: running race times or people's heights)

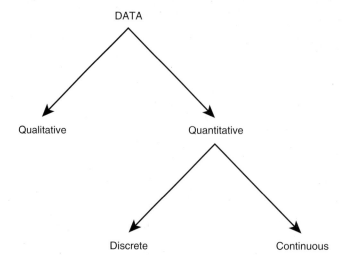

*Example:* Drug Testing

Qualitative drug testing results are measured as positive (drug is present) or negative (absent of the drug)

Quantitative drug test results will give a specific amount of the drug present in the specimen.

*Example:* What data can we determine from this picture and its caption?

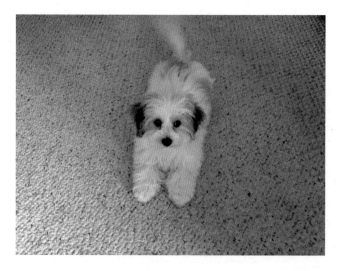

This 15-week-old female puppy is a Lhasa-ton. She was the only female in a 4-puppy litter. Her current weight is 5.4 pounds, and she stands 11 inches tall. When fully grown, she will weigh between 12–15 pounds.

## Qualitative: "What a Cute Dog"

- She is white and brown.
- She has long hair.
- She is wagging her tail.

## Quantitative: "1 dog"

**Discrete:**

- She has 4 legs.
- She has 2 black eyes.
- The liter had 1 female and 3 male puppies.

**Continuous:**
- She weighs 5.4 lbs.
- When grown, she will weigh 12–15 lbs.
- She is 11 inches tall.
- She is 15 weeks old.

Another critical element when analyzing results has to do with the center of the data and the **range** of the data. The range is found by subtracting the largest and smallest values in the number set.

*Example:* 35, 22, 17, 45
$45 - 17 = 28$

However, the range can be skewed by outliers (or extreme values), which is why it is considered a very crude measurement. The use of standard deviation, which will be discussed later in this chapter, is less susceptible to outliers.

## MATH TRIVIA 11-2

A **Census** is data collected from every member of the pre-determined group. It is very accurate if you are able to survey everyone in the group.
A **Sample** is data collection from select members of a pre-determined group.

## OBTAINING SAMPLES

OBJECTIVE 6

Have you ever taken part in a sample poll? Have you ever conducted a sample poll? There is a good chance that the answer is yes to both questions, whether your polling involved sitting on a committee trying to decide what type of food to serve at the fundraiser or (my favorite) asking family members what type of pizza they wanted to order for dinner. Determining the type of sample group to use can be complicated. This section provides basic tools for conducting surveys and gathering data, and refer to Chapter 2 on the different graphs that can be utilized to display your results.

What exactly is a sample group? A sample group is a small subset of the population that is used to draw conclusions about the whole population (or select portions of the population).

Two common techniques for selecting a sample group are random sampling and target sampling. A random sample is selected when you want to get a representative sample in order to draw conclusions about the entire population. Individuals in a random sample group are chosen randomly using methods such as a randomly generated table of numbers or names drawn out of a hat. A target sample group is selected when you desire to draw conclusions about a specific subset of the whole population. To create a target sample, first remove individuals who do not belong to the desired specific population, and then a collect random sample from the remaining population is drawn.

Example: If a teacher wanted to find out what the preferred type of pizza was by the entire school (3000 students), the teacher could poll a random sample of 100 students chosen by drawing names out of a hat. If the teacher wanted to find out the preferred type of pizza of the 4th graders, the teacher could remove all students who are not in 4th grade from the hat, and then draw a sample from the hat that only includes 4th graders. This sample would be a targeted sample.

As careers in biotechnology, research, and quality control increase, so will the opportunity to select sample groups. If you continue your studies in this field, you will encounter many other ways to narrow or determine sample groups. In addition, you will learn how to deal with outliers, data points that lie outside the overall pattern of the set of data, and their effect on the end results.

## MATH IN THE REAL WORLD 11-3
*Examples of Statements Used with Target Sampling*

- "Are you a person between the ages of 25 and 50 who suffers from sleep apnea?"

- "We are looking for young adults between 12 and 22 years old to sample soft drinks."

- "If you are between the ages of 30 and 55 and are not currently taking any prescription allergy or asthma medication, you are eligible to join our study."

- "Please join our focus group."

## MATH IN THE REAL WORLD 11-4
*Examples of Statements Used with Random Sampling*

- "Draw from a hat."

- "This is targeted to people owning specific items."

- "Boy/Girl selected at random"

- "Count off."

## PRACTICE THE SKILL 11-7

Answer the following questions.

Create a chart to visually show your results. Refer to Chapter 2 if needed.

1. Determine two ways to divide your class into groups using target sampling.

   _____

2. Determine three ways to divide your class into groups using simple random sampling.

   _____

3. Conduct a target sampling survey of your choice. Explain how you determined the sampling, or collection of data. Determine the mean, median, and mode based on your data set.

   _____

*(Continued)*

## PRACTICE THE SKILL 11-7
*Continued from p. 272*

Mean: _____

Median: _____

Mode: _____

4. Conduct a random sampling survey of your choice. Explain how you determined the sampling, or collection of data. Determine the mean, median, and mode based on your data set.

Mean: _____

Median: _____

Mode: _____

5. Discuss how information from sample groups affects our society.

_____

## PROBABILITY

OBJECTIVE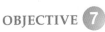

What is the probability of winning the lottery? What is the probability of obtaining a grade of "A" in this class? What is the probability of getting off the night shift at work? Are the answers based on random choices or mathematical predictabilities? When there are equal chances of events occurring, we can figure out probability by dividing the number of desired outcomes by the number of possible outcomes.

$$\text{Probability} = \frac{\text{Number of desired outcomes}}{\text{Number of possible outcomes}}$$

## STRATEGY 11-7
*Determining Probability During One Event*

1. Determine the total number of possible outcomes.

2. Determine the total number of desired outcomes.

3. Input the numbers into the probability equation.

4. Solve the problem.

*Example:*
A jar holds 45 marbles. Fifteen of the marbles are red. What is the probability of selecting a red marble?

1. Determine the total number of possible outcomes.
   45 marbles are in the jar.

*(Continued)*

## STRATEGY 11-7
*Continued from p. 273*

2. Determine the total number of desired outcomes.
   15 red marbles

3. Input the numbers into the probability equation.

$$Probability = \frac{15 \; red \; marbles}{45 \; total \; marbles}$$

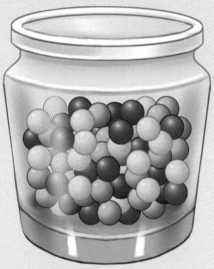

4. Solve the problem.

$$Probability = \frac{15}{45}, \; reduce \; your \; fraction \; to \; \frac{1}{3}$$

*Answer:* The probability of picking a red marble from the jar would be one red marble in every three tries.

## STRATEGY 11-8
*Determining Probability with Two Independent Events*

*Example:*
What is the probability of rolling two dice so the sum of the dice equals 8?

1. Determine how many possible outcomes there are with each event (*on each die*).
   *There are six possible outcomes on each die.*

2. Multiply the total possible outcomes from the two events (*the two dice*).
   *6 outcomes × 6 outcomes = 36 possible outcomes*

3. Determine all the number combinations that will equal the desired outcome (8 on the two dice).
   2 + 6 = 8
   3 + 5 = 8
   4 + 4 = 8
   5 + 3 = 8
   6 + 2 = 8
   *Five combinations will equal 8.*

(Continued)

## STRATEGY 11-8
*Continued from p. 274*

**4.** Input the numbers into the probability equation and solve the problem.

$$Probability = \frac{5 \text{ chances of desired outcome}}{36 \text{ possible outcomes}}$$

**5.** Solve the problem.

$$Probability = \frac{5}{36}$$

*Answer:* The probability of throwing an 8 with the dice is 5 times out of every 36 tries.

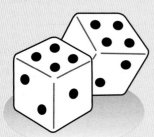

## MATH IN THE REAL WORLD 11-5
*Real World Probability—Games of Chance*

- Bingo
- "Wheel of Fortune"
- "The Price is Right"
- Lottery tickets
- "Deal or No Deal"
- Horse racing

## PRACTICE THE SKILL 11-8

Determine the probability for each question.

**1.** What is the probability of throwing a 5 on a single die?

_____

**2.** What is the probability of drawing a queen out of a regular deck of playing cards? _____

*(Continued)*

## PRACTICE THE SKILL 11-8
*Continued from p. 275*

3. What is the probability of drawing a diamond card out of a regular deck of playing cards? _____

4. What is the probability of throwing exactly one 6 when tossing two dice?

   _____

5. The jar of marbles holds 100 marbles. There are 25 red marbles, 35 blue marbles, 15 yellow marbles, 20 green marbles, and 5 orange marbles. Each selection is random.

   a. What is the probability of selecting a red marble?

   _____

   b. What is the probability of selecting either a green or an orange marble?

   _____

   c. What is the probability of selecting a blue or an orange marble?

   _____

   d. What is the probability of selecting a yellow marble?

OBJECTIVES **8** **9**

## BASIC STATISTICS

Statistics are used in all aspects of our world. For example, statistics can be used to determine how political candidates are viewed in the public eye, the popularity of a TV show, the potential for outbreak of a disease, and the estimated wage for a profession. This section describes how to determine the variance and standard deviation of a data set.

### Variance

The variance of a data set determines how spread out the numbers are within a data set. The smaller the variance, the smaller the difference between data values. Use the following formula* to calculate variance:

$$s^2 = \frac{\Sigma(X_d - \bar{X})^2}{n - 1} \quad \text{Sample Variance}$$

$$s^2 = \frac{\Sigma(X_d - \bar{X})^2}{n} \quad \text{Population variance}$$

where

$s^2$ = variance
$\Sigma$ = sum the numbers within parentheses
$X_d$ = an individual data point within the group
$\bar{X}$ = mean of the group of numbers
$n$ = total quantity of numbers within the group

---

*Variance formula and meanings of abbreviations within formula are from Doucette LJ: *Basic mathematics for the health-related professions*, *Philadelphia, 2000, Saunders*.

With large data sets, computations can be time consuming. The good news is that your scientific calculator has a function that will calculate variance. Of course, you still must understand the formula to input the data correctly.

## STRATEGY 11-9
### *Determining the Variance*

1. Find the mean of your data set.

2. Subtract the mean from each of the numbers in the data set.

3. Square each of the differences found in step 3.

4. Find the sum of all the squared differences.

5. Divide the sum found in step 6 by n – 1, where n is the number of data values in the set.

***Example:***
115, 112, 113, 112, 115, 117, 118, 115

1. Find the mean.
   $112 + 112 + 113 + 115 + 115 + 115 + 117 + 118 = 917$

   $917 \div 8 = 114.625$
   *Mean is 114.625 OR 115 (don't forget to round!).*

2. Subtract the mean from each of the number sets.
   Number set from:

   | Least to highest | Number set – Mean | Difference squared |
   |---|---|---|
   | 112 | $112 - 115 = -3$ | $(-3)^2 = 9$ |
   | 112 | $112 - 115 = -3$ | $(-3)^2 = 9$ |
   | 113 | $113 - 115 = -2$ | $(-2)^2 = 4$ |
   | 115 | $115 - 115 = 0$ | $(0)^2 = 0$ |
   | 115 | $115 - 115 = 0$ | $(0)^2 = 0$ |
   | 115 | $115 - 115 = 0$ | $(0)^2 = 0$ |
   | 117 | $117 - 115 = 2$ | $(2)^2 = 4$ |
   | 118 | $118 - 115 = 3$ | $(3)^2 = 9$ |

3. Square the difference.
   (See above.)

4. $9 + 9 + 4 + 0 + 0 + 0 + 4 + 9 = 35$

5. $s^2 = \dfrac{35}{8-1}$

   $S^2 = \dfrac{35}{7}$

   $S^2 = 5$

   Variance is 5.

## PRACTICE THE SKILL 11-9

Compute the variance for each data set.

1. 22, 35, 67, 99, 108, 151, 223, 67, 59, 42 _____

2. 0.08, 1.09, 2.27, 4.3, 0.007, 0.55, 6.6 _____

3. 325, 130, 65, 95, 128, 42, 140, 35, 240 _____

4. 45, 90, 55, 120, 150, 38, 15 _____

5. 2.25, 4.75, 3.33, 8.92, 6.79, 10.89, 2.02 _____

6. 44.55, 23.55, 89.90, 145.67, 203.11, 571.22 _____

7. 0.003, 1.003, 0.006, 2.27, 0.8907 _____

8. 10, 12, 15, 9, 11, 8, 4, 14, 7, 6, 3, 8 _____

9. 98, 93, 88.5, 84.5, 76, 50, 99, 76.5 _____

10. 444, 333, 555, 666, 222, 111, 888, 999, 777 _____

## Standard Deviation

Standard deviation is another measurement used to describe spread or variation within a set of data points.

Standard deviation is determined by taking the square root of the variance. The standard deviation may be part of the calculation done to find the margin of error, but that is not always the case.

## STRATEGY 11-10
*Determining Standard Deviation*

1. First determine the variance.

2. The standard deviation is the square root of the variance.

   *Example:*
   1.2, 0.9, 0.8, 1.4, 1.5, 0.8
   1. First determine the variance.
      *Variance is 0.096.*
   2. The standard deviation is the square root of the variance.
      $\sqrt{0.096} =$
      *The standard deviation is 0.3.*

# PRACTICE THE SKILL 11-10

Calculate the standard deviation, based on the given variance, for each of the following problems.

1. Variance = 10        Standard deviation = _____
2. Variance = 0.096     Standard deviation = _____
3. Variance = 33.8      Standard deviation = _____
4. Variance = 2.1       Standard deviation = _____
5. Variance = 0.05      Standard deviation = _____
6. Variance = 15        Standard deviation = _____
7. Variance = 0.125     Standard deviation = _____
8. Variance = 0.005     Standard deviation = _____
9. Variance = 1.44      Standard deviation = _____
10. Variance = 6.98     Standard deviation = _____

## Standard Deviation Ranges

For a data set which has a normal distribution, the following describes the approximate percentage of the data set one can expect to fall within the given standard deviation ranges:

±1 standard deviation    68.2% of the data set will be within +/– 1 standard deviation of the mean.

±2 standard deviations   95.5% of the data set will be within +/– 2 standard deviations of the mean.

±3 standard deviations   99.7% of the data set will be within +/– 3 standard deviations of the mean.

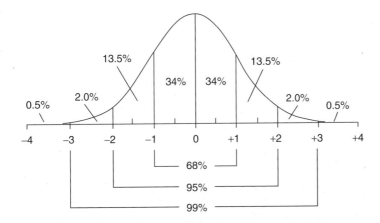

# STRATEGY 11-11
*Determining Standard Deviation Ranges*

1. Determine the mean for the data set.

2. Determine the standard deviation for the data set.

3. Multiply the standard deviation by the standard deviation ranges (1, 2 and 3).

4. Add and subtract respective multiples of the standard deviation to the mean.

5. Determine the ranges.

*(Continued)*

## STRATEGY 11-11
*Continued from p. 279*

*Example:*

If the mean for a group is 220 and the standard deviation is 4, what are the ±1, ±2, and ±3 standard deviation ranges?

1. Determine the mean for the data set.
   *220*

2. Determine the standard deviation for the data set.
   *4*

3. Multiply the standard deviation by 1, 2, and 3.

   | | |
   |---|---|
   | *± 1 x Standard Deviation* | *+4, −4* |
   | *± 2 x Standard Deviation* | *+8, −8* |
   | *± 3 x Standard Deviation* | *+12, −12* |

4. Add and subtract the respective multiples of the standard deviation to the mean.

   | | | |
   |---|---|---|
   | *mean ± 1 x Standard Deviation* | *220 + 4 = 224* | *220 − 4 = 216* |
   | *mean ± 2 x Standard Deviation* | *220 + 8 = 228* | *220 − 8 = 212* |
   | *mean ± 3 x Standard Deviation* | *220 + 12 = 232* | *220 − 12 = 208* |

5. Determine the ranges.

   | | |
   |---|---|
   | *± 1 standard deviation range* | *216-224* |
   | *± 2 standard deviation range* | *212-228* |
   | *± 3 standard deviation range* | *208-232* |

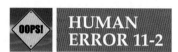

## HUMAN ERROR 11-2

*Remember to always write the standard deviation ranges with the smaller of the two numbers on the left. This will always be the mean <u>minus</u> the multiple of the standard deviation.*

## PRACTICE THE SKILL 11-11

**Determine the standard deviation range for the following questions.**

1. What is the probability that a quality control result from a normal distribution will fall within ±1 standard deviation from the mean?

   _____

2. What is the probability that a quality control result from a normal distribution will fall outside of ±2 standard deviations from the mean?

   _____

3. What is the probability that a quality control result from a normal distribution will fall within the ±3 standard deviation range?

   _____

4. Mean = 37.0          Standard deviation = 1.4
   Find the following standard deviation ranges.

   ±1 _____

   ±2 _____

   ±3 _____

*(Continued)*

# PRACTICE THE SKILL 11-11
*Continued from p. 280*

5. Mean = 17.0          Standard deviation = 2.6
   Find the following standard deviation ranges.

   ±1 _____

   ±2 _____

   ±3 _____

6. Mean = 4          Standard deviation = 0.004
   Find the following standard deviation ranges.

   ±1 _____

   ±2 _____

   ±3 _____

7. Mean = 15          Standard deviation = 0.4
   Find the following standard deviation ranges.

   ±1 _____

   ±2 _____

   ±3 _____

8. Mean = 22          Standard deviation = 7.9
   Find the following standard deviation ranges.

   ±1 _____

   ±2 _____

   ±3 _____

9. Mean = 327          Standard deviation = 21.4
   Find the following standard deviation ranges.

   ±1 _____

   ±2 _____

   ±3 _____

10. Mean = 117          Standard deviation = 11.8
    Find the following standard deviation ranges.

    ±1 _____

    ±2 _____

    ±3 _____

## BUILDING CONFIDENCE WITH THE SKILL 11-3

**Answer the following questions for each set of numbers.**

**1.** 23, 44, 36, 88, 71, 65, 83, 43, 27, 30

     a. Calculate the mean of the set. _____

     b. Calculate the median number in the set. _____

     c. Calculate the mode in the set. _____

     d. Calculate the variance for the set. _____

     e. Calculate the standard deviation of the set. _____

     f. Find the following standard deviation ranges.

        ±1 _____

        ±2 _____

        ±3 _____

**2.** 32.1, 46.5, 87.6, 76.3, 98.9, 101.9, 110.4, 115.3, 112.9

     a. Calculate the mean of the set. _____

     b. Calculate the median number in the set. _____

     c. Calculate the mode in the set. _____

     d. Calculate the variance for the set. _____

     e. Calculate the standard deviation of the set. _____

     f. Find the following standard deviation ranges.

        ±1 _____

        ±2 _____

        ±3 _____

**3.** 0.012, 0.003, 0.987, 0.056, 0.547, 0.022, 0.113, 0.055

     a. Calculate the mean of the set. _____

     b. Calculate the median number in the set. _____

     c. Calculate the mode in the set. _____

     d. Calculate the variance for the set. _____

*(Continued)*

## BUILDING CONFIDENCE WITH THE SKILL 11-3
*Continued from p. 282*

   e. Calculate the standard deviation of the set.

   _____

   f. Find the following standard deviation ranges.

     ±1 _____

     ±2 _____

     ±3 _____

**4.** 2.0, 1.8, 1.6, 1.4, 1.2, 0.9, 0.7, 0.5, 0.3, 0.1, −1, −1.2, −1.4, −1.6, −1.8, −2

   a. Calculate the mean of the set. _____

   b. Calculate the median number in the set. _____

   c. Calculate the mode in the set. _____

   d. Calculate the variance for the set. _____

   e. Calculate the standard deviation of the set. _____

   f. Find the following standard deviation ranges.

     ±1 _____

     ±2 _____

     ±3 _____

**5.** −5, −3, −2, −7, −11, 14, 28, 17, 15, 13, 2

   a. Calculate the mean of the set. _____

   b. Calculate the median number in the set. _____

   c. Calculate the mode in the set. _____

   d. Calculate the variance for the set. _____

   e. Calculate the standard deviation of the set. _____

   f. Find the following standard deviation ranges.

     ±1 _____

     ±2 _____

     ±3 _____

## CONCLUSION

The goal of this chapter is to expose you to basic formulas used in obtaining statistical data in the health care environment. Not everyone will be involved in selecting sample groups or drawing conclusions from research data; however, we are all affected by the results. Quality control standards for equipment, acceptable medication dosages, and laboratory values are all based on statistical information. Understanding the necessary data and the use of a scientific calculator will make calculations of large data sets more obtainable. I hope this chapter increases your knowledge level regarding statistical computations and bolsters your confidence with these types of calculations.

OBJECTIVES ③ ④ ⑤ ⑥ ⑦ ⑧ ⑨

## MASTER THE SKILL

Throughout, write your answers using significant figures.

Determine the mean for each data set.

1. 14, 18, 16, 13, 11, 19, 20, 10, 18, 13 _____

2. 25.7, 26.8, 32.2, 40.4, 29.1, 26.8 _____

3. 2.62, 2.62, 2.56, 2.58, 2.60, 2.61, 2.64 _____

Determine the median number for each data set.

4. 85, 77, 87, 78, 79, 80, 82 _____

5. 258, 237, 241, 250, 260, 248, 238, 245, 256, 246 _____

6. 135, 128, 132, 134, 129, 131 _____

Determine the mode for each data set.

7. 498, 480, 484, 479, 488, 487, 482, 487, 487, 490, 492, 491

_____

8. 53, 56, 57, 53, 52, 58, 57, 53, 56, 53 _____

9. 0.01, 0.98, 0.75, 0.44, 0.75, 0.97, 0.75, 0.001, 0.43, 0.99, 0.75, 0.98

_____

Calculate the variance of the following data sets.

10. 295, 290, 298, 287, 291, 301, 303, 300 _____

11. 35.5, 40.0, 37.5, 36.0, 35.0, 38.0, 39.5, 34.5 _____

Calculate the standard deviation for each data set.

12. 290, 287, 301, 300, 295, 298, 291, 303 _____

13. 40.0, 36.0, 38.0, 34.5, 39.5, 35.0, 37.5, 35.5 _____

(Continued)

## MASTER THE SKILL
*Continued from p. 284*

**Answer the following questions.**

14. What is the probability that a quality control result from a normal distribution will fall within ±1 standard deviation from the mean?

_____

_____

_____

15. What is the probability that a quality control result from a normal distribution will fall outside of ±2 standard deviations from the mean?

_____

_____

_____

16. What is the probability that a quality control result from a normal distribution will fall within the ±3 standard deviation range?

_____

_____

_____

17. Calculate the ±2 standard deviation range for the mean of 37.0 and standard deviation of 1.5. _____

18. Calculate the ±3 standard deviation range for the mean of 15.7 and standard deviation of 4.2. _____

19. Calculate the ±1 standard deviation range for the mean of 21.5 and standard deviation of 2.2. _____

20. The mean value for cholesterol is 224 mg/dl. The laboratory has determined that the standard deviation is 4 mg/dl. Calculate the standard deviation ranges for the following:

   a. ±1 standard deviation: _____

   b. ±2 standard deviations: _____

   c. ±3 standard deviations: _____

21. The mean value for Hematocrit is 15.5 mg/dl. The laboratory has determined that the standard deviation is 2.1 mg/dl. Calculate the standard deviation ranges for the following:

   a. ±1 standard deviation: _____

   b. ±2 standard deviations: _____

   c. ±3 standard deviations: _____

*(Continued)*

## MASTER THE SKILL
*Continued from p. 285*

22. The mean value for glucose is 450 mg/dl. The laboratory has determined that the standard deviation is 15 mg/dl. Calculate the standard deviation ranges for the following:

   a. ±1 standard deviation: _____

   b. ±2 standard deviations: _____

   c. ±3 standard deviations: _____

23. Use the data set to answer the following questions:
   23, 24, 25, 23, 25, 26, 25, 27, 28, 24, 25, 23, 25

   a. Compute the mean value. _____

   b. Compute the median value. _____

   c. Compute the mode value. _____

   d. Compute the variance value. _____

   e. Compute the standard deviation. _____

   f. Compute the standard deviation range for ±1 standard deviation.

   _____

24. Use the data set to answer the following questions:
   12.3, 12.5, 13.2, 13.5, 12.5, 13.6, 12.4, 12.5, 13.2, 12.5

   a. Compute the mean value. _____

   b. Compute the median value. _____

   c. Compute the mode value. _____

   d. Compute the variance value. _____

   e. Compute the standard deviation. _____

   f. Compute the standard deviation range for ±2 standard deviations.

   _____

25. Use the data set to answer the following questions:
   112, 110, 114, 89, 96, 112, 112, 115, 97, 96, 95, 88, 112, 112, 114

   a. Compute the mean value. _____

   b. Compute the median value. _____

   c. Compute the mode value. _____

*(Continued)*

## MASTER THE SKILL
*Continued from p. 286*

   d. Compute the variance value. _____

   e. Compute the standard deviation. _____

   f. Compute the standard deviation range for ±3 standard deviations.

   _____

26. Mr. Smith's blood sugar tests had the following results:
107, 116, 109, 109, 113, 121, 114, 132, 109, 115, 87

   a. What is Mr. Smith's average blood sugar reading? _____

   b. What is the mode of Mr. Smith's blood sugar readings? _____

27. The supply drawer has the following syringe combinations:

   1 cc TB syringe:     5
   3 cc syringe:      10
   1 cc insulin syringe:   8

   a. What is the possibility of choosing a 3 cc syringe? _____

   b. What is the possibility of choosing a 1 cc insulin syringe? _____

   c. What is the possibility of choosing a 1 cc TB syringe? _____

28. In the closet, there are 8 scrub pants, 4 scrub jackets, and 5 scrub tops.

   a. What is the possibility of choosing a pair of scrub pants? _____

   b. What is the possibility of choosing a scrub top? _____

   c. What is the possibility of choosing a scrub jacket? _____

   Solve the linear equations:
   For problems 29-35 and 39-49, solve the equation for the unknown
     variable.

29. $2\ 1/5\ h = 2$ _____

30. $3/8\ d = 24$ _____

31. $1/2\ b = 21$ _____

32. $-2 = 1/6\ y$ _____

33. $21 = (-2)/3\ g$ _____

34. $y/6 = 6/9$ _____

35. $(x - 15)/4 = -6$ _____

*(Continued)*

## MASTER THE SKILL
*Continued from p. 287*

**36.** Solve $3/5\ c = 1/5\ b + 10$ for b _____

**37.** Solve $1/3\ b - 6 = 5c$ for b _____

**38.** Solve $(5x)^2 + 5y^2 - 2z = 5 + 3z$ for z _____

**39.** $12 - 3(w + 7) = 15$ _____

**40.** $-(7 - w) - 22 + 4(8 - w) = 0$ _____

**41.** $3(x - 2) = 2(x + 4)$ _____

**42.** $4(2y - 8) = 14 + 6y$ _____

**43.** $8 + 18c = -2(6c + 5)$ _____

**44.** $4(2x - 5) - 3 = 5x + 1$ _____

**45.** $2(3y + 3) - 9 = 16$ _____

**46.** $3(x + 5) - 20 = 8(x - 3)$ _____

**47.** $2(x + 6) = 7x - 3$ _____

**48.** $7y - 2(5 + 3y/2) = 5y - 17$ _____

**49.** $4(v - 1) = -(4v + 5) - 32$ _____

**50.** Solve $C = \dfrac{5}{9}(F - 32)$ for F _____

# Solutions and IV Calculations

## CHAPTER OUTLINE

## LEARNING OBJECTIVES

*Upon completion of this chapter, the learner will be able to:*

1. Define the key terms in the chapter.
2. Identify the tonicity of a solution.
3. Compute concentration levels.
4. Calculate molality and molarity levels
5. Compute IV drip factors
6. Calculate intake and output
7. Graph intake and output data

## KEY TERMS

| | |
|---|---|
| Colloids | Molarity |
| Concentration | Mole |
| Drop Factor | Osmosis |
| Flow Rate | Solute |
| Hypertonic | Solution |
| Hypotonic | Solvent |
| Intravenous | Suspensions |
| Isotonic | Tonicity |
| Molality | |

With the changes of job responsibilities, more health care careers are requiring chemistry as part of the curriculum. This chapter will primarily discuss concepts of osmolality, moles, molarity, molality, and drip rate computations and how math can become a factor in the study of chemistry. This chapter is purely an overview of the important concepts; you will receive additional instruction in your specialty classes.

## SOLUTIONS

OBJECTIVE 1

**Solution** is a broad term used to describe anything from reconstituted amoxicillin to a combination of gases. A solution is simply a mixture of two or more substances with the same composition throughout and can be separated by a physical means such as distillation. To make a solution, two components are needed, a **solute** and a **solvent**. The solute is a substance that dissolves into the solvent, and the solvent thus, dissolves the solute. A handy way to remember this is that *solute rhymes with cute and gets hugged by the larger word solvent*. Meaning the larger word solvent takes the cute solute into it. Kool-Aid drink is a classic example of a solution made by the Kool-Aid powder (the solute) and water (the solvent). There are other types of solutions beyond this solid in liquid type of solution. Solutions can be a liquid in liquid such as alcohol dissolved in water; a gas dissolved in a liquid such as oxygen in the blood; a liquid dissolved in a gas such as water vapor or humidity; a solid dissolved into another solid such as brass. In fact, a solution can be any combination of a solid, liquid, or gas dissolved into a solid, liquid, or a gas.

Similar to and often confused with solutions are **suspensions** and **colloids**. Suspensions are mixtures that are not the same composition throughout the mixture and that if allowed to rest, the parts of the mixture will separate. A colloid is also a heterogeneous mixture similar to suspensions in that their composition is not uniformed, but with larger particles. Like suspensions, many colloids can appear cloudy or milky in appearance. In addition, like suspensions, the more diluted the colloid is, the clearer it becomes.

## REAL WORLD BOX 12-1
*Examples of Colloids*

Mayonnaise

milk

marshmallow

whipped cream (from a can)

aerosols

paint

gelatin

blood

## CONCENTRATIONS

When working with a solution it is important to remember that all solutions are not created equally; some are strong and some are weak. The strength of a solution is determined by the relative amount of solute dissolved in the solvent and is referred to as concentration. Concentration can be thought of as how strong a glass of Kool-Aid is, the more powder, the more intense the taste. The stronger the taste, the higher the concentration. At the same time, if there is very little Kool-Aid powder, the taste will be very watery and have a low concentration.

OBJECTIVE 2    ## TONICITY

Problem solving for diseases and illnesses are affected by the concentration of fluids and the interaction of cells in the body. The solute can often travel into or out of the cell through **osmosis**, causing the relative concentrations of the cell and the solutions to change. This phenomenon is known as **tonicity**. Tonicity is based on how much water moves in and out of the cell when in a solution. Ideally, we would like the body to be balanced: no water moving in or out of the cell. Movement will only occur if there is a difference in concentration. Tonicity can best be examined by placing a cell into a salt-water solution. Water will enter or exit the cell depending upon the concentration in the cell and the concentration of the solution. The general saying is that things flow from a higher concentration to a low concentration. What that means is if you have a 75% solution and a cell with 25%, water will move out from the cell to the solution until both are at a 50% solution. There are three terms involved with tonicity: hypertonic, hypotonic, and isotonic.

- **Hypertonic** is where the concentration in the cell is lower than the solution; thus water leaves the cell and goes into the solution, causing the cell to shrink.
- **Hypotonic** is where the concentration in the cell is higher than the solution; thus water enters the cell and leaves the solution, causing the cell to grow and become engorged. Sometimes the cell can grow so large that it will burst or lyse.
- **Isotonic** is where the cell and the solution have the same concentration and thus water does not flow into or out of the cell.

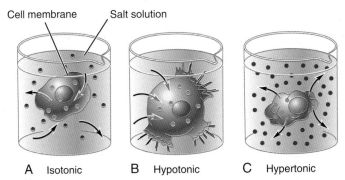

Osmosis in cells. A, Cells placed in an isotonic solution maintain a constant volume because the fluid within the cell and the fluid around the cell are equal. B, A cell placed in a hypotonic solution may swell because the solution surrounding the cell diffuses inward. C, A cell placed in a hypertonic solution will shrink because the solution inside the cell diffuses outward. (Modified from Herlihy B, Maebius NK: *The human body in health and illness,* ed 3, St Louis, 2007, Saunders.)

## MATH QUICK TIPS 12-1

Percentages are used to indicate the amount (concentration) of something in a solution. Concentration is indicated by either volume to volume or weight to volume. All measurements are based on 100 mililiter.

Volume to volume: ml/100 ml

Weight to volume: g/100 ml

*Example #1:* The physician orders 60% dextrose in 1000 mL NS. How many grams of dextrose are in the bag?

OBJECTIVE ③

Examples on how to set up the problem:

**1.** First change the percentage to grams.     60% = 60 grams
**2.** Xg/1000 mL = 60 g/100 mL     Proportion Method

OR

Xg : 1000 mL :: 60 g : 100 mL    FOIL method

OR

Xg = 1000 mL × 60 g/100 mL    Dimensional analysis

OR

60% × 1000 = 0.6 × 1000 = X grams

0.6 g × 1000 ml    Converting percent to a decimal

*Answer:* 600 g of dextrose are in each 1000 mL bag.

*Example #2:* The physician orders 50% dextrose in 1000 mL of NS. How many mL will give you 10 g of Dextrose?

Examples on how to set up the problem:

X ml/10 g = 100 mL/50 g              Proportion Method

X ml : 10 g :: 100 mL : 50 g          FOIL Method

X ml = 10 g × 100 mL/50 g            Dimensional analysis

*Answer:* 20 mL of 50% solution contains 10 g of dextrose.

OBJECTIVE 2

| Common intravenous solutions | Hypertonic | Hypotonic | Isotonic |
|---|---|---|---|
| Saline Solutions | 3-5% sodium chloride Commonly known as: 3-5% NS | 0.45% sodium chloride Commonly known as: 0.45% NS Half Normal Saline | 0.9% sodium chloride Also known as: 0.9% NaCl Normal Saline |
| Dextrose in Saline | 5% dextrose in 0.9% sodium chloride Also known as: $D_5$ 0.9% NaCl | | 5% dextrose in 0.225% sodium chloride Also known as: $D_5$ 0.225% NaCl |
| Dextrose in Water | 10% dextrose in water Commonly known as: $D_{10}W$ | | 5% dextrose in water Commonly known as: $D_5W$ |
| Electrolyte Solutions | 5% dextrose in lactated Ringer's Also known as $D_5LR$ | | Lactated Ringer's Also known as LR |

## MEASURING CONCENTRATION

Concentration of a solution is simply a measurement of how much solute is dissolved in the solvent and can be measured in a variety of different ways. One type of concentration is percent volume to volume; for example, alcohol often comes in a 70% solution, which means that of the total volume 70% is alcohol and the remaining 30% would be water. A similar type of concentration is percent mass to mass, for example ammonium hydroxide (ammonia) in a strong form is 35% solution, which means that for a total mass of 100 g, 35% would be the mass of the ammonium hydroxide. Another type of percent concentration is mass to volume, which is found by dividing the mass of the solute by the volume of the solution and multiplying by 100 to represent it as a percent. It should be noted that often weight is used instead of mass, but they are actually very different scientific concepts. Mass to volume is also represented simply with units of mass/volume. For example, if 40 mg of NaCl is dissolved into 100 ml of water, it could be represented as 40 mg/100 ml or simplified to just 0.4 mg/ml.

## PRACTICE THE SKILL 12-1

1. You have 70% dextrose solution. How many grams are in 20 mL of solution?

2. You have 70% dextrose solution. How many grams are in 75 mL of solution?

3. You have 70% dextrose solution. How many grams are in 50 mL of solution?

4. You have a 50% dextrose solution. How many ml will give you 10 g of dextrose?

5. You have a 50% dextrose solution. How many mL will give your 35 g of dextrose?

6. You have a 50% dextrose solution. How many mL will give you 25 g of dextrose?

7. If 200 g of dextrose is ordered using a 50% dextrose solution, how many mL are needed?

8. If 40 g of dextrose is ordered using a 50% dextrose solution, how many mL are needed?

9. If 80 g of dextrose is ordered using a 50% dextrose solution, how many mL are needed?

10. Lactated Ringers is considered what type of tonicity?

11. $D_5$ 0.9%NaCl (normal saline) is considered what type of tonicity?

12. $D_5W$ is considered what type of tonicity?

## REAL WORLD 12-2

Corn syrup: Hypertonic

Contact lens cleaner: Hypertonic

Ocean Habitat: Hypertonic

Tap water: Hypertonic or Hypotonic depending on the concentration of the ions.

Sports Drinks: Hypertonic if contains increased levels of sodium (Na) or Sugar (dextrose). Drinks used to prevent dehydration are hypertonic.

Distilled Water: Hypotonic

Freshwater Habitat: Hypotonic

OBJECTIVE 3

*Example Problems with Concentrations:*

1. A 100 mL of 5% saline is diluted to 1250 mL, what is the new concentration?
   - Concentration × Volume = Concentration × Volume
   - Since both concentrations are %'s and volumes are in mL, no conversions are needed
   - $100 \times 5 = X\% \times 1250$
   - Answer is 0.4%

2. A 100 ml of 5% solution is left open and 80 ml of water evaporate creating a more concentrated solution; what is the new concentration?
   - Concentration × Volume = Concentration × Volume
   - Since both concentrations are %'s and volumes are in ml, no conversions are needed
   - $100 \times 5 = X\% \times 20$
   - Answer is 25%

3. To create 100 ml of 5% solution from a stock supply of 25% solution how much of the stock supply must be used?
   - Concentration × Volume = Concentration × Volume
   - Since both concentrations are %'s and volumes are in mL, no conversions are needed
   - $100 \times 5\% = \text{volume} \times 25\%$
   - Answer is 20 mL

OBJECTIVE 3

## PRACTICE THE SKILL 12-2

1. An injection of a drug is made by dissolving 0.68 g of the drug into 8 mL of water. What is the percent strength of the drug in mass/volume?

2. 35 mL of a drug is mixed with 452 mL of water; what is the percent by volume of the drug?

3. 200 mL of 15% saline is diluted to 1250 mL; what is the new concentration?

4. 1 L of 5% solution is left open and 80 mL of water evaporate; creating a more concentrated solution; what is the new concentration?

5. To create 1.75 L of 5% solution from a stock supply of 70%, how much of the stock supply must be used?

OBJECTIVE 4

## CHEMISTRY CONCENTRATIONS

The realm of chemistry has its own methods for measuring concentration of chemical solutes in solutions based on the **mole**. The mole is a grouping of atoms or molecules to make them easier to work with in calculations. Individual atoms or molecules are too small to actually handle, so chemists group a very large number of them together and then perform calculations with those groupings called moles. A mole, abbreviated mol, contains 602,200,000,000,000,000,000,000 atoms or molecules. The mole is similar in concept to a dozen, just on a much larger scale. When ordering donuts most people would order 8 dozen because 8 (dozen) is a more manageable number than 96 (individual donuts). Similarly, a chemist uses 1 mole because it is more manageable than $6.022 \times 10^{23}$ or 602,200,000,000,000,000, 000,000. There are two major ways that chemists use the mole to calculate concentration molarity (abbreviated M) and molality (abbreviated m). **Molarity** is the number of moles per liter of solution. For example, 12 M means that for every 1 liter of solution there are 12 moles dissolved in that solution. **Molality** is the number of moles per kilogram of solvent. For example, 12 m means that for every 1 kg of solvent 12 moles of solute was dissolved. Molality can be very useful when dealing with calculations where total volume of solution is not as important as the amount of solute. Both molarity and molality are forms of concentrations. While very useful in the realm of chemistry, as it applies to research, they are rarely used in other areas of health care. In areas of research and development, molar mass can become very useful. Molar mass occurs when converting moles to grams. The molar mass is simply the mass in grams of one mole of a given substance.

$$\text{Molarity (M)} = \frac{\text{Moles}}{\text{Liters of solution}} \qquad \text{Molality (m)} = \frac{\text{moles of solute}}{\text{kg of solvent}}$$

*Example 1:*
A researcher creates a test solution using 2 kilograms of water and 12.5 moles of the test chemical. What is the molality of the solution?
- Formula: m = moles/kg solvent
  12.5 moles/2 kg
- Answer: 6.25 molality or m = 6.25 mol/kg

*Example 2:*
A 12 M solution is used in a given research; if 50 ml are used, how many moles are actually being used?
- 50 ml converted to liters is 0.05 L
- 0.05 L × 12 mol/L
- Answer: 0.6 moles

*Example 3:*
The molar mass of sodium chloride is 58.4 g/mol; if a solution is made containing 394.2 grams of sodium chloride and has a total volume of 1225 ml, what is the molarity of the sodium chloride solution?
- Convert grams sodium chloride to moles by dividing by molar mass

$$394.2g \times \frac{1\ mol}{58.4\ g} = 6.75\ moles$$

- Convert ml of solution to L of solution
  1225 mL –> 1.225 L
- M = moles solute/liters of solution
  6.75 mol/1.225 L
*Answer:* M = 5.51 moles/liter or 5.51 mol/L

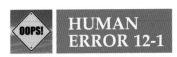

**HUMAN ERROR 12-1**

*The abbreviation M or m can stand for different measurements:*

*Meter (M or m), molarity (M), molality (m)*

*Make sure you are using the correct formula based on the information and measurement you are trying to solve. Does your answer make sense, and does it answer the question?*

 **PRACTICE THE SKILL 12-3**          OBJECTIVES

1. A solution is prepared using 245 grams of water and $1.25 \times 10^{-3}$ moles of the sulfuric acid; what is the molality of the solution?

2. 65 mL of a 4.25 Molar solution is to needed; how many moles are actually needed?

3. 35 mL of a 5.25 Molar solution is needed; how many moles are actually needed?

4. How many grams of solute are needed to create 750 ml of a 3 molar NaOH solution if the molar mass of sodium hydroxide is 40.0 g/mol?

5. How many grams of solute are needed to create 500 ml of a 12 molar HCL solution if the molar mass of hydrochloric acid is 36.5 g/mol?

## CHANGING CONCENTRATIONS

There are some instances when a technician may need to convert a solution with one concentration to a solution with a different concentration. This frequently occurs when preparing hyperalimentation or total parenteral nutrition for patients who need to be fed completely through IVs. Solving this type of problem can be done by using the following formula:

$$\frac{X \text{ volume wanted}}{\% \text{ Wanted}} = \frac{\text{volume prescribed}}{\% \text{ Have}}$$

The most common solution used to change the concentration from one level to another is sterile water.

*Example 1:*
If a physician orders 25% dextrose 1000 mL and the only available solution is 70% dextrose in 1000 mL, how much of the 70% dextrose would you use and how much sterile water would you use?

$$\frac{X}{25} = \frac{1000}{70}$$

$$70 X = 25,000$$

$$\frac{70X}{70} = \frac{25,000}{70}$$

X = 357 mL of 70% dextrose
To find out how much sterile water you would use:
1000 ml (total volume) – 357 ml (70% dextrose) = 643 ml of sterile water.
*Remember both quantities have to add up to the total amount of fluid being used. In this case it was 1000 ml.

---

### REAL WORLD BOX 12-3
*How Temperature Affects a Solution*

Temperature influences the rate at which a solute dissolves. The higher the solution temperature, the quicker the solute will dissolve. This reaction occurs because there is an increase in surface area.

**Example:** Sugar in hot tea.

---

OBJECTIVE **3**        ## PRACTICE THE SKILL 12-4

1. If a physician orders 20% dextrose 1000 mL and the only available solution is 70% dextrose in 1000 mL:

   a. How much of the dextrose will you use?

   b. How much of the sterile water will you use?

*(Continued)*

## PRACTICE THE SKILL 12-4
*Continued from p. 296*

2. If a physician orders 40% dextrose in 1000 mL and the only available solution is 70% dextrose in 1000 mL:

   a. How much of the dextrose will you use?

   b. How much of the sterile water will you use?

3. If a physician orders 25% dextrose 500 mL and the only available solution is 50% dextrose in 1000 mL:

   a. How much dextrose will you use?

   b. How much of the sterile water will you use?

4. The physician orders 50% dextrose 500 mL and the only available solution is 70% dextrose in 1000 mL.

   a. How much dextrose will you use?

   b. How much of the sterile water will you use?

5. The physician orders 20% dextrose in 500 mL and the only available solution is 50% in 500 mL.

   a. How much dextrose will you use?

   b. How much of the sterile water will you use?

## BUILDING CONFIDENCE WITH THE SKILL 12-1

OBJECTIVES ② ③ ④

**Solve the following problems:**

1. The container of liquid contains 12 mg/10 mL. What percent is this liquid?

2. The container of solution contains 15 mg/20 mL. What percent is this solution?

3. The container label reads 75 mg/15 mL. What percent is this liquid?

4. If a physician orders 40% dextrose in 1000 mL and the only available solution is 70% dextrose in 1000 mL:

   a. How much dextrose would you use?

   b. How much sterile water would you use?

*(Continued)*

## BUILDING CONFIDENCE WITH THE SKILL 12-1
*Continued from p. 297*

5. The physician orders 35% dextrose in 1000 mL and the only available solution is 50% in 1000 mL.

   a. How much dextrose would you use?

   b. How much sterile water would you use?

6. The physician orders 50% dextrose in 100 mL and you only have available 50% in 1000 mL.

   a. How much dextrose would you use?

   b. How much sterile water would you use?

7. A solution has a total mass of 400 g. If the solvent has a mass of 236 g of the total mass, what is the strength of the drug?

8. An injection is made by dissolving 2.68 g of the drug into 15 mL of water, what is the percent strength of the drug in mass/volume?

9. 50 ml of a chemical is mixed with 450 mL of alcohol; what is the percent by volume of the chemical?

10. A 10 ml of 12 M saline is diluted to 1000 mL; what is the new concentration?

11. A 5-gallon stock supply of 90% rubbing alcohol is accidentally used to finish filling a 1000-gallon drinking water tank. What is the concentration of alcohol in the drinking water?

12. An ointment has a total mass of 50 g if the solvent has a mass of 35.6 g of the total mass; what is the strength of the ointment?

13. A solution is prepared using 245 grams of water and $1.25 \times 10^{-3}$ moles of the sulfuric acid; what is the molality of the solution?

14. 65 ml of a 4.25 Molar solution is needed; how many moles are actually needed?

15. How many grams of solute are needed to create 750 ml of a 3 molar NaOH solution if the molar mass of sodium hydroxide is 40.0 g/mol?

OBJECTIVE 5

## INTRAVENOUS (IV) AND FLOW RATE

Tonicity is very important in terms of medication or other liquids being put into a living organism because it could cause water to enter or exit the cells of the living organism, which could have serious consequences. Such medications or liquids can be given as a shot or an injection. Another way to administer the medications or liquids is to have an IV, which administers directly into a vein. IVs deliver a set volume of medication or liquids to a patient over a length of time. The rate at which the IV delivers the medication is known as the flow or **flow rate**. Flow rate as a formula is $F = V/T$, where F represents flow, V represents volume, and T represents time.

*Example:* 2 liters of normal saline delivered over 8 hours would have a flow rate of ¼ L/h (liter per hour). With some simple conversions that same flow rate would be 250 ml/h. Depending on the situation, you might need to calculate volume, time, or the flow. Remember to make sure that your units are appropriate. For example, to find the time it takes to administer a volume of 2 liters with a flow of 100 ml/h, a conversion must first be completed because the volumes are not in the same units; 2 liters would need to be converted to 2000 ml. The time could then be found by dividing the volume, 2000 ml, by the flow rate 100 ml/h resulting in a time of 20 hours.

## MATH QUICK TIPS 12-2

Formulas for solving Flow Rate with Intravenous solutions:

| | |
|---|---|
| Flow = Volume/Time | $F = V/T$ |
| Volume = Flow × Time | $V = F \times T$ |
| Time: Volume/Flow | $T = V/F$ |

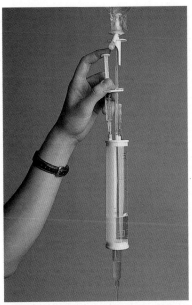

Example of medication being added to an intravenous solution. (From Potter PA, Perry AG: *Fundamentals of nursing,* ed 6, St Louis, 2005, Mosby.)

Another way to look at the formula is:
Amount of fluid (ml)/Total time of infusion (minutes) × Set up drop factor = gtt/min

Depending on the amount and type of fluids being administered, a health care professional may need to figure out the infusion rate based on the manufacturer predetermined **drop factor**. This information can be located on the packaging. Drop factors are based on the number of drops/milliliters. Microdrip infusion sets can deliver a larger quantity of drops/milliliter than Macro drip sets. Special administration sets (blood, TPN) have their own unique drop factors. For safety, always check the drop factor on the packaging when calculating flow rate. When working with drops/min, the solution must be given in whole numbers. Use the rules for rounding to determine the flow rate.

*Example #1:*
The physician orders 500 mL of IV fluids to infuse over 12 hours. The micro set-up packaging indicates the drop factor is 60 gtt/mL. What would be the flow rate? What would be the drop factor?

$F = V/T$

$F = 500 \text{ mL} / 12 \text{ hours}$

$F = 42 \text{ mL/hour}$ (1 mL is equal to 60 gtt)

Using Dimensional Analysis to solve the above equation:

T gtt/min = 500 mL/12 hours

$$T \text{ gtt/min} = \frac{500 \text{ mL}}{12 \text{ hours}} \times \frac{1 \text{ hour}}{60 \text{ min}} \quad \text{Change hour to minutes since your answer is in minutes.}$$

$$T \text{ gtt/min} = \frac{500 \text{ mL}}{12 \text{ hours}} \times \frac{1 \text{ hour}}{60 \text{ min}} \times \frac{60 \text{ gtts}}{1 \text{ ml}} \quad \text{Multiply by the drop factor}$$

$$T \text{ gtt/min} = \frac{500 \; \cancel{\text{ml}}}{12 \; \cancel{\text{hours}}} \times \frac{1 \; \cancel{\text{hour}}}{\cancel{60} \text{ min}} \times \frac{\cancel{60} \text{ gtts}}{1 \; \cancel{\text{ml}}} \quad \text{Cross Cancellation}$$

T gtt/min = 500 gtt/ 12 min

*Answer:* The nurse would infuse at 42 gtt/min.

*Example #2:*
How long will an IV last if 500 ml of a 30% solution are given at a flow rate of 2.5 ml/min?

- $T = V/F$
- $T = 500 \text{ mL}/(2.5 \text{ ml/min}) = 200 \text{ mins}$

*Answer:* 200 mins or 3 hours 20 mins

*Example #3:*
A patient is started on a 2 L IV with a flow rate of 250 ml/hour, but because of complications the IV is removed after 1 hour and 45 minutes. How much of the IV did the patient receive?

- $V = T*F$
- 1 H45 min is 1.75 hours
- 1.75 hours × 250 ml/hour = 437.5 ml

*Answer:* The patient received 437.5 mL or 438 mL.

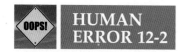

## HUMAN ERROR 12-2

*Many facilities only use electronic pumps to administer IV solutions. Be aware that some machines will administer the flow rate in ml/hour and some will administer the flow rate in ml/minute.*

*Be familiar with your machine and have someone verify your machine setup prior to starting all infusions.*

## REAL WORLD BOX 12-3

| | |
|---|---|
| Microdrip setup | 60 gtt/mL |
| Standard setup | Range from 10, 15 or 20 gtt/mL |
| Blood setup | 10 gtt/mL |

## PRACTICE THE SKILL 12-5

1. What is the flow rate, in L/H, of an IV if a patient is to be given 2 L of solution in 3 hours?

2. How long will an IV last if 0.75 L of a 5% saline solution is given at 2.5 mL/min?

3. A patient is started on a 9 L IV with a flow rate of 175 mL/hour, but because of complications the IV is removed after 45 mins. How much of the IV did the patient receive?

4. What is the drop factor that will deliver 1.25 L of fluids to a patient over 4 hours?

5. When should an IV be replaced it the patient is receiving 2000 mL of antivirals at 3.5 mL/min, assuming the patient is supposed to be continuously receiving the antiviral IV?

6. The physician orders 1000 ml of NS to be infused over 8 hours. The setup drop factor is 10 gtt/mL. Determine the drops/min.

7. The physician orders 550 ml of D5W to be infused over 5 hours. The setup drop factor is 20 gtt/mL. Determine the drops/min.

8. The setup drop factor is 20 gtt/mL. The doctor has order 150 mL of LR over the next 24 hours. Determine the drops/min.

9. The nurse is to give an IV bolus of 250 mL of normal saline over the next 2 hours. How many mL will the patient receive each hour?

10. The physician ordered 1000 mL of D5 0.45% NaCl solution to be given over the next 8 hours. Determine the flow rate.

Depending on your field of study, health care workers will receive orders to administer other fluids through an IV. Total Parenteral Nutrition (TPN), lipids, and blood products must be infused with special IV setups. Determining flow rate will be based on specific IV manufacturers' instruction and will be discussed in depth in specialty classes.

## INTAKE AND OUTPUT GRAPHS

Measurement of the body's intake of fluids and output of fluids is very important in monitoring how the body is dealing with disease, trauma, and illnesses. The heart must work harder if there is a retention of fluids. This can be evaluated by observing for edema or swelling in the extremities. Kidney function can be observed based on the amount of urine excreted from the body.

Cell and tissue repair is based on nutritional intake. Health care workers will evaluate the amount of consumption of solid foods in the form of percentage. Patients who only consume 25% of their diet over a period of time could lead to decrease in body weight, and is an indicator that there is a change in the body's condition.

Intake and Output graphs are used to help measure the amount of liquids which are going into and out of the body in a 24-hour period. This might be kept at the bedside for easy access. At the end of the day, totals are recorded in the EHR.

Looking at Figure 12-1, the lower section includes the intake—liquids that are taken into the body via mouth, IV, feeding tubes, and irrigation. The output section

Med-Forms, Inc.
FORM #MF37079 (Rev 9/95)

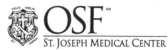

OSF
ST. JOSEPH MEDICAL CENTER
Bloomington, Illinois 61701

**DAILY SUMMARY AND GRAPHIC**

**TEMPERATURE**
Write in 105¹ or over

| DATE | 5 – 7 | | | | | | 5 – 8 | | | | | | | | | | | | | | | | | |
|---|---|---|---|---|---|---|---|---|---|---|---|---|---|---|---|---|---|---|---|---|---|---|---|---|
| HOSPITAL DAY | 4 | | | | | | 5 | | | | | | | | | | | | | | | | | |
| POST OP DAY | | | | | | | | | | | | | | | | | | | | | | | | |
| HOUR | 2400 | 0400 | 0800 | 1200 | 1600 | 2000 | 2400 | 0400 | 0800 | 1200 | 1600 | 2000 | 2400 | 0400 | 0800 | 1200 | 1600 | 2000 | 2400 | 0400 | 0800 | 1200 | 1600 | 2000 |
| B/P | | | 130/80 | 120/76 | 130/76 | 130/80 | | | 120/72 | 120/80 | 130/80 | 130/82 | | | | | | | | | | | | |

TEMPERATURE scale: 104 / 40, 102.2 / 39, 100.4 / 38, 98.6 / 37, 96.6 / 36

| PULSE | | | 74 | 80 | 76 | 74 | | | 74 | 74 | 76 | 72 | | | | | | | | | | | | |
| RESPIRATION | | | 18 | 18 | 16 | 16 | | | 18 | 20 | 18 | 16 | | | | | | | | | | | | |
| WEIGHT | | | | | | | | | | | | | | | | | | | | | | | | |
| DR. VISIT | @ 0900 | | | | | | | | | | | | | | | | | | | | | | | |

| INTAKE | 2300-0700 | 0700-1500 | 1500-2300 | TOTAL | 2300-0700 | 0700-1500 | 1500-2300 | TOTAL | 2300-0700 | 0700-1500 | 1500-2300 | TOTAL | 2300-0700 | 0700-1500 | 1500-2300 | TOTAL |
|---|---|---|---|---|---|---|---|---|---|---|---|---|---|---|---|---|
| Oral | 100 | 1200 | 800 | 2100 | 100 | 1050 | 820 | 1970 | | | | | | | | |
| IV | | | | | | | | | | | | | | | | |
| Tube Feedings | | | | | | | | | | | | | | | | |
| PPN/TPN/Lipids | | | | | | | | | | | | | | | | |
| Blood/Blood Products | | | | | | | | | | | | | | | | |
| IV Meds | | | | | | | | | | | | | | | | |
| Chemotherapy | | | | | | | | | | | | | | | | |
| Unreturned irr. sol. | | | | | | | | | | | | | | | | |
| TOTAL INTAKE | 100 | 1200 | 800 | 2100 | 100 | 1050 | 820 | 1970 | | | | | | | | |
| OUTPUT | 2300-0700 | 0700-1500 | 1500-2300 | TOTAL | 2300-0700 | 0700-1500 | 1500-2300 | TOTAL | 2300-0700 | 0700-1500 | 1500-2300 | TOTAL | 2300-0700 | 0700-1500 | 1500-2300 | TOTAL |
| Urine | 0 | 1050 | 800 | 1850 | 200 | 850 | 750 | 1800 | | | | | | | | |
| GI | | | | | | | | | | | | | | | | |
| Emesis | 100 | | | 100 | | | | | | | | | | | | |
| Drains | | | | | | | | | | | | | | | | |
| | | | | | | | | | | | | | | | | |
| TOTAL OUTPUT | 100 | 1050 | 800 | 1950 | 200 | 850 | 750 | 1800 | | | | | | | | |
| Feces | | ✓ | | | | ✓ | | | | | | | | | | |

**Figure 12-1** Vital sign graphic sheet. (Courtesy OSF St. Joseph Medical Center, Bloomington, Ill.)

records urine, emesis (vomit, drains, and bowel movements) for each time of the day. This information can be critical to the physician regarding the treatment of the patient.

## PRACTICE THE SKILL 12-6

Determine the total amount of Intake and/or Output for each scenario.

1. The patient consumed the following liquids during his breakfast:

   240 mL of coffee, 4 oz of OJ, 4 oz of milk, and 180 ml of supplemental shake.

2. The patient care assistant recorded the following values for an 8-hour shift. Determine the correct intake and output for this shift:

   0600 Patient urinated 600 mL

   0800 Patient consumed 4 oz of soda, 6 oz of coffee, and 180 mL of broth

   1030 Patient received 150 mL of IV antibiotics

   1230 Patient experienced emesis of 500 mL

   1330 Nurse recorded that the patient had received 780 mL of IV fluid

   1400 Patient urinated 450 mL

3. Determine the total intake and output based on the following data:

   1700 350 mL of blood

   1930 250 mL of IV antibiotics

   2030 500 mL bolus of IV fluids

   2100 Urinated 650 mL

   2330 Urinated 400 mL

   2345 IV fluid 750 mL

4. Use an Intake and Output Graph sheet or your computer to record the data.

| Time | 0600 | 0800 | 1200 | 1400 | 1600 | 1800 | 2000 | 2300 |
|------|------|------|------|------|------|------|------|------|
| PO Fluids | 240 mL | 120 mL | 500 mL | 180 mL | 120 mL | 480 mL | 240 mL | 120 mL |
| IV | 500 mL | 400 mL | 500 mL | 475 mL | 525 mL | 500 mL | 475 mL | 480 mL |
| IVPB | | 100 mL | | 100 mL | | | 100 mL | |
| Urine | 600 mL | 300 mL | 400 mL | 180 mL | 300 mL | 180 mL | 240 mL | 250 mL |
| Drains | 10 mL | 5 mL | 3 mL | 2 mL | | 5 mL | | 5 mL |

5. Determine the difference between the intake and output from the above data.

## CONCLUSION

This ends our exploration of the way math is used in health care settings. I hope you've increased your confidence in working mathematical computations and have a few new tools to put in your educational toolbox.

Some final reminders:

- There is more than one way to solve a math problem.
- Common errors have to do with addition or subtraction.
- Conversion problems are just proportions worded in a different way.
- Make sure your answer makes sense.
- When in doubt, have someone else check your answer.

OBJECTIVES ② ③ ④
⑤

# MASTER THE SKILL

1. How many ml of an IV bag will a patient receive if the IV was set to 2 mL/min and the bag lasted for 3 hours?

2. What is the flow of an IV that lasted 8 hours and contained 1.75 L of solution?

3. What is the flow mL/H of an IV that lasted 8 hours and contained 1.75 L of solution?

4. What is the flow mL/min of an IV that lasted 8 hours and contained 1.75 L of solution?

5. If a patients IV is not checked for 4 hours, will it still have fluid left if the IV has 500 mL of fluid given at a flow rate of 3 mL/min?

6. A 3 mole of glucose solution is to be made with 1.5 kg of water. How many grams are required if the molar mass of glucose is 180.2 g/mol?

7. A solution has a concentration of 12 molar or 12 mols/liter; if half of the solvent evaporates, what will the new concentration be?

8. The molar mass of Methylamine is 31.06 g/mol. If 2.5 L of a solution of Methylamine is made containing 994.2 grams of Methylamine, what is the molarity of the Methylamine solution?

9. How many grams of solute are needed to create 2500 mL of a 9 molar HCL solution if the molar mass of hydrochloric acid is 36.5 g/mol?

10. A 2.5 M solution is used in a given research; if 5 ml are used, how many moles are actually being used?

11. The physician orders a 750 mL IV fluid to be run over 8 hours. The setup drop factor is 60 gtt/mL Calculate the gtt/mL.

12. The physician orders 125 ml antibiotic piggy back to be run over 4 hours. The setup drop factor is 10 gtt/mL Calculate the gtt/mL.

*(Continued)*

## MASTER THE SKILL
*Continued from p. 304*

13. The physician orders 1000 ml to be infused at 100 mL/hour. How long will it take for the infusion to be complete?

14. The physician orders a 500 mL bolus to be infused at 125 mL/hour. How long will it take for the infusion to be complete?

15. How many milliliters will be infused at a flow rate of 42 mL/hour and the infusion time of 12 hours?

Using the information below answer questions 16-20.

| Time | 0600 | 0800 | 1200 | 1400 | 1600 | 1800 | 2000 | 2300 |
|---|---|---|---|---|---|---|---|---|
| PO Fluids | 4 oz | 320 mL | 500 mL | 100 mL | 220 mL | 600 mL | 8 oz | 4 oz |
| IV | 500 mL | 400 mL | 500 mL | 475 mL | 525 mL | 500 mL | 475 mL | 480 mL |
| IVPB | | 250 mL | | 100 mL | | | 150 mL | |
| Urine | 300 mL | 600 mL | 200 mL | 180 mL | 400 mL | 180 mL | 240 mL | 250 mL |
| Drains | 10 mL | 5 mL | 3 mL | 2 mL | 4 mL | 5 mL | 3 mL | 5 mL |

16. What was the total oral fluid intake? _____

17. What was the total IV and IVPB intake? _____

18. What was the total urine output? _____

19. What was the total drain output? _____

20. Which was greater: Intake or Output? _____

APPENDIX

# Answers to Odd-Numbered Practice the Skill and Building Confidence with the Skill Questions

## CHAPTER 1

### Practice the Skill 1-1

1. 9,612
3. 78,005
5. 123,122
7. 7,189
9. 2,183
11. 1,278
13. 34,382
15. Thousand
17. Billion
19. Ten thousand

### Practice the Skill 1-2

1. 72,065
3. 641,387
5. 3,712,108
7. 629
9. 7,049

### Practice the Skill 1-3

1. 98
3. 180
5. 3,456
7. 9,000
9. 7,938
11. 40,016

### Practice the Skill 1-4

1. 8 remainder 5
3. 50
5. 10 remainder 4
7. 5,473 remainder 7
9. 790 remainder 31
11. 9

### Practice the Skill 1-5

1. 8
3. −389
5. 123,410
7. −1,449
9. 20
11. −8
13. −138
15. −82
17. −7,590
19. −1,794
21. −6 remainder 2
23. −257 remainder 20
25. −29,747 remainder 2

### Practice the Skill 1-6

1. $2^3 \times 3^2$
3. $5^5$
5. $2^3 \times 3^2 \times 4^2$
7. $10^3 \times 12^3$
9. $60^2 \times 30^3 \times 10^2$

### Practice the Skill 1-7

1. 1,024
3. 1,000,000
5. 7,776
7. 4,096
9. 72
11. 0.04

### Practice the Skill 1-8

1. 24
3. 2,401
5. $5.77 \times 10^{21}$
7. $2.06 \times 10^{24}$
9. 20,480,000
11. 0.04

### Practice the Skill 1-9

1. 18
3. 75
5. 144
7. 480
9. 5
11. 43,890
13. 44,672
15. 81
17. 2
19. 2.5
21. 25
23. 76
25. 46

### Practice the Skill 1-10

1. 4,320
3. 13,017
5. 68.57
7. −169
9. 301

### Practice the Skill 1-11

1. True
3. False
5. False
7. True
9. True

### Practice the Skill 1-12

1. 1, 3, 5, 9, 15, 45
3. 1, 2, 4, 5, 10, 20, 25, 50, 100
5. 1, 3, 9, 27
7. 1, 2, 3, 5, 6, 7, 10, 14, 15, 21, 30, 35, 42, 70, 105, 210
9. 1, 2, 3, 4, 6, 9, 12, 18, 36

### Practice the Skill 1-13

1. 5
3. 7
5. 11
7. 2
9. 8
11. 12
13. 4
15. 1

### Practice the Skill 1-14

1. 8
3. 60
5. 60
7. 40
9. 26
11. 75
13. 576
15. 120

### Building Confidence with the Skill 1-1

1. 8
3. 290 remainder 2
5. 898 remainder 1
7. 448
9. 11,730
11. 1,450
13. 1,571
15. 7,508
17. −16
19. −133
21. 6
23. 1
25. 5

306

## Building Confidence with the Skill 1-2

1. 28
3. 75
5. 75
7. 144
9. 42

11. 384
13. 1,800
15. 3,120
17. 5
19. 35

21. 1
23. 60
25. 8

# CHAPTER 2

## Practice the Skill 2-1

1. VII
3. VIII
5. XV
7. LXV
9. MMVI
11. 4
13. 30
15. 1008
17. 8
19. 16

## Practice the Skill 2-2

1. 32.569
3. 1986.201
5. 89.205
7. 210.11
9. 4476.57
11. 2.6
13. 1.2
15. 0.1

## Practice the Skill 2-3

1.

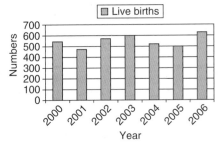

5. a. April, September, and December; b. July and October; c. March, July, September, and December; d. September; e. April and September

3.

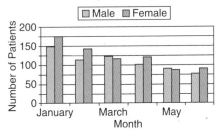

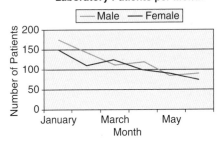

## Practice the Skill 2-4

1.

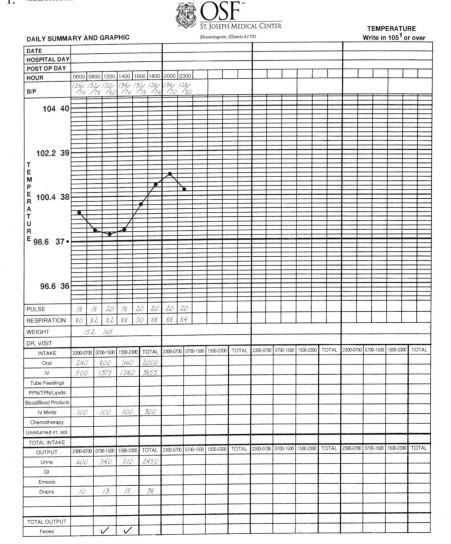

3. Intake 6,155 mL; output 2,488 mL

## Building Confidence with the Skill 2-1

| | | |
|---|---|---|
| **1.** 2100 | **15.** 6:00 a.m. | **29.** MCMLXV |
| **3.** 0700 | **17.** 9:00 p.m. | **31.** XXIII |
| **5.** 1200 | **19.** 2:00 p.m. | **33.** XXXI |
| **7.** 0300 | **21.** XIX | **35.** XXIX |
| **9.** 1345 | **23.** XLI | **37.** VI |
| **11.** 7:00 a.m. | **25.** CX | **39.** xviss |
| **13.** 11:30 p.m. | **27.** IV | |

## Building Confidence with the Skill 2-2

| Problem | Ones | Thousandths | Tenths | Hundredths |
|---|---|---|---|---|
| **1.** 0.97341 | 1 | 0.973 | 1.0 | 0.97 |
| **3.** 15.97523 | 16 | 15.975 | 16.0 | 15.98 |
| **5.** 12.20914 | 12 | 12.209 | 12.2 | 12.21 |
| **7.** 0.55645 | 1 | 0.556 | 0.6 | 0.56 |
| **9.** 0.27743 | 0 | 0.277 | 0.3 | 0.28 |

| | |
|---|---|
| **11.** C | **17.** G |
| **13.** B | **19.** J |
| **15.** I | |

## Building Confidence with the Skill 2-3

**1.**

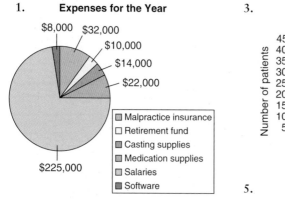

Expenses for the Year

$8,000  $32,000
$10,000
$14,000
$22,000
$225,000

☐ Malpractice insurance
☐ Retirement fund
☐ Casting supplies
☐ Medication supplies
☐ Salaries
☐ Software

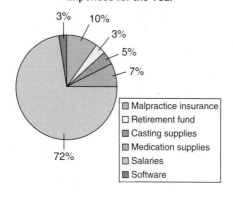

Expenses for the Year

3%  10%
3%
5%
7%
72%

☐ Malpractice insurance
☐ Retirement fund
☐ Casting supplies
☐ Medication supplies
☐ Salaries
☐ Software

**3.**

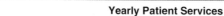
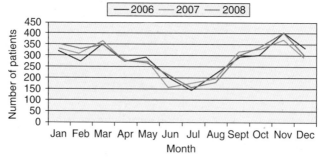

Yearly Patient Services

— 2006 — 2007 — 2008

**5.**

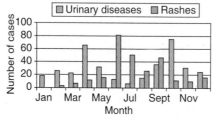

Diseases per Year

☐ Urinary diseases  ☐ Rashes

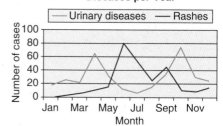

Diseases per Year

— Urinary diseases — Rashes

# CHAPTER 3

## Practice the Skill 3-1

1. $\frac{2}{3}$
3. $\frac{1}{2}$
5. $\frac{1}{10}$

## Practice the Skill 3-2

1. 3
3. 3
5. 5
7. Yes
9. No

## Practice the Skill 3-3

1. $6\frac{3}{4}$
3. $1\frac{2}{10}$, reduce to $1\frac{1}{5}$
5. $10\frac{3}{6}$ or $10\frac{1}{2}$
7. $6\frac{3}{7}$
9. $11\frac{1}{2}$

## Practice the Skill 3-4

1. $\frac{15}{4}$
3. $\frac{11}{2}$
5. $\frac{93}{8}$
7. $\frac{38}{3}$
9. $\frac{39}{8}$

## Practice the Skill 3-5

1. $\frac{3}{5}$
3. $\frac{11}{13}$
5. 1
7. $\frac{11}{14}$
9. $\frac{12}{35}$

## Practice the Skill 3-6

1. $\frac{3}{10}$
3. $\frac{3}{5}$
5. $\frac{1}{8}$
7. $\frac{26}{75}$
9. 1

## Practice the Skill 3-7

1. 6
3. 45
5. 18
7. 30
9. 12

## Practice the Skill 3-8

1. $1\frac{3}{14}$
3. $1\frac{1}{16}$
5. $\frac{7}{8}$
7. $1\frac{1}{9}$
9. $1\frac{9}{20}$

## Practice the Skill 3-9

1. $1\frac{7}{15}$
3. $1\frac{23}{42}$
5. $1\frac{22}{45}$
7. $1\frac{1}{60}$
9. $1\frac{17}{24}$
11. $\frac{1}{4}$

## Practice the Skill 3-10

1. $7\frac{11}{12}$
3. $21\frac{5}{24}$
5. $44\frac{21}{22}$
7. $17\frac{2}{9}$
9. $19\frac{7}{15}$

## Practice the Skill 3-11

1. $\frac{2}{9}$
3. $\frac{7}{20}$
5. $\frac{13}{24}$
7. $\frac{3}{40}$
9. $\frac{1}{12}$

## Practice the Skill 3-12

1. 11
3. $3\frac{47}{48}$
5. $3\frac{7}{10}$
7. $2\frac{4}{5}$
9. $6\frac{1}{6}$
11. $12\frac{11}{24}$

## Practice the Skill 3-13

1. $\frac{7}{10}$
3. $\frac{1}{4}$
5. $\frac{8}{21}$
7. $\frac{5}{96}$
9. $\frac{14}{25}$

## Practice the Skill 3-14

1. $14\frac{5}{24}$
3. $55\frac{1}{8}$
5. $35\frac{7}{9}$
7. $30\frac{11}{12}$
9. $97\frac{7}{8}$

## Practice the Skill 3-15

1. $2\frac{2}{3}$
3. $4\frac{2}{7}$
5. $\frac{27}{64}$
7. $1\frac{1}{5}$
9. $2\frac{1}{2}$

## Practice the Skill 3-16

1. $1\frac{1}{3}$

3. $1\frac{31}{99}$

5. $1\frac{23}{51}$

7. $1\frac{23}{25}$

9. $1\frac{17}{75}$

## Building Confidence with the Skill 3-1

1. Yes
3. No
5. No
7. No
9. Yes
11. $\frac{1}{2}$
13. $\frac{2}{3}$
15. $\frac{3}{5}$
17. $\frac{1}{4}$
19. $\frac{3}{4}$
21. a. $\frac{1}{4}$; b. $\frac{1}{3}$

## Building Confidence with the Skill 3-2

1. $\frac{1}{24}$, $\frac{1}{16}$, $\frac{1}{12}$
3. $\frac{5}{36}$, $\frac{5}{24}$, $\frac{5}{15}$
5. $\frac{1}{8}$, $\frac{2}{3}$, $\frac{3}{4}$
7. $3\frac{3}{4}$
9. $1\frac{1}{4}$
11. $\frac{1}{3}$
13. $\frac{1}{3}$
15. $\frac{1}{8}$
17. $\frac{93}{10}$
19. $\frac{79}{10}$
21. $\frac{12}{18}$
23. $\frac{15}{20}$
25. $\frac{9}{48}$
27. $\frac{1}{5}$
29. Least hours worked: Wednesday
Most hours worked: Friday

## Building Confidence with the Skill 3-3

1. $1\frac{7}{11}$

3. $1\frac{5}{12}$

5. $1\frac{5}{12}$

7. $\frac{23}{24}$

9. $1\frac{1}{16}$

11. $\frac{2}{11}$

13. $\frac{3}{16}$

15. $\frac{3}{4}$

17. $\frac{1}{4}$

19. 0

21. $9\frac{7}{8}$

23. $21\frac{13}{32}$

25. $16\frac{11}{16}$

27. $31\frac{24}{55}$

29. $2\frac{5}{6}$

31. 1

33. $\frac{3}{4}$ cup

35. $2\frac{1}{6}$ cups

## Building Confidence with the Skill 3-4

1. $\frac{8}{15}$

3. $\frac{10}{21}$

5. $\frac{16}{27}$

7. $\frac{35}{72}$

9. $\frac{1}{11}$

11. $1\frac{1}{9}$

13. $1\frac{2}{7}$

15. $1\frac{3}{32}$

17. $\frac{10}{21}$

19. $25\frac{14}{27}$

21. $131\frac{1}{4}$

23. $\frac{104}{123}$

25. $\frac{679}{775}$

27. $14\frac{7}{40}$

29. $7\frac{2}{5}$ hours per day

# CHAPTER 4

## Practice the Skill 4-1

1. 64 miles
3. 15,000 mg
5. 6.67 hours
7. 17 cc
9. 4.5 hours

## Practice the Skill 4-2

1. 2.358
3. 12.972
5. 7.132
7. 12.37
9. 14.33
11. 13.5
13. 1.0
15. 109.9
17. 89
19. 1

## Practice the Skill 4-3

1. 103.554
3. 20.226
5. 148.28
7. 15.1731
9. 1.89
11. 12.5
13. 5
15. 400
17. 721.871
19. 0.932

## Practice the Skill 4-4

1. 24.221
3. 7891.00
5. 63
7. 5.035
9. 100

## Practice the Skill 4-5

1. 170.6
3. 5
5. 1301
7. 300
9. 2.9126875

## Practice the Skill 4-6

1. $\frac{15}{100}$ (reduced: $\frac{3}{20}$)
3. $\frac{75}{100}$ (reduced: $\frac{3}{4}$)
5. $\frac{66}{100}$ (reduced: $\frac{33}{50}$)
7. $\frac{45}{100}$ (reduced: $\frac{9}{20}$)
9. $\frac{12}{100}$ (reduced: $\frac{3}{25}$)
11. 75%
13. 20%
15. 25%
17. 525%
19. 166.67%

## Practice the Skill 4-7

1. $18.75
3. $4.84
5. 375
7. 33.3%
9. 8.57%
11. $127.75
13. $138.94
15. $610.52

## Practice the Skill 4-8

1. 75%
3. 12.5%
5. 462.5%
7. 20%
9. 25%
11. 0.16666666667
13. 0.375
15. 0.75
17. 0.4166666
19. 0.7142857

## Building Confidence with the Skill 4-1

1. 10.13
3. $95.03
5. $2680.70
7. 22 mL
9. 13.63
11. 14.5
13. 13.53
15. 10.79
17. 600
19. $28.68
21. 30,000 mg
23. 166.67 mL per hour
25. a. $366.31; b. $91.58

## Building Confidence with the Skill 4-2

| Problem number | Fraction | Percentage | Decimal |
| --- | --- | --- | --- |
| 1. | $\frac{1}{2}$ | 50% | .5 |
| 3. | $\frac{9}{20}$ | 45% | .45 |
| 5. | $\frac{3}{4}$ | 75% | .75 |
| 7. | $\frac{33}{50}$ | 66% | .66 |
| 9. | $\frac{3}{5}$ | 60% | .60 |
| 11. | $\frac{2}{3}$ | $66\frac{2}{3}$% | .67 |
| 13. | $\frac{4}{5}$ | 80% | .80 |
| 15. | $\frac{2}{5}$ | 40% | .40 |

17. $692.34; $173.08
19. 3.1 mL

# CHAPTER 5

## Practice the Skill 5-1

1. 200:5
3. 0.4:2
5. 50:1
7. 2:3 and 3:5
9. 25:1
11. 2:17
13. 25:5
15. 20:1000
17. 1:158
19. 150:50

## Practice the Skill 5-2

1. X = 4
3. X = 168
5. X = 8
7. X = 0.2
9. X = 44
11. X = 22.22
13. X = 7.1
15. X = 33.3
17. X = 45
19. X = 1.7
21. X = 2.4
23. X = 36
25. X = 35

## Practice the Skill 5-3

1. 15 mL
3. 3,500 mL
5. 375 mL
7. 2.5 tablets
9. 40 mg
11. .75 mL

## Building Confidence with the Skill 5-1

1. X = 12
3. X = 22.7
5. X = 3
7. X = 4
9. X = 5
11. X = 4
13. X = 168
15. X = 8
17. X = $\frac{1}{5}$ or 0.2
19. X = 44
21. 18 carnations
23. 1.9 or 2 teachers
25. 10 minutes of commercials
27. 12 children
29. 108 cookies
31. 7 sedans
33. 25 gallons of gas
35. 105 bushels
37. 56 tickets
39. 450 minutes

# CHAPTER 6

## Practice the Skill 6-1

1. copayment
3. coinsurance
5. copayment
7. deductible
9. deductible; coinsurance

## Practice the Skill 6-2

1. No
3. Yes
5. $15.00

## Practice the Skill 6-3

1. a. 35%; b. $22.89; c. $42.51
3. a. 55%; b. $173.11; c. 141.63

## Practice the Skill 6-4

1. a. $134.00; b. $95.00; c. No, $39.00; d. $39.00; e. Yes, $11.20; f. $50.20; g. $44.80

## Building Confidence with the Skill 6-1

1. $25.00
3. a. $68.20; b. $66.80
5. a. $69.56; b. $105.44; c. $3.95
7. a. $505.00; b. 5323.50; c. 5828.50; d. 12421.50
9. a. $285.00; b. $95.00

## Practice the Skill 6-5

| 1. Payment methods | Total amount |
|---|---|
| Beginning Cash Balance | $135.00 |
| Total Amount of Cash | $479.00 |
| Total Amount of Coins | $5.68 |
| Total Amount of Checks | $130.62 |
| Total Amount of Credit Card | $135.00 |
| Total Amount of Refunds | $480.00 |
| Total Amount from Calculations | $479.00 + $5.68 + $130.62 + $135.00 − $135.00 − $480 = $135.30 |
| Do you have a Net Profit OR Net Loss? | Net Profit |

| 3. Payment methods | Total amount |
|---|---|
| Beginning Cash Balance | $525.00 |
| Total Amount of Cash | $414.00 |
| Total Amount of Coins | $8.21 |
| Total Amount of Checks | $30.62 |
| Total Amount of Credit Card | $535.00 |
| Total Amount of Refunds | $340.00 |
| Total Amount from Calculations | $122.83 |
| Do you have a Net Profit OR Net Loss? | Net Profit |

| 5. Payment methods | Total amount |
|---|---|
| Beginning Cash Balance | $600.00 |
| Total Amount of Cash | $239.00 |
| Total Amount of Coins | $1.73 |
| Total Amount of Checks | $454.43 |
| Total Amount of Credit Card | $685.00 |
| Total Amount of Refunds | $0.00 |
| Total Amount from Calculations | $780.16 |
| Do you have a Net Profit OR Net Loss? | Net Profit |

## Practice the Skill 6-6

**1.**

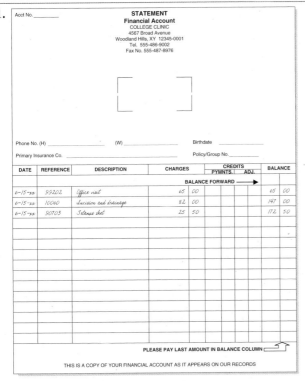

a. $172.50; b. $147.50; c. $0.00

**3.** a. $312.00; b. 78.00

| | DATE | PROFESSIONAL SERVICE | FEE | PAYMENT | ADJUST-MENT | NEW BALANCE | OLD BALANCE | PATIENT'S NAME | |
|---|---|---|---|---|---|---|---|---|---|
| 1 | | | | 25 00 | | | | Nathan Smith | 1 |
| 2 | | | | 45 00 | | | | Lori Hosty check 3354 | 2 |
| 3 | | | | 145 00 | | | | M.R. Jones | 3 |
| 4 | | | | 32 67 | | | | Nathan Smith pd by Nebi Health | 4 |
| 5 | | | | 436 58 | | | | M.R. Jones pd by Community Health | 5 |
| 6 | | | | | -20 00 | | | Lori Hosty over charge | 6 |
| 7 | | | | | | | | | 7 |
| 8 | | | | | | | | | 8 |
| 9 | | | | | | | | | 9 |
| 10 | | | | | | | | | 10 |
| 11 | | | | | | | | | 11 |
| 12 | | | | | | | | | 12 |
| 13 | | | | | | | | | 13 |
| 14 | | | | | | | | | 14 |
| 15 | | | | | | | | | 15 |
| 16 | | | | | | | | | 16 |
| 17 | | | | | | | | | 17 |
| 18 | | | | | | | | | 18 |
| 19 | | | | | | | | | 19 |
| 20 | | | | | | | | | 20 |
| 21 | | | | | | | | | 21 |
| 22 | | | | | | | | | 22 |
| 23 | | | | | | | | | 23 |
| 24 | | | | | | | | | 24 |
| 25 | | | | | | | | | 25 |
| 26 | | | | | | | | | 26 |
| 27 | | | | | | | | | 27 |
| 28 | | | | | | | | | 28 |
| 29 | | | | | | | | | 29 |
| 30 | | | | | | | | | 30 |
| 31 | | | | 686 25 | -20 00 | | | TOTALS THIS PAGE | 31 |
| 32 | | | | | | | | TOTAL PREVIOUS PAGE | 32 |
| 33 | | | | | | | | TOTALS MONTH TO DATE | 33 |

### JOURNAL OF DAILY CHARGES & PAYMENTS

d. $664.25

## Practice the Skill 6-7

1. $18.02
3. a. No, $35.00 from the IOU is unaccounted for; b. $74.42

## Practice the Skill 6-8

1. 1:30 p.m.; 1330; $116.00
3. 7:30 p.m.; 1930; $265.85
5. 6:30 a.m.; 0630; $205.38
7. a. Weekday: $20.97. Weekend: $21.47/hour; b. Weekday: $167.76, Weekend: $171.76; c. $846.80
9. a. Weekday: $16.35, Weekend: $16.85; b. Weekday: $15.60, Weekend: $16.35; c. Weekday: $130.80, Weekend: $118.80; d. $187.20; e. $698.40

## Practice the Skill 6-9

1. a. $598.40; b. $151.02; c. $447.38
3. a. $1,395.72; b. $397.69; c. $998.01
5. a. 1,596.00; b. $205.38; c. $1,269.08

## Building Confidence with the Skill 6-2

1. a. $142.84; b. $35.71
3. $35.00
5. a. $432.80; b. $93.20; c. $118.20
7. a. $738.00; b. $438.00; c. $300.00
9. a. $138.00/day; b. $282.00/day; c. $978.00
11. a. $1,946.40; b. $516.82; c. $1429.56
13. a. $1,728.00; b. $350.19; c. $1,377.81
15. a. $340.80; b. $2385.60; c. $611.85; d. $1773.75

## Practice the Skill 6-10

1.

| Item | Description | Unit price | Total price |
|---|---|---|---|
| 5 each | Gloves Medium unsterile | $5.10 | $25.50 |
| 3 each | Gloves XL unsterile | $5.60 | $16.80 |
| 5 boxes | Alcohol Swabs | $1.99 | $9.95 |
| 2 packages | Cotton balls | $1.00 | $2.00 |
| 4 boxes | Face Shields 25/box | $11.54 | $46.16 |
| | | Subtotal Price | 100.41 |
| | | Tax 5.5% | 5.53 |
| | | Shipping | 17.00 |
| | | Total Price | 122.94 |

3.

| Item | Description | Unit price | Total price |
|---|---|---|---|
| 10 each | Post-it Notes | $1.99 | $19.90 |
| 5 each | Staples | $3.99 | $19.95 |
| 5 boxes | Copy paper 12 packages/box | $56.79 | $283.95 |
| 8 dozen | Coffee Cups | $5.09 | $40.72 |
| 9 packages | Black Pens/3 per package | $3.75 | $33.75 |
| 3 Bags | Cotton 100/bag | $1.00 | $3.00 |
| 2 Boxes | Alcohol Pads | $1.99 | $3.98 |
| 12 each | Band-Aids assorted sizes | $4.12 | $49.44 |
| 3 boxes | Face Shields 25/box | $11.54 | $34.62 |
| | | Subtotal Price | $489.31 |
| | | Credit | $213.45 |
| | | New Total | $275.86 |
| | | Tax 5.5% | $15.18 |
| | | Shipping/Handling | $30.00 |
| | | Total Price | $321.04 |

# CHAPTER 7

## Practice the Skill 7-1

1. liter
3. meter
5. gram
7. kilo-
9. centi-

## Practice the Skill 7-2

| | Millimeters | Centimeters | Meters | Kilometers |
|---|---|---|---|---|
| 1. | 20,000 | 2,000 | 20 | 0.02 |
| 3. | 6,000,000 | 600,000 | 6000 | 6 |
| 5. | 750 | 75 | 0.75 | 0.00075 |
| 7. | 4000 | 400 | 4 | 0.004 |
| 9. | 12,500 | 1250 | 12.5 | 0.0125 |
| 11. | 37,000,000 | 3,700,000 | 37,000 | 37 |

## Practice the Skill 7-3

| | Milliliters | Deciliters | Liters |
|---|---|---|---|
| 1. | 500 | 5 | 0.5 |
| 3. | 4,000 | 40 | 4 |
| 5. | 750 | 7.5 | 0.75 |
| 7. | 2,000 | 20 | 2 |
| 9. | 50 | 0.5 | 0.05 |
| 11. | 0.008 | 0.00008 | 0.000008 |

## Practice the Skill 7-4

1. 200 mg
3. 1600 mg
5. 40 mg

| | Micrograms | Milligrams | Grams |
|---|---|---|---|
| 13. | 20,000 | 20 | 0.02 |
| 15. | 3,500,000 | 3,500 | 3.5 |
| 17. | 2,500 | 2.5 | 0.0025 |
| 19. | 125 | 0.125 | 0.000125 |

7. 2,000 mcg
9. 1,800 mcg
11. 0.5 G

## Practice the Skill 7-5

1. 50 mg
3. 2 mL
5. 750 mg
7. 6 mL
9. 105 mg

## Building Confidence with the Skill 7-1

1. a. 100 centimeters
3. d. 0.01 meter
5. a. 0.1 meter
7. hecto-
9. deci-
11. milli-
13. 2.5 cm
15. 750 mm
17. 0.2 cm
19. 400,000 m

## Building Confidence with the Skill 7-2

1. L
3. kl
5. 980 mL
7. 3.6 kiloliters
9. 2,750 mL
11. 30 deciliters
13. 30 liters
15. 475 mL
17. 1 dal and 30 L bottles
19. 200 mL

## Building Confidence with the Skill 7-3

1. 0.275 G
3. 3.5 G
5. 3.4 kg
7. 7 G
9. 7000 G
11. 4 dag
13. 0.003675 kg
15. 14,000,000 mcg
17. 4000G
19. 9G

## Building Confidence with the Skill 7-4

1. 25,000 mcg
3. 0.25 g
5. 1.5 mg
7. 10 m
9. 250 mg/L
11. 12,000 mg/L
13. 20 mm
15. 0.03 L
17. 10,000 m
19. 0.035 km

# CHAPTER 8

## Practice the Skill 8-1

1. 2000 mg
3. $\frac{1}{3}$ G
5. 900 mg
7. .24 G
9. 15 mL
11. 90.9 kg
13. 68.2 kg
15. 19.1 kg
17. 8.03 pounds
19. 220 pounds

## Practice the Skill 8-2

1. 18 tsp
3. 4 pt
5. 4 gallons
7. 2 Tbsp
9. 1 Tbsp
11. 24 cups
13. 21 ft
15. 5 yd
17. 9 T and 4.5 oz
19. 6 ft, 5 inches or 6'5"

## Building Confidence with the Skill 8-1

1. $\frac{1}{4}$ tsp
3. 5 Tbsp
5. 3 qt
7. 5 ft
9. 704 oz
11. 1 tsp
13. 3 pt
15. 3 feet 3 inches
17. 3 oz
19. 40 oz
21. $1\frac{1}{4}$ tsp
23. 2 pt
25. 56 oz
27. 10 feet 5 inches
29. 1.1875 gallons or 1.2 gallons

# CHAPTER 9

## Practice the Skill 9-1

1. D
3. F
5. A
7. R
9. T
11. Q
13. H
15. G
17. J
19. P

## Practice the Skill 9-2

1. Vital signs every 1 hour times 6 hours
3. Epinephrine immediately
5. Complete blood count every 12 hours
7. Amoxil 500 milligrams three times a day times 10 days
9. Aspirin (ASA) 500 milligrams twice a day as needed

## Practice the Skill 9-3

1. −4°F
3. 89.6°F
5. 113°F
7. 167°F
9. 212°F
11. −21.7°C
13. 0°C
15. 21.1°C
17. 36.1°C
19. 40.6°C
21. 36.1° − 37.2°C
23. 26.6° − 32°F
25. a. 104°F; b. 41.1°C

## Building Confidence with the Skill 9-1

1. Penicillin 250 milligram by mouth four times a day for 10 days
3. Diuril 0.25 milligrams one tablet every morning as needed for swelling
5. a) Atorvastatin 10 mg
   b) 10 mg
   c) PO or by mouth
   d) 30
   e) 1 tablet every bedtime or 1 tablet every night at bedtime.
7. a) Premarin 0.625 mg
   b) 0.625 mg
   c) by mouth or per oral
   d) 30
   e) 1 tablet daily at approximatively the same hour
9. 4000 mL
11. a) 225 mg

## Building Confidence with the Skill 9-2

1. 304.8 mm
3. 176 lbs
5. Any of the following answers are accepted: 1.37795, 1.377, 1.378, 1.4 inches
7. 5,500,000 mcg
9. Any of the following answers are accepted: 30.283 L, 30.28 L, 30.3 L
11. 132 lbs
13. Any of the following answers are accepted: 27.432 M, 27.43 M, 27.4 M
15. $1,080
17. 84 phlebotomists
19. 75 mL

# CHAPTER 10

## Practice the Skill 10-1

1. $10^2$
3. $10^6$
5. $10^5$
7. $10^{-6}$
9. $10^{-2}$

## Practice the Skill 10-2

1. $10^3$
3. $10^7$
5. $10^9$
7. $10^{-4}$
9. $10^{-9}$
11. $10^3$
13. $10^4$
15. $10^{-2}$
17. $10^{-3}$
19. $10^5$

## Practice the Skill 10-3

| Problem | Which direction is the decimal moving? | How many places will the decimal move? | Answer |
|---|---|---|---|
| 1. $892.0491 \times 100$ | Right | Two | 89,204.91 |
| 3. $275632.1 \div 100,000$ | Left | Five | 2.756321 |
| 5. $11.44 \times 10$ | Right | One | 114.4 |
| 7. $621.3589 \times 100$ | Right | Two | 62,135.89 |
| 9. $321.557 \times 10$ | Right | One | 3215.57 |

11. 456,000
13. 7.893,100
15. 20,000
17. $8.971 \times 10^{-9}$
19. $3.4521 \times 10^{-9}$

## Practice the Skill 10-4

1. 7
3. 4
5. 5
7. 3
9. 3
11. 5
13. 3
15. 7

## Practice the Skill 10-5

1. a. 15.77; b. 15.77
3. a. 2.4; b. 2.5
5. a. 4,736.45; b. 4,736.46
7. a. 0.890; b. 0.891
9. a. 21.9; b. 21.9
11. a. 0.11; b. 0.12
13. a. 1.21; b. 1.22
15. a. 0.022; b. 0.023
17. a. 1,364; b. 1,400
19. a. 0.3; b. 0.30

## Practice the Skill 10-6

1. $3.5 \times 10^3$
3. $5.67 \times 10^6$
5. $6.7 \times 10^9$
7. $5.6 \times 10^{-2}$
9. $3.7 \times 10^{-4}$

## Practice the Skill 10-7

1. 0.000356
3. 0.00009
5. 0.304
7. 15,727,500
9. 3,086.9136
11. 0.0028048780
13. 50
15. 45,200,000.8

## Building Confidence with the Skill 10-1

| Problem | Movement of decimal: right or left | Mathematical operation: multiplication or division |
|---|---|---|
| 1. 0.15 g to mg | Right | Multiplication |
| 3. 500 mg to G | Left | Division |
| 5. 5 mm to m | Left | Division |
| 7. 3,500 mL to L | Left | Division |
| 9. 2.5 G to mg | Right | Multiplication |
| 11. 300 hm to m | Right | Multiplication |
| 13. 750 mg to G | Left | Division |
| 15. 2 L to mL | Right | Multiplication |

## Building Confidence with the Skill 10-2

1. 9,620
3. 567
5. 13,452
7. 9.8
9. 0.0000000089
11. 4,675
13. 1,200.000002
15. 409,090.9091
17. 204,545.4545
19. 3,000,000

## Building Confidence with the Skill 10-3

1. a. 77,080,000;
   b. $7.708 \times 10^7$
3. a. 96,100;
   b. $9.61 \times 10^4$
5. a. 17.94117647;
   b. $1.794117647 \times 10^1$
7. a. 10,020;
   b. $1.002 \times 10^4$
9. a. −6,500;
   b. $-6.5 \times 10^3$
11. a. 277.4193548;
    b. $2.774193548 \times 10^2$
13. a. 5.090959206
    b. $5.090959206 \times 10^0$
15. a. 291.6;
    b. $2.916 \times 10^2$
17. a. 4,500
    b. $4.5 \times 10^3$
19. a. 0.035
    b. $3.5 \times 10^{-2}$

## CHAPTER 11

### Practice the Skill 11-1

1. 7
3. 21
5. 1
7. 5
9. 37.5
11. 17
13. −9
15. 512
17. 84
19. d = 7

### Practice the Skill 11-2

1. 0.75 or $\frac{3}{4}$
3. 36
5. 2

### Practice the Skill 11-3

1. x = (y-b)/m
3. y = (C-Ax)/B
5. F = 9/5 C + 32
7. b = 2A/h
9. h = 3V/(4πr²)

### Practice the Skill 11-4

1. 87.3
3. 133
5. 5.56
7. 1.54
9. 83

### Practice the Skill 11-5

1. 5
3. 21.5
5. 2.255
7. −7
9. 430

### Practice the Skill 11-6

1. 31
3. 95
5. 33
7. 9.99
9. −2 and −6

### Practice the Skill 11-7

*Note: Answers will vary.*
1. Boys/girls, birthday, grade level, age
3. *Answer will vary based on data.*
5. *Answer will vary based on data.*

### Practice the Skill 11-8

1. $\frac{1}{6}$
3. $\frac{1}{4}$
5. a. $\frac{1}{4}$ ; b. $\frac{1}{4}$ ; c. $\frac{2}{5}$ ; d. $\frac{3}{20}$

### Practice the Skill 11-9

1. Variance: 3746.56
3. Variance: 9043.5
5. Variance: 11.72
7. Variance: 0.868
9. Variance: 256.21

### Practice the Skill 11-10

1. Standard deviation = 3.16227766
3. Standard deviation = 5.813776741
5. Standard deviation = 0.2236067977
7. Standard deviation = 0.3535533906
9. Standard deviation = 1.2

### Practice the Skill 11-11

1. 68.2%
3. 99.7%
5. ±1: 14.4-19.6
   ±2: 11.8-22.2
   ±3: 9.2-24.8
7. ±1: 14.6-15.4
   ±2: 14.2-15.8
   ±3: 13.8-16.2
9. ±1: 305.6-348.4
   ±2: 284.2-369.8
   ±3: 262.8-391.2

## Building Confidence with the Skill 11-1

1. b = −1.5 or $-1\frac{1}{2}$ or $-\frac{3}{2}$
3. x = 0
5. d = 64
7. y = −12
9. y = 4
11. m = 25
13. d = $-21\frac{1}{3}$ OR −21.3 OR (−64)/3
15. k = −4
17. l = (P − 2w)/2 OR P/2 − w
19. Solve V = $\frac{1}{3}$ lhw for w. w = 3V/(lh)

## Building Confidence with the Skill 11-2

1. Mean: 33
   Median: 33
   Mode: 33
3. Mean: 1.0
   Median: 0.85
   Mode: 0.8
5. Mean: 2.62
   Median: 2.62
   Mode: 2.62
7. Mode: Youngest
9. Mean: 3.34
   Median: 3
   Mode: 3

## Building Confidence with the Skill 11-3

1. a. 51; b. 43.5; c. There is no mode;
   d. 569.78; e. 23.9; f. ±1: 27.1-74.9,
   ±2: 3.2-98.8, ±3: −20.7-122.7
3. a. 0.2244; b. 0.0555; c. No mode;
   d. 0.1272; e. 0.3566; f. ±1:
   −0.1322-0.581, ±2: −0.4888-0.936,
   ±3: −0.8454-1.2942
5. a. 5.55; b. 2; c. No mode; d. 153.7;
   e. 12.4; f. ±1: −6.85-17.95, ±2:
   −19.25-30.35, ±3: −31.65-42.75

## CHAPTER 12

### Practice the Skill 12-1

1. 14 g
3. 35 g
5. 70 mL
7. 400 mL
9. 160 mL
11. Hypertonic

### Practice the Skill 12-2

1. 8.5%
3. 2.4%
5. 0.125 L

## Practice the Skill 12-3

1. 0.0051 molal or m = 0.0051 mol/kg
3. M = 0.0005 moles/liter or 0.18375 mol/L
5. 219 grams of HCl

## Practice the Skill 12-4

1. a. 286 mL 70% dextrose; b. 714 mL of sterile water
3. a. 250 mL 50% dextrose and 250 mL of sterile water
5. a. 200 mL of 70% dextrose and 300 mL of sterile water.

## Practice the Skill 12-5

1. 0.667 L/h or 0.7 L/h
3. 131.25 mL or 131 mL
5. 571 min or 9 hours and 31 min.
7. 37gtts/min
9. 125 mL/hour

## Practice the Skill 12-6

1. 660 mL
3. 1850 mL intake and 1050 mL output
5. 3675 mL

## Building Confidence with the Skill 12-1

1. 0.12%
3. 5%
5. a. 700 of dextrose; b. 300 of sterile water
7. 16% by mass
9. 0.1 or 10%
11. 0.45%
13. m = 0.0051 mol/kg
15. 90 grams of HCl

# Glossary

**Addend:** Any number being added.

**Addition:** To combine two or more numbers.

**Algebra:** A branch of mathematics that uses letters to represent an unknown amount.

**Apothecary System:** One of the oldest measurement systems used to calculate medications based on grains and minims.

**Arabic Numerals:** The number system used in the Western Hemisphere, related to the English system of measurement.

**Arithmetic:** Calculation using addition, subtraction, multiplication, and division.

**Arithmetic Average:** A single number that is determined by adding a series of numbers and dividing the sum by the total number added.

**Associative Property of Addition:** The sum stays the same when the grouping of addends is changed.

**Associative Property of Multiplication:** The product stays the same when the grouping of factors is changed.

**Avoirdupois System:** The English system for measuring weight, in which 1 pound is 16 ounces; also used in the United States.

**Bar Graph:** Graph that compares measurements by using vertical or horizontal bars.

**Base of an Exponent:** The repeated factor that is to be multiplied by itself.

**Base Unit:** Three base units are commonly used for metric measurement of medications to indicate weight, volume, and length.

**Borrow:** Regroup from one place value to a lower place value in order to subtract.

**Bimodal:** When there are 2 modes that appear in a sample set.

**Carry:** Move an extra digit from one place value column to the next higher place value column.

**Celsius (or Centigrade):** The measurement of temperature with 0 degrees representing the freezing point and 100 degrees representing the boiling point of water.

**Census:** Data collection for every member of the group.

**Circle Graph (Pie Graph):** Graph that indicates the proportion or percentage in relation to the whole.

**Coefficients:** a number or letter used to multiple a variable.

**Coinsurance:** The patient assumes a percentage of the fee for covered services; also known as cost-sharing. This amount is usually collected at the end of a visit.

**Colloid:** A heterogeneous mixture similar to suspensions, in that their composition is not uniform. The particles are generally larger than those in a solution, and smaller than those in a suspension.

**Common Factor:** A number that is a factor of two or more numbers.

**Common Multiple:** A number that is a multiple of two or more numbers.

**Commutative Property of Addition:** The sum stays the same when the order of the addends is changed.

**Commutative Property of Multiplication:** The product stays the same when the order of the factors is changed.

**Computation:** The process of computing.

**Compute:** To find a numerical result, usually by adding, subtracting, multiplying, or dividing.

**Concentration:** The strength of a solution determined by the relative amount of solute dissolved in the the solvent.

**Continuous Data:** any value within a range.

**Copayment:** Predetermined amount that usually must be paid before the patient sees the physician. Copayments are used primarily in managed care plans.

**Cross Multiplication:** A mathematical computation in which the numerator of one ratio is multiplied by the denominator of the second ratio.

**Day Sheet:** A register for recording daily business transactions (charges, payments, or adjustments); also known as a daybook, daily log, or daily record sheet.

**Decimal:** A number system based on the number 10. Each unit is measured by how far to the right of the decimal point its place value represents.

**Decimal Fraction:** A fraction whose denominator is a power of 10; it expresses the position by units to the right of the decimal point.

**Decimal Point:** Used to distinguish decimal fractions or to distinguish the whole number from a decimal fraction.

**Deductible:** Specific amount of money for health care that must be paid by the patient each year before insurance policy benefits begin. This amount is usually collected at the end of a visit.

**Denominator:** The number of equal parts in a whole. It is the bottom number of a fraction.

**Difference:** The amount that remains after one quantity is subtracted from another.

**Digit:** Any one of the 10 symbols used in mathematical computations: 0, 1, 2, 3, 4, 5, 6, 7, 8, 9.

**Dimensional Analysis:** An advanced form of ratios and proportions that cancels unwanted units in the conversion to establish the desired unit of measurement.

**Directed Number:** A number with a positive or negative sign to show the direction it lies from 0. A specific value; usually a whole number.

**Distributive Property:** When one of the factors of a product is written as a sum, multiplying each addend before adding does not change the product.

**Divide:** To separate into equal groups.

**Dividend:** A quantity to be divided.

**Divisible:** One number is divisible by another if its quotient is an integer.

**Division:** The operation of making equal groups.

**Divisor:** The quantity by which another quantity is to be divided.

**Dosage Strength:** Weight of medication in a dose (mEq, mcg, mg, G).

**Drop Factor:** Infusion rate based on the number of drops/milliliters.

**Encounter Form:** An all-encompassing billing form used by physicians to communicate to the billing department what services were performed during the patient's visit; also known as a fee schedule, fee slip, or superbill.

**Equation:** A statement that two mathematical expressions are equal.

**Equivalent:** Equal in value.

**Equivalent Fraction:** Fractions that represent the same relationship of part to the whole. The fractions are equal even though there are variations in the size of the pieces or the number of parts of the total.

**Evaluate:** To find the value of a mathematical expression.

**Exponent:** A number that indicates to what power the factor is being raised; the number that determines how many times the base will be multiplied.

**Extremes:** First and last numbers found in a proportion.

**Factor:** The number being multiplied; an integer that divides evenly into another.

**Fahrenheit:** The measurement of temperature with 32 degrees representing the freezing point and 212 degrees representing the boiling point of water.

**Flow rate:** The rate at which an IV delivers medication or fluid.

**Fraction:** A ratio that represents part of something in comparison to the total number of parts.

**Fractions with Common Denominators:** Fractions that have the same denominator.

**Graph:** Visual chart of how data sets compare.

**Greatest Common Factor (GCF):** The largest factor of two or more numbers; the largest number that divides evenly into two or more numbers.

**Gross Income:** The amount of pay received before taxes and withholding are deducted.

**Hypertonic:** The concentration in the cell is lower than the solution; thus water leaves the cell and goes into the solution causing the cell to shrink.

**Hypotonic:** The concentration in the cell is higher than the solution; thus water enters the cell and leaves the solution, causing the cell to grow and become engorged.

**Identity Property of Addition:** If you add 0 to a number, the sum is the same as the given number.

**Identity Property of Multiplication:** If you multiply a number by 1, the product is the same as the given number.

**IM:** The abbreviation for intramuscular.

**Improper Fraction:** A fraction in which the numerator is greater than the denominator.

**Inscription:** The part of the prescription that identifies the medication and dosage.

**Intake and Output Graph:** Graph or chart used to record fluid intake and output over several days on one page.

**Integers:** Whole numbers and their opposites.

**Intravenous:** Within a vein.

**Isotonic:** The cell and the solution have the same concentration and thus water does not flow into or out of the cell.

**IV:** The abbreviation for intravenous.

**Least Common Denominator (LCD):** The smallest common multiple of the denominators of two or more fractions.

**Least Common Multiple (LCM):** The smallest common multiple of a set of two or more numbers.

**Ledger Card:** An individual record indicating charges, payments, adjustments, and balances owed for services rendered; also known as a ledger.

**Mean:** A single number that is determined by adding a series of numbers and dividing the sum by the total number added; also known as the average.

**Means:** Second and third numbers found in a proportion.

**Measurement Graph:** Graph to record growth and development at specific age intervals; height and weight are recorded.

**Median:** The middle number(s) in a set of data that is arranged in either ascending or descending order.

**Medication Order:** Directions for administration of medication; these may be written or verbal orders.

**Mental Math:** The process of performing mathematical calculations in one's head without paper and pencil or physical aids.

**Metric System:** Standardized international system of units and measurements based on powers of 10, also known as the International System of Units; used for most medication doses in the United States.

**Military Time:** Time based on a 24-hour clock.

**Milliequivalent:** Another way to describe contents of medication in a solution.

**Minuend:** In subtraction, the number from which you subtract.

**Mixed Number:** A number expression that consists of a whole number and a fraction.

**Mode:** A number that appears most frequently in a series of numbers. Depending on the amount of data, there can be more than one mode. If more than one number appears the same amount of times, there is "no mode."

**Molality:** Number of moles per kilogram of solvent.

**Molarity:** Number of moles per liter of solution.

**Mole:** Basic unit of measure used in chemistry representing the amount of a substance expressed in grams containing as many atoms, molecules, or ions as the number of atoms in 12 grams of carbon-12.

**Multidose Vial:** A container that holds multiple doses of a specific medication in liquid format; the label reads mg/ml.

**Multiple:** The product of a whole number and any other whole number.

**Multiplicand:** In multiplication, the factor being multiplied by another (the multiplier).

**Multiplication:** The operation of repeated addition.

**Multiplicative Inverse:** When you multiple a number by its multiplicative inverse you get 1. Also known as *reciprocal*.

**Multiplier:** In multiplication, the factor by which another (the multiplicand) is multiplied.

**Negative Numbers:** Numbers less than 0.

**Net Income:** The amount of pay received after taxes and withholding have been deducted; also referred to as take home pay.

**Net Loss:** Less than the amount needed to maintain a solvent business.

**Net Profit:** Actual profits after all deductions have been paid.

**Number Sentence:** An equation or inequality with numbers.

**Numerator:** The number of parts to which the problem is referring. It is the top number of a fraction.

**Operation:** Addition, subtraction, multiplication, division, raising to a power, and taking a root are mathematical operations.

**Order of Operations:** Rules describing what sequence to use in evaluating expressions.

**Osmosis:** The tendency of a fluid to pass through a semipermeable membrane.

**Outlier:** A number that is much larger or smaller than the other numbers in the data set; a data point outside of the statistically acceptable range.

**Percentage, or Percent:** A representation of a proportion based on 100. Percentage can represent the amount of change (positive or negative) based on the total amount involved.

**Place Value:** The value of the position of a digit in a number.

**PO:** The abbreviation for medication given by mouth.

**Polymodal:** When there is greater than 2 sets of modes in a sample set.

**Positive Numbers:** Numbers that are greater than 0.

**Power:** An exponent.

**Power of 10:** A number with 10 as a base and a whole number exponent.

**Prefix:** Found at the beginning of a word to adjust or qualify its meaning.

**Prescription:** Orders written by a physician that outline the medication dose, frequency, and length of time for treatment.

**Prime Number:** A number that has exactly two different positive factors, itself and 1.

**Probability:** The chance of an event occurring.

**Product:** The result of multiplication.

**Proper Fraction:** A fraction in which the denominator is greater than the numerator.

**Proportion:** Comparative relationship between the parts; one or more ratios that are compared.

**Purchase Order:** Form used to order equipment, medications, and supplies from outside vendors.

**Qualitative Data:** descriptive information using words.

**Quantitative Data:** descriptive information using numbers.

**Quantity:** The amount of medication that is to be dispensed.

**Quotient:** The result of division.

**Random Sampling:** Equal chance for the number, object, event, or person to be included in the study.

**Range:** The difference between the greatest and least value found within the data set.

**Ratio:** Means of describing the relationship between two numbers.

**Reciprocal:** To get the reciprocal divide the number by 1. Also known as *Multiplicative Inverse*.

**Reduce or Simplify Fractions:** Finding the lowest equivalent fraction by dividing the numerator into the denominator. This is done by finding the greatest common factor of the numerator and the denominator.

**Refills:** The number of times the physician will allow the prescription to be repeated.

**Remainder:** In whole number division, when you have divided as far as you can without using decimals, what has not been divided yet is the remainder.

**Roman Numerals:** Letter symbols used by the ancient Romans to represent numbers.

**Rounding Down:** Leaving the number being rounded as it currently appears; done when the digit to the right of the number is a 4 or lower digit.

**Rounding Numbers:** Approximating a large number to a specific place value or whole number.

**Rounding Up:** Increasing the value the number being rounded by 1; done when the digit to the right of the number is a 5 or higher digit.

**Route:** How the medication is to be given.

**Sample:** Select member of a group.

**Signa (Sig):** The part of the prescription that indicates the dosage and frequency with which the medication is to be given.

**Significant Figures:** A prescribed decimal place, which determines the amount of rounding off to be done; this is usually based on the degree of accuracy needed in measurement.

**Solute:** A substance that dissolves into the solvent.

**Solution:** A mixture of two or more substances (with the same composition throughout) that can be separated by a physical means.

**Solvent:** Maintaining enough money to meet one's liabilities (Chapter 6); a substance that dissolves another to form a solution (Chapter 12).

**Standard Deviation:** The most common measurement used to determine how widely spread the values are in a statistical calculation.

**Standard Scientific Notation:** A method of writing or displaying numbers in terms of a decimal number between 1 and 10 multiplied by a power of 10.

**Statistics:** The study of data sets and their distribution within the set.

**Subtraction:** An operation that gives the difference between two numbers. Subtraction is also used to compare two numbers.

**Subtrahend:** In subtraction, the number being subtracted.

**Sum:** The result of addition.

**Suspension:** Mixtures that are not the same composition throughout and if allowed to rest, the parts of the mixture will separate.

**Symbol:** Something that represents something else. Examples include: $+$, $-$, $\times$, $\div$.

**Target Sampling:** A sample that closely represents the characteristics of the population being studied.

**Tonicity:** Osmotic pressure or tension of a solution; causing the relative concentrations of the cell and the solutions to change.

**Traditional Time:** The use of a.m. and p.m. to determine 24-hour cycle on a 12-hour clock.

**U.S. Customary System (Household Measurements):** System of measurement based on common kitchen measuring utensils.

**Units:** Basic measurement used to determine the strength of medications; in the metric system, a dimension, such as weight (or mass), volume, and length.

**Variables:** a symbol for a number that is unknown. Most common letters that are used as variables are x or y.

**Variance:** Common measurement used to determine precision of the population.

**Vital Sign Graph:** Graph or chart used to record temperature, pulse, respirations, and blood pressure over several days on one page.

**Whole Number:** Any number that does not include a fraction, decimal, or negative sign, for example, 0, 1, 2, 3; part of a mixed number that is not in fractional form.

**Word Root:** Place of origin; base unit.

**Zero Pair:** Two numbers whose sum is 0.

**Zero Property:** The product of any number and 0 is 0.

# Index

Page numbers followed by "*f*" indicate figures, "*t*" indicate tables, and "*b*" indicate boxes.